# Advanced Pharmacy Practice for Technicians

**SECOND EDITION**

**SECOND EDITION**

# Advanced Pharmacy Practice for Technicians

...

**Anita A. Lambert, RPh**

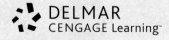
DELMAR
CENGAGE Learning

Australia • Brazil • Japan • Korea • Mexico • Singapore • Spain • United Kingdom • United States

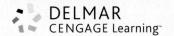

**Advanced Pharmacy Practice for Technicians, Second Edition**
**Anita A. Lambert, RPh**

Vice President, Health Care Business Unit:
William Brottmiller

Editorial Director: Matthew Kane

Acquisitions Editor: Kalen Conerly

Senior Product Manager: Darcy M. Scelsi

Editorial Assistant: Meaghan O'Brien

Marketing Director: Jennifer McAvey

Marketing Channel Manager:
Christopher Manion

Marketing Coordinator: Andrea Eobstel

Production Director: Carolyn Miller

Senior Art Director: Jack Pendleton

Content Project Manager: Katie Wachtl

For product information and technology assistance, contact us at
**Cengage Learning Customer & Sales Support, 1-800-354-9706**
For permission to use material from this text or product,
submit all requests online **www.cengage.com/permissions**
Further permissions questions can be emailed to
**permissionrequest@cengage.com**

Library of Congress Control Number: 2007023876

ISBN-13: 978-1-4180-5539-4

ISBN-10: 1-4180-5539-5

**Delmar**
Executive Woods
5 Maxwell Drive
Clifton Park, NY 12065
USA

Cengage Learning is a leading provider of customized learning solutions with office locations around the globe, including Singapore, the United Kingdom, Australia, Mexico, Brazil, and Japan. Locate your local office at
**www.cengage.com/global**

Cengage Learning products are represented in Canada by Nelson Education, Ltd.

To learn more about Delmar, visit **www.cengage.com/delmar**

Purchase any of our products at your local college store or at our preferred online store **www.cengagebrain.com**

Printed in the United States of America
6 7 15 14 13 12

# Contents

## 1   Pharmacy and the U.S. Health Care System   1

## 6   Home Health Care    133

## 7   Home Infusion Pharmacy    147

## 10   Nuclear Pharmacy        235

## 11    Hospice Pharmacy    269

## 12   Federal Pharmacy     287

## 13   Pharmaceutical Industry     305

## 15   Advanced Pharmacy Technician Roles   341

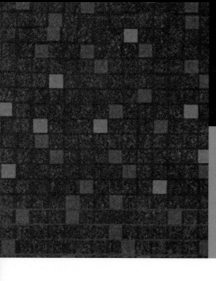

# Preface

Pharmacy practice has expanded over the years into nontraditional areas such as long-term care, home health care, managed care, and hospice care, as well as other less familiar pharmacy practice areas such as nuclear pharmacy, federal pharmacy, and telepharmacy. Each of these settings is unique and offers advanced pharmaceutical services to patients. Pharmacy technicians are found in all of these pharmacy practice areas. These areas offer expanded roles and increased levels of responsibility for the pharmacy technician based on advanced knowledge and skills that go beyond the knowledge and skills required in the traditional community or hospital pharmacy setting.

As a practicing pharmacist in some of these nontraditional pharmacy areas and as a pharmacy technician instructor, I have had difficulty in locating educational materials concerning these areas. Most pharmacy technician training texts are basic in nature and do not cover the nontraditional pharmacy practice areas. Of those that discuss one or two nontraditional areas, none discusses these areas in depth and detail. Thus, there has been a need for an advanced pharmacy technician training textbook of this type that deals not with basic pharmacy knowledge and skills as practiced in traditional pharmacy settings, but with specific and unique knowledge and skills used in nontraditional pharmacy areas. *Advanced Pharmacy Practice for Technicians* was developed to go beyond the basic pharmacy technician training text that covers the traditional community retail and hospital areas of pharmacy. It was intended to discuss the specific and unique knowledge and skills used in nontraditional pharmacy areas. Today it remains the only advanced pharmacy technician training text on the market. This textbook builds upon the basic training requirements for pharmacy technicians to provide the pharmacy technician with knowledge and training that are complete.

*Advanced Pharmacy Practice for Technicians* continues to be a teaching tool and an information resource. It is intended for pharmacy technician students, pharmacy technician instructors, practicing pharmacists, and practicing pharmacy technicians. It is a tool for teaching purposes, especially for pharmacy technicians in advanced educational programs, and it is an excellent source of information on the various nontraditional pharmacy areas. Pharmacy technicians approaching this text should already possess basic pharmacy knowledge and skills as practiced in traditional community and hospital pharmacies as a prerequisite to the material in this text. This basic knowledge and skills can be applied to these advanced pharmacy practices and built upon through the use of this book.

In an easy-to-read fashion, this text describes pharmacy services in depth in each advanced pharmacy practice area. Because most pharmacy technicians have limited exposure to the U.S. health care system, the book begins with a discussion of our system of health care, the roles of managed care and pharmaceutical care, and the changes in the way pharmacy is being practiced today. There are several chapters dedicated to the discussion of long-term care and home health care, as these are dominant and growing nontraditional pharmacy practice areas. The remainder of the book is organized into separate chapters, each dealing with a different nontraditional area. The text concludes with appendices, an extensive glossary, and an index.

The discussion of each nontraditional pharmacy practice area starts with an overview of the area, along with any necessary background information. The elements that make up the pharmacy are discussed, some of them being the same as in a traditional pharmacy but many of them unique to the type of nontraditional practice area being discussed. The text then discusses the prescription-filling process in that practice area, followed by the various services of the pharmacy. The legislation and regulations that pertain to each area are presented. Finally, the roles of the pharmacist and the pharmacy technician are defined. The discussion of the pharmacist's role in each area is essential to the pharmacy technician's understanding of his duties.

Features include:

- *Learning Objectives* give the students an outline of the knowledge and skills they will learn by reading and studying the chapter.

- *Key Terms*, listed at the beginning of each chapter as well as highlighted and defined within the chapter, present the terminology used in the particular pharmacy area and topics.

- *Key Concepts*, found at the end of the chapter text, are tied to the Learning Objectives. They summarize and review the material presented in the chapter.

- *Self-Assessment Questions,* with answers found in Appendix E, include multiple choice, true/false, fill in the blanks, and critical thinking questions and allow students to evaluate their learning.

- *A Bibliography* is provided for further information and research.

In addition, throughout the book, **bold** type is used to identify key terms and *italics* are used to emphasize key points. The text is enhanced through the extensive use of photographs, drawings, diagrams, tables, and forms.

Changes in pharmacy practice, equipment, legislation and regulations, and pharmacist and pharmacy technician roles within the various pharmacy practice areas have come about since the initial writing of *Advanced Pharmacy Practice for Technicians*. New and additional topics of interest that relate to each practice area have been included in this edition, as well as new technologies that have emerged in these areas.

New to this edition:

- Long-Term Care Pharmacy includes new topics, such as electronic medical records, e-prescribing, bar coding, the Medicare Prescription Drug Benefit, and medication therapy management.

- Home Infusion Pharmacy also discusses the impact of the Medicare Prescription Drug Benefit, other new legislation and regulations, as well as new pump technologies.

- Nuclear Pharmacy includes a discussion of USP Chapter <797> regulations.

- Hospice Pharmacy also discusses the impact of USP Chapter <797> standards on specialized compounding, as well as the creation of the Pharmacy Compounding Accreditation Board.

- Pharmaceutical Industry adds several new topics, including "authorized generics," generic biotechnology, and drug pedigree laws.

- Telepharmacy is identified as a new nontraditional pharmacy practice area and is added as a new chapter.

As more and more nontraditional career opportunities for pharmacy technicians open in all practice settings, and as pharmacy technicians' roles continue to expand, there will be a greater need for well-trained and knowledgeable pharmacy technicians. *Advanced Pharmacy Practice for Technicians* has helped to meet these greater training needs and, with its updated and enhanced content and instructor's package, will continue to find an important place in the curriculums for pharmacy technician training.

Anita A. Lambert, RPh, author
*Advanced Pharmacy Practice for Technicians*

## SUPPLEMENTS

An *Electronic Classroom Manager* accompanies *Advanced Pharmacy Practice for Technicians*. This instructor resource is divided into three major sections:

- An Instructor's Manual
- A Testbank
- Power Point Presentations

The *Instructor's Manual* is a valuable resource to aid the instructor in presentation of the material discussed in the text, and offers suggestions for additional activities for students who want to gain a better understanding of the content outside the classroom setting. The *Instructor's Manual* includes additional topics for in-class discussion, additional critical thinking questions to encourage student application of knowledge, and activities for students to do outside the classroom to become better acquainted with various practice settings.

The *Testbank* contains 300 questions, consisting of a 20-question multiple-choice test for each chapter. These chapters tests can be printed and distributed as chapter tests, or the questions can be used to create larger tests or final examinations.

The *Power Point Presentations* correlate to each chapter. They highlight the key points of the chapter and provide a foundation for the instructor to use in building lectures.

All components of the *Electronic Classroom Manager* are fully customizable. The instructor is able to add or edit any of the materials to tailor the materials to his or her own curriculum.

# Acknowledgments

I would like to sincerely thank all of those who have provided me with their assistance in producing this text. Among them are the following: my husband, Kevin, and my sons, Brian and David, for their love and support; Sidney J. Kahn, a mentor and friend, for his encouragement of this project and his advice; my personal friends and professional colleagues for their support; the pharmacists and pharmacy technicians who opened their doors to me and shared their pharmacy experiences and operations; and the individuals and companies who contributed materials to this text.

In particular I would like to acknowledge:

Jeffrey L. Stauffer, PharmD, FASCP, Stauffer's Drug Store, New Holland, Pennsylvania

Todd Ross, Artromick International, Inc.

Doug Harlow, MED-PASS, Inc.

Michael Stotz, AutoMed Technologies, Inc.

Elaine A. Allegrucci, RNBS, Moses Taylor Home Health, Scranton, Pennsylvania

Terri Servais, Smiths Medical

Samuel R. Wachsman, RPh, Horizon Healthcare Services, Lancaster, Pennsylvania

P.J. Ortman, RPh, MBA, Novartis Pharmaceuticals Corporation

I would also like to thank the reviewers of my manuscript. Their comments and suggestions were invaluable.

Second Edition

Cheryl Aiken, PharmD
Adjunct Faculty
Vermont Technical College
Randolph Center, VT

Denise Anderson, CPhT
Instructor
United Education Institute
Fontana, CA

Aniruddh Hathi, BS, MS
Associate Professor
Texas State Technical College
Waco, TX

Troy McColley, CPhT
Instructor
Pennsylvania Institute of Technology
Philadelphia, PA

Earl McKinstry, RPh
Program Director
Western Dakota Technical Institute
Rapid City, SD

James Mizner, RPh, MBA
Pharmacy Technician Program Director
Applied Career Training
Reston, VA

Karen Snipe, CPhT, AS, BA, MAEd
Pharmacy Technician Program Coordinator
Trident Technical College
Charleston, SC

Mary Ann Stuhan, RPh
Pharmacy Program Manager
Cuyahoga Community College
Highland Hills, OH

Sandi Tschritter, BA, CPhT
Director of Pharmacy Technician Program
Spokane Community College
Spokane, WA

Judy Weisbard, MPA, CPhT
Coordinator Pharmacy Technician Program
Chaffey College
Rancho Cucamonga, CA

First Edition

Barbara Donahue, RN, MSN
Professor
Southern West Virginia Community and Technical College
Mount Gay, West Virginia

Laurel Dugan, BS, CPhT
Instructor, Pharmacy Technology
North Central State College
Mansfield, Ohio

Thomas George, RPh, JD
Chair, Pharmacy Technician Program
Mount Aloysius College
Cresson, Pennsylvania
President
Drug Key LLC

Daniel Hussar, PhD
Remington Professor of Pharmacy
The Philadelphia College of Pharmacy
Philadelphia, Pennsylvania

Earl McKinstry, RPh
Instructor, Pharmacology Technology
Western Dakota Technical Institute
Rapid City, South Dakota

Katherine Ricossa, MS, RN
Business Management/Development Specialist, Regional Health Occupations
Resource Center, an EdNet Initiative
Mission College
Santa Clara, California

Janet B. Wakelin, MR Pharm., CPhT
Retired, Program Manager, Pharmacy Technology
Cuyahoga Community College
Cleveland, Ohio

# About the Author

**Anita A. Lambert, RPh,** is a practicing pharmacist with over 30 years of experience and expertise in several areas of pharmacy, including community retail pharmacy practice, long-term care pharmacy practice, hospital pharmacy practice, and home infusion pharmacy practice. She has also been involved in pharmacy technician education, teaching students in associate degree and certificate programs. Ms. Lambert holds a Bachelor of Science degree in Chemistry from Marywood University and a Bachelor of Science degree in Pharmacy from the University of the Sciences in Philadelphia. She is active in local and national pharmacy and pharmacy technician organizations.

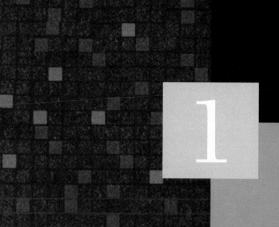

# 1

# Pharmacy and the
# U.S. Health Care System

Upon completion of this chapter, the student should be able to:

- Describe the components of any health care system.
- List the types of health care systems found throughout the world.
- Describe the different types of health care personnel.
- Explain the differences among health care institutions.
- Describe the types of health care services available.
- Explain the financing of health care in the United States.
- Recognize some of the problems in the U.S. health care system.
- Explain the need for health care reform.
- Describe managed care.
- Explain the importance of outcomes-based therapy.
- Discuss pharmaceutical care.

## Key Terms

| | | |
|---|---|---|
| capitation | interdisciplinary | pharmaceutical care |
| continuity of care | managed care | process |
| drug-related problem | managed care organization | structure |
| fee-for-service | network | |
| gatekeeper | outcomes | |

## Introduction

The U.S. health care system has many facets. It has evolved over time and still is evolving. Pharmacists play a vital role in our health care system. The expertise provided by pharmacists helps to provide affordable, comprehensive, and quality health care. Because of their important role in the delivery of health care, pharmacists and pharmacy technicians must be aware of the changes in the health care system and how they affect the pharmacy profession. This chapter examines the health care delivery system in the United States, and its present problems and concerns, and discusses opportunities for improving the system. It also highlights pharmacy's new role in our evolving health care system. ∎

## INTRODUCTION TO HEALTH CARE SYSTEMS

Health is an ideal all people strive for. Health care deals with the promotion of health and the treatment of disease. The goals of any health care system are to maintain healthy lives and to improve the quality of life through health care services. These services should be high-quality, cost-effective, and accessible to all citizens. The health care system in the United States has encountered problems in trying to provide quality health care to all Americans. In an attempt to achieve a more effective health care system, health care is being restructured and extensively managed. However, our health care system continues to be a combination of health care providers, institutions, and payers working together to produce health care services.

### COMPONENTS OF A HEALTH CARE SYSTEM

There are three components to any health care system: cost, access, and quality. Cost exerts the most pressure on a health care system. It forces changes and innovations aimed at delivering more cost-effective health care services. It is, however, the most difficult to control. Access is the most political aspect of a health care system. Access is a patient's ability to obtain medical care. Good public health relies on the availability and affordability of health care services for all people. Finally, quality is the most complex aspect. It is not well defined, and it is difficult to measure. Quality implies value, worth, and excellence. It requires setting standards for health care services, standards that can be measured so as to be improved. Quality must be ensured in any health care system.

### TYPES OF HEALTH CARE SYSTEMS

Although all health care systems are different in some way, there are three basic types: socialized programs, decentralized programs, and voluntary programs. Socialized programs, as in Canada and the United Kingdom, have government involvement through the provision of mandatory health insurance, ownership of health care institutions, and the administration of health care services. Decentralized programs, as in Germany and Japan, also provide mandatory insurance for everyone, but there are many different health care providers. Voluntary programs, as in the United States and South Africa, do not offer health coverage to everyone and have many different systems of health care delivery and payment.

Although no two health care systems are alike, they do share common features. Most try to make health care services accessible to everyone, and most have some structure at the center of their health care system that allows them to produce health care services for their people. The U.S. health care system is unique compared with other health care systems throughout the world. It is a complicated arrangement of health care providers and payers. In terms of accessibility, almost any service is available as long as there is money for payment. Those patients having a payer, that is, health insurance, have a wide range of services available, whereas those without health insurance have few options available. Health care is not a right in the United States but a privilege, in that it is not available to everyone. Although the *concept* of health care for everyone is endorsed, it is not put into effect in this country.

As for structure, there is no central structure within the health care system in the United States. The U.S. government has less involvement with its health care system than any other industrialized country in the world. What role the government has in the health care system is limited owing to the strength of physicians, hospitals, and insurance companies and, now, managed care organizations, which oppose government control and interference for a variety of reasons. Thus, there is no central system for organizing, delivering, and paying for health care services or for providing every American with access to health care.

## HEALTH CARE PERSONNEL

Health care services in this country are provided by different types of health care personnel and the institutions in which they work. Health care personnel are the backbone of the health care system. The health care field has enjoyed a long period of expansion. The number and types of health care workers have greatly increased since World War II. The development of new occupations, such as physician assistants and nurse practitioners, has been stimulated by the development of new techniques and services. The increase in health care workers has led to an increase in the supply of health care services and, therefore, to an increase in overall health care costs. Each type of health care worker is needed and has a defined area of expertise involving detailed education, training, and experience. Although most health care personnel have well-defined roles, there is now some overlap among some health professionals, with managed care requiring more collaboration. Today, the largest groups of health care personnel are nurses, physicians, and pharmacists. In keeping with the focus of this book, we begin our discussion of health care personnel with the pharmacist.

### PHARMACISTS

Pharmacists are the third largest group of health care personnel. In the early twentieth century, pharmacists provided medications and compounded formulations when appropriate. In those days, although their technical skills were important, pharmacists were known for their patient care, that is, their ability to listen to a patient's problems and provide solutions. In the 1950s, 1960s, and 1970s, with the availability of commercially prepared medications, the role of the pharmacist evolved mostly into a dispensing function. The focus was on getting the correct medication to the patient as quickly and efficiently as possible. Compounding of medications was an exception rather than the norm. Patient consultation often was not provided for many reasons.

Pharmacy has seen many changes over the years. Like other professions, pharmacy has become much more specialized. Areas of practice now include retail pharmacy, hospital pharmacy, long-term care pharmacy, home care pharmacy, managed care pharmacy, nuclear pharmacy, hospice pharmacy, industrial pharmacy, public health, telepharmacy, and Internet pharmacy. Educational requirements for the profession have been increased. Pharmacists are now required to complete a professional degree program that leads to the Doctor of Pharmacy, or PharmD, degree. Today, in addition to dispensing services, pharmacists are again involved in providing patient care services, which take many forms within the various practice areas. Overall, patient counseling requirements, such as those mandated by the Omnibus Budget Reconciliation Act of 1990 (OBRA 90), combined with the increasing number and complexity of medications, have made patient counseling and education an important component of pharmacy practice. In addition, automation and the use of pharmacy technicians have allowed pharmacists to move from dispensing functions into patient care functions. Pharmacists provide a type of patient care that is unique to pharmacy—pharmaceutical care. The role of the pharmacist has thus evolved from compounding and patient care, to dispensing, and back again to patient-centered care.

## PHARMACY TECHNICIANS

Pharmacy technicians play a role in today's health care system owing to the expansion of the pharmacy profession. A pharmacy technician is an individual working in a pharmacy, who, under the supervision of a licensed pharmacist, assists in pharmacy activities that do not require the professional judgment of the pharmacist (PTCB, 2005). Technicians assist the pharmacist in medication-dispensing functions but cannot consult with physicians, counsel patients, or perform clinical functions. Specific pharmacy technician functions and responsibilities are governed by state laws called pharmacy practice acts. Pharmacists have the responsibility of checking and verifying all work performed by pharmacy technicians and are ultimately responsible for that work.

Pharmacy technicians are trained in several ways. Many technicians receive on-the-job training only. Formal education and training can be obtained through certificate programs or up to 2-year associate degree programs at universities, local community colleges, or career schools. There is no academic degree for pharmacy technicians because they work under the supervision of the pharmacist, not independent of the pharmacist. However, more and more pharmacy technicians, especially those who are more highly trained, are seeking certification, CPhT, which is formal *recognition* of meeting certain qualifications. Certified pharmacy technicians must still work under the supervision of a licensed pharmacist.

As do pharmacists, pharmacy technicians work in different pharmacy practice areas, and they have different roles in each of those areas. These practice areas and the roles of the pharmacist and pharmacy technician are discussed throughout this book.

## PHYSICIANS

The medical profession is only one of many health care professions required to make the health care system work. It is, however, the dominant profession in the health care system, although changes in the system are transforming the physician's role from that of the dominant player to a member of the health care team. Physicians serve patients directly without the authority of another health care professional. All other health care personnel work on the orders of or under the general supervision of physicians.

The majority of physicians are involved in patient care. A small percentage of physicians work in administration, education, research, and industry. Of the physicians working in patient care, most are involved in private practice. A physician in private practice provides a service directly to a patient in return for a fee. There are three types of private practice: solo practice, partnership practice, and group practice. A group practice is defined as three or more physicians who practice together, sharing space, staff, equipment, and the workload. The majority of group practices are made up of physicians in the same medical specialty; these are called single-specialty group practice. Less common is the multispecialty group practice, in which physicians in different medical specialties work together. The appeal of group practice comes from higher incomes (due to sharing), intellectual stimulation, the ease of consultation with a colleague, and coverage. The remainder of physicians involved in patient care but not in private practice work on salary for hospitals, health maintenance organizations, industries, and schools or colleges. Examples of hospital-based physicians are anesthesiologists, radiologists, and pathologists. In addition to a regular salary and benefits such as malpractice insurance, they enjoy more regular hours and are spared the high cost of starting and maintaining a private practice. Physicians are not evenly distributed across the United States. The majority of physicians are concentrated in urban areas.

Specialization is a prominent feature of American medical practice. It allows a physician to focus on a narrow range of knowledge and skill and provides a higher degree of compensation. Specialization has advantages for patients. It results in a greater depth of knowledge and skill in the specialist's area of expertise. But specialization has some disadvantages. Specialists tend to concentrate on one organ or organ system or disease rather than on the whole person. They often have trouble coordinating care with other specialists when the patient has complaints that originate in different organ systems. Often there is poor communication with other specialists. All of these can lead to less than optimum care for the patient. A better approach to specialists is through a primary care physician, which is discussed later in the chapter.

In addition to physicians, there are a variety of other professionals educated in advanced professional degree programs who use the title "doctor." They specialize in specific areas of the body. Each has his own body of knowledge, skills, and educational requirements. These specialists include the following:

- Dentists are specialists in dental medicine.
- Podiatrists diagnose, treat, and prevent abnormal foot conditions.
- Chiropractors treat problems of the body's skeletal and neurologic systems by chiropractic manipulation, that is, adjustment of the skeletal system.
- Optometrists diagnose and selectively treat eye problems.

## NURSES

Nurses are the largest group of health personnel. The nursing profession has many "tiers." There are registered nurses, licensed practical nurses, and other nursing personnel.

A registered nurse, or RN, has the highest level of education, the most responsibility, and the most authority. There are three types of RN educational programs: a 2-year associate degree program, a 3-year hospital-based diploma program, and a 4-year baccalaureate degree program. In addition, graduate nursing education is found in university master's and doctoral degree programs. About half of all registered nurses work in hospitals. The remainder work in long-term care facilities, private medical or dental practices, schools, public health clinics, industries, and private-duty positions. Registered nurses have assumed expanded roles also. They have moved into the area of advanced clinical practice as clinical nurse specialists, nurse practitioners, nurse midwives, and nurse anesthetists. A clinical nurse specialist has skills in a particular area, such as mental health or women's health. A nurse practitioner performs primary care services, such as routine physicals. A nurse midwife provides prenatal and postnatal care, family planning, and routine gynecology care, and performs uncomplicated deliveries. A nurse anesthetist administers anesthetics during surgery under the supervision of an anesthesiologist. Registered nurses have also moved into other areas, such as teaching, administration, and management. Preparation for these expanded roles is usually achieved through graduate education.

A licensed practical nurse, or LPN, has a lower level of knowledge and skill than does a registered nurse. LPNs perform more hands-on caregiving tasks and work under the supervision of an RN. Their training usually consists of 12 to 18 months of study in a state-approved program found in trade, technical, or vocational schools. Other nursing personnel include certified nurses' aides as well as orderlies and attendants. They perform simple tasks and also work under the supervision of a registered nurse.

## PHYSICIAN ASSISTANTS

Physician assistants are a group of health care personnel that developed in the United States around the time of the Vietnam War. A physician assistant, or PA, also referred to as a physician extender, performs many of the routine functions of a primary care physician, such as physical exams and basic treatment of a variety of common illnesses. Physician assistants are intended to be an *extension* of the physician and work under the general supervision of the physician. Training is through accredited physician assistant programs in a number of academic settings, most being 2 years long. Most physician assistants work in outpatient settings such as physician offices and clinics. With the emphasis on primary care, physician assistants, as well as nurse practitioners, are playing a larger role in the health care system and are allowed to write prescriptions in many states.

## ALLIED HEALTH CARE PERSONNEL

Allied health personnel include workers in health-related areas who assist, facilitate, or complement the work of a physician. They work either on the orders of or under the general supervision of a physician. Examples of allied health personnel are found in Box 1–1.

There are also many types of practitioners of alternative and complementary medicine. Alternative and complementary medicine are defined as treatments and practices outside of traditional medicine that promote health and well-being.

## BOX 1–1  Allied Health Personnel

Dietician
Occupational therapist
Physical therapist
Respiratory therapist
Speech therapist
Social worker
Optician
Audiologist
Radiologic technologist
Cardiovascular technologist
Surgical technician
Laboratory technician
Nuclear medicine technologist
Emergency medical technician
Dental hygienist
Diagnostic medical sonographer

Among these types of health practitioners are acupuncturists, homeopaths, aromatherapists, herbalists, massage therapists, and music therapists. Finally, there are miscellaneous workers who are employed in the health care industry. Health care administrators manage health care institutions. Other personnel include clerical workers, maintenance workers, housekeeping staff, and food services staff.

From this discussion of health care personnel, it is clear that much expertise is brought to the patient. Health care in this country has been multidisciplinary; that is, many different health care personnel work somewhat independently. However, health care is moving toward being **interdisciplinary;** that is, many different health care personnel work together and communicate for the good of the patient. All health care personnel make up the interdisciplinary health care team.

## HEALTH CARE INSTITUTIONS

Health care institutions are the locations or places where health care services are provided to patients and where health care personnel work. Hospitals are the most visible and well known health care institutions. However, various other types of health care institutions provide health care services, including long-term care facilities, home health care organizations, hospices, physician practices, clinics, and pharmacies.

### OUTPATIENT CARE INSTITUTIONS

An outpatient care institution is a health care institution that provides health care services to a patient without an overnight stay. The patient is outside a traditional health care institution, such as a hospital, and is considered an *out-patient*. Because the patient is ambulatory, this type of health care institution is also referred to as an ambulatory care institution. Most of the need for health care services and the corresponding provision of care are in the ambulatory care or outpatient care setting. In fact, care has been shifting from inpatient care to outpatient care because it is a more cost-efficient way to provide health care services. There are three types of outpatient care institutions: physician medical practices, organized ambulatory care settings, and community pharmacies. It is important to recognize that different services are provided in each of these institutions.

## Physician Medical Practices

Private physician practices are the largest type of outpatient care institution. Physicians may see patients in a solo practice, partnership practice, or group practice.

## Organized Ambulatory Care Setting

An organized ambulatory care setting is an outpatient care institution where there is a medical practice that is identified by the type of service provided rather than by the physicians working in it. There are two types of health care services that may be provided in this setting: clinic services and emergency services.

### ■ Clinic Services

Clinic services provide ongoing care for routine or nonemergency medical problems in what is referred to as an outpatient clinic or "walk-in" clinic. Examples include outpatient hospital departments, community health centers including mental health clinics, surgery centers, diagnostic imaging centers, renal dialysis centers, clinical laboratories, public health clinics, occupational health clinics, school health clinics, and voluntary health agencies. Hospital outpatient clinics can be medical, surgical, or other specialty clinics, such as diabetes or asthma clinics. Community health centers, formerly called neighborhood health centers, deliver primary care services. Surgery centers, diagnostic imaging centers, renal dialysis centers, and clinical laboratories all provide health care services that once required inpatient hospital stays but now can be safely provided in an outpatient setting owing to advances in medical practice and technology. Public health clinics concentrate on disease prevention and are provided by local government health departments. In contrast to some hospital outpatient clinics, public health clinics offer their services to all persons regardless of their ability to pay. Services provided by public health clinics include family planning, tuberculosis care, mental health care, AIDS care, child health care, prenatal care, and sexually transmitted diseases care. Occupational health clinics treat job-related disorders as well as promote wellness. They are usually located "in plant" and staffed with trained industrial nurses and part- or full-time physicians. School health clinics are found in primary schools, secondary schools, and universities. They are usually run by boards of education or local health departments. Examples of services provided are vision and hearing screenings, immunizations, and first aid care. Volunteer or voluntary health agencies operate local chapters and focus on a specific disease. They provide education and financing for needed services and research and are usually funded through charitable donations. Examples include the American Heart Association, American Cancer Society, American Lung Association, and American Red Cross.

### ■ Emergency Services

Emergency services provide immediate treatment for serious or acute illness or injury that may be life-threatening. Emergency services are also used to assess a patient with a medical problem that may lead to a hospital admission or that requires health care personnel or diagnostic equipment not usually available in a physician's office. Emergency services may be provided in a hospital emergency department, in a freestanding emergency care center, or in a prehospital emergency situation, such as an ambulance. Hospital emergency departments, also referred to as "emergency rooms," are staffed by health care personnel trained in emergency care. A trauma center is a highly specialized hospital emergency department that handles the severest emergency cases. Freestanding emergency care centers, also referred to as "emergi-centers," are emergency departments located outside of a hospital. They provide emergency services but do not receive severe cases or cases that arrive by ambulance. Advantages to this type of emergency care are lower cost (than in a hospital emergency department), access, and convenience. Emergency services in a prehospital emergency situation usually begin with the 911 national emergency response system. These services consist of highly trained emergency personnel, such as emergency medical technicians, advanced equipment, transportation in the form of an ambulance, and communication with a hospital emergency department. The goal here is to preserve life by providing treatment and transportation to a hospital emergency department.

### Community Pharmacies

Community pharmacies are the third type of outpatient care institution. A community pharmacy is a pharmacy that provides pharmaceutical products and services to outpatients or ambulatory patients; that is, those capable of "walking in" to the pharmacy for service. It refers to a pharmacy located outside of a hospital or other institutional setting or a pharmacy that does not provide services to inpatients in any institutional setting. It usually refers to a pharmacy in a retail setting.

## INPATIENT CARE INSTITUTIONS

An inpatient care institution is a health care institution that provides health care services to a patient who is admitted to and assigned a bed in that institution. The patient is considered to be inside a traditional health care institution and is referred to as an *inpatient*. There are several types of inpatient care institutions.

### Hospitals

Begun as charitable institutions, hospitals have become the institutional center and the most visible part of the health care system. The hospital is the meeting center for the health care needs of a community. It has been referred to as the "physician's workshop," and physicians are indeed the driving force behind hospitals. Physicians are the only health care personnel who can admit patients to a hospital, and all other health care personnel must act on their orders. However, hospitals generally function reasonably well with each group of health care personnel knowing their roles, responsibilities, and authority.

Hospitals provide health care services to inpatients who are admitted and assigned a bed, as well as to outpatients who come to the hospital for a health care service that does not require admission. Owing to the shift from inpatient to outpatient services, hospitals are shifting from being the *center* of the health care system to being an important *part* of the health care system.

Hospitals are classified in several ways: type of service provided, size, length of patient stays, and ownership (AHA, 2006). A hospital can be classified by the types of services provided. The most commonly used classifications are general hospital, specialty hospital, refined specialty hospital, psychiatric hospital, teaching hospital, and critical access hospital. A general hospital provides medical, surgical, diagnostic, and treatment services for a wide variety of medical conditions. A specialty hospital provides medical, surgical, diagnostic, and treatment services for specific medical conditions or segments of the population. Examples of specialty hospitals are found in Box 1–2.

A refined specialty hospital specializes in the treatment of a specific chronic disease, examples being cancer hospitals and respiratory hospitals. Mental or psychiatric hospitals provide diagnosis and treatment services to patients with mental illness and alcoholism and other chemical dependencies. A teaching hospital provides education and training for physicians and research in addition to patient care. Relative to nonteaching hospitals, they are usually large, located in large metropolitan areas, offer more specialized services, and provide more charity or unpaid care. Finally, a critical access hospital is a small hospital that is located quite a distance from a full-service hospital and provides limited services, mostly evaluation of a patient's needs.

Another method of hospital classification is by size, that is, the number of beds regularly available for inpatient care. The size of a hospital depends on the population it serves, the range of health care services offered, and whether it is used as a referral hospital by other hospitals. The average hospital in the United States has between 100 and 199 beds. About 20 percent of U.S. hospitals have 300 or more beds (AHA, 2006).

## BOX 1–2   Specialty Hospitals

Maternity or women's hospital
Rehabilitation hospital
Orthopedic hospital
Children's hospital
Burn hospital
Eye hospital
Psychiatric hospital
Cancer hospital
Drug and alcohol treatment hospital
Long-term acute care hospital

Another method of classification involves the length of the patient's stay in the hospital. A short-term hospital is one in which the average length of stay is less than 30 days. A long-term hospital is defined as one in which the average length of stay is 30 days or more.

Finally, hospitals are classified by ownership, either public or private. A public hospital is owned by the federal, state, or local government. Public hospitals do not strive to make a profit. Funding comes from tax revenues, and they handle many charity cases. Examples of public hospitals are Veterans Administration (VA) hospitals (federal), state mental hospitals (state), and city and county hospitals (local). A private hospital is not owned by the government. Private hospitals may be further characterized as for-profit or not-for-profit. A for-profit hospital is owned by investors, and revenues are distributed among shareholders as profits. A not-for-profit hospital, also called a nonprofit hospital, is owned by a not-for-profit group, and revenues are reinvested for improvements and charity care. Not-for-profit hospitals are given tax advantages and are allowed to receive donations. Examples of not-for-profit hospitals are those run by religious groups, such as Catholic hospitals. Other terms are also used to describe hospitals. A general hospital includes the bulk of U.S. hospitals, but the term *community hospital* is used as the all-inclusive term for the majority of them. A community hospital is defined as a nonfederal, short-term general, or other special hospital whose facilities and services are available to the public. Increasingly, hospitals are becoming part of multihospital systems and larger health care delivery systems through mergers and acquisitions.

## Long-Term Care Institutions

The long-term care facility, generally referred to as a nursing home, is another example of an inpatient care institution. Long-term care describes a range of health and personal care, social services, and housing services provided to people of all ages with chronic health conditions that limit their ability to carry out normal functions without assistance (Kovner & Jonas, 2005). A long-term care facility provides inpatient care for those who need care over longer periods of time than would be provided in an acute care hospital. Nursing homes are only one type of long-term care facility. Other examples include psychiatric hospitals, chronic disease hospitals, rehabilitation hospitals, and correctional facilities.

## Home Health Care Institutions

Home health care is defined as health care services provided to patients in their homes. Home health care patients cannot receive health care services on an ambulatory basis owing to some type of functional disability or medical problem. As an alternative, these patients can be cared for as successfully in the home as in the hospital or long-term care facility because of new and improved technology. In this sense, home care can be considered a health care institution. The services offered by home health care organizations are many and varied and are discussed in depth in Chapters 6 and 7.

## Hospice

Hospice involves palliative care and support services for the dying patient. It can be extended to patients in their homes if they so choose or in inpatient hospice facilities as well as in hospitals or long-term care facilities. Hospice care is covered in Chapter 11.

## HEALTH CARE SERVICES

There are three basic types of health care services produced in our health care system: primary care, secondary care, and tertiary care. Simply stated, primary care is basic general care; secondary care involves more specialized care; and tertiary care is the most advanced and expensive care of all.

Primary care is defined as preventative health care and routine medical care. It involves meeting an individual's health care needs over a long period of time. Primary care addresses the most common health problems and is the level of care that most people need and use. It is comprehensive; that is, it includes everything from the diagnosis and treatment of medical problems to health promotion and disease prevention activities. Primary care is provided by a primary care practitioner who may refer the patient to a specialist when appropriate. The primary care practitioner may be one of four types of health care personnel: physicians, nurse practitioners, nurse midwives, and physician assistants. Among physicians, family practitioners, pediatricians, internal medicine physicians, and obstetrician/gynecologists all provide primary care services. Most primary care is provided in outpatient or ambulatory care institutions. However, primary care may extend into the inpatient setting, where a primary care physician can continue to care for the patient now as an inpatient. This continuation of care from one health care setting to another is referred to as **continuity of care.**

Secondary care consists of specialized health care services beyond primary care services. Secondary care is arranged after a primary care evaluation. It includes specialist physician care, surgery, and advanced diagnostic services. Secondary care services are available in private physician offices and other outpatient institutions and in hospitals.

Tertiary care involves highly specialized services for diagnosis, treatment, or rehabilitation. The highly trained health care personnel and equipment for this type of care normally are not found at the level of the average community hospital but in major medical centers and teaching hospitals. Examples of tertiary care include open-heart surgery, organ transplant surgery, bone marrow transplant, and other complex procedures.

## HEALTH CARE FINANCING

The gross domestic product (GDP), the dollar value of all goods and services produced in the United States in any one year, is used as a rough measure of the nation's economy. The health care industry accounts for one of the largest shares of the GDP. In 2003, total spending for health care services was $1.7 trillion, or 15.3 percent of the GDP (Centers for Medicare and Medicaid Services, 2005). The health care industry has captured a growing share of the GDP over the years, and that share is expected to rise. The Centers for Medicare and Medicaid Services (CMS) estimates that health care spending will reach $3.6 trillion, or 18.7 percent of the GDP, by the year 2014 (Table 1–1).

**TABLE 1–1** National Health Care Expenditures as a Percentage of the Gross Domestic Product

| YEAR | PERCENTAGE OF GDP |
| --- | --- |
| 1980 | 8.8 |
| 1985 | 10.5 |
| 1990 | 12.0 |
| 1995 | 13.4 |
| 2000 | 13.3 |
| 2003 | 15.3 |
| 2014 | 18.7 |

From "Highlights—National Health Care Expenditures Projections: 2000–2014," CMS, Office of the Actuary, National Health Statistics Group, 2005, www.cms.gov.

The rise in the share of the GDP for health care can be attributed to many factors, including the following:

- Inflation, which affects all areas of the economy including health care
- The growth in the population, which increases the demand for health care services
- The aging of the population, which likewise increases the demand for services
- Increased spending for prescription drugs
- The use of expensive new medical technology
- The overall increased utilization of health care services
- The Medicare Part D prescription drug benefit, which took effect in 2006

## HEALTH CARE EXPENDITURES

National health care expenditures are grouped into two categories: personal health care expenditures and nonpersonal health care expenditures. Personal health care expenditures make up the majority of health care spending and go for personal health care services and supplies. These include hospital care, physician services, nursing home care, prescription drugs, other professional services such as dental services, home health care, eyeglasses, and other related medical products. Nonpersonal health care expenditures go toward program administration, research, construction, and government public health activities. The biggest share of health care spending is on hospitals and physicians. In 2003, spending on hospitals and physicians accounted for 53 percent of total U.S. health care spending, physician services accounting for 22 percent, and hospital care accounting for 31 percent. Nursing home care accounted for another 7 percent. In 2003, prescription drugs alone accounted for 11 percent of national health care expenditures (CMS, 2005). These figures are summarized in Figure 1–1.

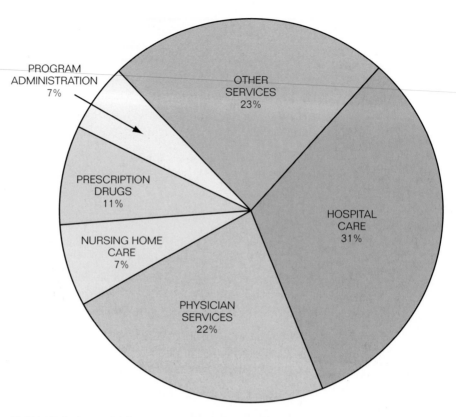

**FIGURE 1–1**  Health Care Expenditures: 2003. (From "The Nation's Health Care Dollar: 2003," CMS, Office of the Actuary, National Health Statistics Group, 2005, www.cms.gov.)

## SOURCES OF FUNDING

The lack of a single national health care financing system in the United States complicates how health care providers are paid for their services. Ultimately, the people of the United States pay all health care costs:

- From tax revenues, which fund government programs
- From charitable donations, which fund voluntary agencies and not-for-profit institutions
- From insurance premiums and co-pays, which fund managed care organizations and insurance companies
- From direct payments from patients to health care providers

Thus, financing for the U.S. health care system comes from public and private sources. This system contrasts with health care financing in many other countries, where money comes largely from public sources. Private funding represented 55 percent of health care expenditures in 2003 (CMS, 2005). Private funding comes from two sources: private health insurance companies and patients. Private health insurance companies make payments to health care providers on behalf of patients. There are two types of private health insurance: employment-based plans and direct-purchase plans. An employment-based plan is health care coverage provided through an employer or union. A direct-purchase plan is coverage purchased by an individual from a private health insurance company. The patient receiving health care services is the other source of private health care funding in what is referred to as a direct "out-of-pocket" payment. An out-of-pocket payment refers to a direct payment made to a health care provider by a patient. This payment may be for a noncovered service, that is, a service not paid for by any other source of funds, or for a deductible, co-payment, or coinsurance of some type.

Public funding refers to government health insurance. Government health insurance includes plans at the federal, state, and local levels. Medicare and Medicaid are the two largest government programs. Medicare is a federal program that was enacted in 1965 to finance health care services for the elderly and disabled. A prescription drug benefit was added in 2006. Medicaid is administered by the states within federal guidelines and was enacted in 1965 to finance health care services for the poor. Another state health care program is the State Children's Health Insurance Program, which provides health care services for low-income children whose parents do not qualify for Medicaid. It is known by different names in different states. Additionally, other government health insurance plans take care of the health care needs of veterans (through the Veterans Administration), the military (through TRICARE), Native Americans (through the Indian Health Service), and residents of federal or state mental hospitals and correctional facilities.

Since the 1980s, managed care organizations have entered the health care financing market. They may be not-for-profit or for-profit, owned by a private insurance company, or independently owned. Managed care combines health care financing with health care delivery. Managed care is discussed further in this chapter.

It would be helpful to briefly discuss the health care payment system referred to as a three-party payment system. This system consists of three parties or groups. The first party is the patient; the second party is the health care provider; and the third party is the payer. The third party, or payer, is the party who is responsible for the payment for the health care services provided by the health care provider to the patient. From our discussion, a third-party payer can be a private health care insurance company, the government, or, more recently, a managed care organization.

## HEALTH CARE REIMBURSEMENT

There are two types of health care provider reimbursement. Money is paid for health care services on the basis of fee-for-service or capitation. Physicians and health care institutions have been paid on a **fee-for-service** basis. It is a simple system in which a separate fee is paid for each type of health care service performed. The fee is set, and the patient or third party pays *after* the service is rendered. Because payment is made after the service is provided, it is a retrospective payment system. This system offers little financial incentive for the health care provider to control costs. The alternative method of payment is called **capitation.** Capitation refers to paying a fixed, prepaid fee per person, or per "capita," to provide a range of health care services to a patient for a specified period of time, usually a year. This fee, called the *capitation fee,* is paid *before* the services are rendered and is the same regardless of how many health care services a patient receives during the designated period of time. Because payment is prearranged and made before the service is provided, it is a prospective payment system. This system offers financial incentives to control health care costs and manage resources effectively. Managed care is changing how reimbursement is made to health care providers by shifting from a fee-for-service payment system to a capitation system of payment.

## PROBLEMS IN THE U.S. HEALTH CARE SYSTEM

The United States has the most technologically advanced health care in the world. The United States spends a higher proportion of its GDP on health care and also spends more per capita on health care than any other country in the world. However, despite the large degree of spending on health care, the United States does not have the best health levels in the world, measured in terms of increased life expectancy and decreased infant mortality, as compared with other countries that spend less on health care.

The U.S. government is less involved in health care than the government of any other industrialized nation in the world. What involvement there is is split among federal, state, and local governments, each having responsibility and authority for different health care services. Thus, there is no centralized structure in our health care system. What strength there is in the U.S. health care system comes from the private medical sector. Physicians practice in a free-enterprise system, which is based on individual economic gain. It is driven by profit (the private incomes of physicians), not by social values. Although the system is being influenced by managed care, medical care is still provided by private and direct contact between patient and physician.

Serious and widespread health care problems continue to exist in our country, contributing to less than optimal health care. Some specific problems (relating to cost, access, and quality) include:

- It is difficult to keep rising health care costs under control.
- Millions of Americans have inadequate health care coverage.
- Of all Americans, 45.8 million, or 15.7 percent, have no health insurance (U.S. Census Bureau, 2005).
- Health care resources are being wasted due to the fragmented and disorganized way they are delivered.
- There is an undersupply of primary care physicians in some areas of the country.
- There is an oversupply of specialist physicians.
- Health care services are unevenly distributed on the basis of geography and income levels.
- Physicians practice independently and are not trained to work on health care teams or to coordinate care.
- Many practicing physicians do not use the most current scientific knowledge or the latest in medical technology in treating patients.
- Ambulatory health care settings, where the majority of health care is delivered, lack quality improvement systems.
- Medical errors are occurring at an alarming rate, including medication errors.
- Few safety systems are in place to prevent medical errors.
- Many people make questionable lifestyle choices without considering their impact on the nation's health care system.
- Many people do not actively participate in their own health care because they often lack the necessary information to make health care decisions.
- The focus of health care is still on the treatment of disease rather than on health promotion and disease prevention.

## HEALTH CARE REFORM

According to the Institute of Medicine (IOM) Committee on the Quality of Health Care in America, the U.S. health care system is in need of change. Examining the problems in our health care system has led to questions such as (1) How can health care costs be controlled? (2) How can access to health care for everyone be improved? and (3) How can high-quality health care be consistently provided? The answers again are related to cost, access, and quality. Reforms have been proposed, and changes are being made in the way the United States organizes, delivers, and pays for the advanced health care we have. The goal of health care reform then is to control health care costs while improving access to high-quality health care services for all Americans. Specific health care reforms include:

- Controlling costs by incorporating managed care systems into the entire health care system
- Providing health care services through an interdisciplinary health care team, including pharmacists, where possible
- Using the latest in information and life-saving technology
- Encouraging physicians to practice in groups, especially multispecialty groups, to provide continuity of care
- Putting safety systems in place in all health care settings to prevent medical errors and reporting medical errors to determine their causes rather than to punish
- Focusing on the outcome of any health care service delivered
- Stressing healthy lifestyle choices
- Involving patients in their own health and the health care services they receive by giving them necessary medical information
- Stressing health promotion and disease prevention rather than the treatment of disease

## THE ROLE OF MANAGED CARE

If health care personnel, health care institutions, and financing are to be brought together to provide quality health care services, they must be *managed*. It is believed that health care costs can be controlled by managing delivery of services without limiting access or sacrificing quality. The concept of managing health care can be traced to the early twentieth century, when prepaid health insurance plans appeared in the United States. Managed care itself originated in 1973, when then President Nixon signed the Health Maintenance Organization Act into law. It encouraged the use of low-cost delivery systems and provided financial assistance for these early health maintenance organizations. This was the government's first attempt at replacing the fee-for-service payment system and changing reimbursement. The U.S. health care system has moved into managed care at an accelerated rate in response to the demands for health care reform. Managed care has changed the way health care services are delivered and paid for.

What is managed care? There is no single definition. **Managed care** is a system that provides both the financing *and* delivery of health care for its members. This financing is accomplished through prearranged, or *prospective,* payment contracts with a limited number of health care providers. In fact, the defining feature of managed care is the use of health care provider networks. A **network** is defined as a group of health care providers linked through a contract to provide a range of health care services. Managed care then is a network of providers formed to offer cost-effective health care services. It is a planned and coordinated approach to providing health care.

The foundation of the managed care system is the primary care physician or provider. He is often referred to as the **gatekeeper.** The primary care physician is the first health care professional a patient sees for a medical condition. He is responsible for a patient's treatment. He coordinates and authorizes all health care services, including lab tests, specialist referrals, and hospitalization. Careful screening can eliminate costly and needless health care services. Equally important is the primary care physician's stress on health promotion and disease prevention, which have been shown to decrease health care costs.

## MANAGED CARE ORGANIZATIONS

A **managed care organization**, or MCO, is defined as a health care organization that both insures and provides health care services. It provides health care services for a fixed amount of money, negotiated and paid in advance. There are several types of managed care organizations.

### Health Maintenance Organizations

A health maintenance organization, or HMO, is a managed care organization that provides health care services to enrolled members for a capitation fee, that is, a fixed, prepaid fee. There is a pool of physicians, as well as hospitals and pharmacies, that agree to provide health care services. There are advantages for the patient, such as predictable cost in the form of a small co-payment, no paperwork, and broad coverage for routine inpatient and outpatient care. The disadvantages are that members must usually choose a physician affiliated with the HMO, and a referral is required from the primary care physician for a specialist visit. There are also advantages for physicians in HMOs. Advantages include a guaranteed income and the possibility of expanding their patient base. Some disadvantages for physicians include outside interference, loss of independence, and reduced income. There are several types of health maintenance organizations:

- Staff model. The HMO employs its own physicians, usually in a central site. They see only HMO patients.
- Group model. The HMO enters an exclusive contract with large physician groups. The physicians see only HMO patients.
- Network model. The HMO enters a nonexclusive contract with a large physician group. The physicians can see non-HMO, or private, patients as well as HMO patients.
- Independent practice association (IPA) model. The HMO enters a nonexclusive contract with individual physicians. The physicians can see non-HMO as well as HMO patients.

## Preferred Provider Organizations

A preferred provider organization (PPO) is a managed care organization that provides health care services to enrolled members on a discounted fee-for-service basis. A discounted payment is made to the health care provider according to the number and type of health care services provided rather than on a capitation basis. The PPO enters a nonexclusive contract with a network of providers who can see non-PPO, or private, patients as well as PPO patients. No referral is needed for a specialist visit if he is also a PPO provider. A member may select a non-PPO health care provider, but the member is responsible for the balance of the fee above what the discounted fee would be. A hybrid of the PPO is the "exclusive preferred provider organization," in which no payment is made by the PPO for health care services received outside of the network of providers.

## Point-of-Service Plans

A point-of-service plan, or POS plan, can be considered an HMO/PPO hybrid. It is called a "point-of-service" plan because members may choose an option, either an HMO or PPO, whenever they need health care. Like an HMO and a PPO, a POS plan has a contracted network of physicians. As in a traditional HMO, the primary care physician acts as a gatekeeper and makes referrals. As in a traditional PPO, members are not required to choose a primary care physician or to obtain a referral. A POS plan allows its members to choose a physician not contracted by the plan as well as a physician contracted by the plan, with or without a referral, although the costs for the member are higher when seeing a physician outside of the plan or without a referral. POS plans offer flexibility and freedom of choice. The types of managed care organizations are summarized in Table 1–2.

## Pharmacy Benefit Management Company

A pharmacy benefit management company, or PBM company, is another type of managed care organization. It is a company that focuses only on the pharmacy

**TABLE 1–2    Comparison of Managed Care Organizations**

|  | PHYSICIANS | TYPE OF CONTRACT | MCO PATIENTS? | PRIVATE PATIENTS? | PAYMENT MCO SYSTEM |
|---|---|---|---|---|---|
| **Staff Model HMO** | Individual | Exclusive | Yes | No | Capitation |
| **Group Model HMO** | Group | Exclusive | Yes | No | Capitation |
| **Network Model HMO** | Group | Non-exclusive | Yes | Yes | Capitation |
| **IPA Model HMO** | Individual | Non-exclusive | Yes | Yes | Capitation |
| **PPO** | Individual + group | Non-exclusive | Yes | Yes | Fee for service |
| **POS Plan** | Individual + group | Exclusive | Yes | No | Capitation |

component of health care. The PBM company contracts with an insurer to provide prescription drugs to members, usually using existing community pharmacies. Pharmacy services, initially an afterthought, have become a major benefit that a managed care organization can offer its members and is now the fastest-growing component of managed care (Sanofi Aventis Pharmaceuticals, 2006). The prescription drug benefit is now being removed from, or "carved out" of, traditional health insurance plans for several reasons. It is a very visible benefit to members; it can be negotiated easily; and it can be aggressively managed to reduce drug costs. Managed care pharmacy and PBM companies are discussed in depth in Chapter 8.

Managed care is an established form of health care delivery in this country. It has challenged our health care system to reduce the unnecessary use of health care resources, to improve how health care services are delivered, and, in general, to become more efficient. Managed care's involvement in our health care system will continue to evolve, with more changes to come in the future.

## OUTCOMES-BASED THERAPY

In the late 1980s, there was a call for assessment of health care services when Arnold Relman, editor-in-chief emeritus of the *New England Journal of Medicine,* stated: "We can no longer afford to provide health care without knowing more about its successes and failures" (Relman, 1988). Managed care has focused on controlling costs while emphasizing quality care. A major difficulty in measuring quality is that there is no universal definition of quality. What variables should be measured and how? In 1978, Avedis Donabedian, a health services researcher, identified three variables that should be measured to ensure quality and that are still used today: structure, process, and outcomes (Donabedian, 1978). Simply stated, **structure** refers to the resources, personnel, and policies and procedures available to provide care. **Process** refers to how well the structures are used to provide care. **Outcomes** are defined as a change in the patient's health status resulting from the health care service. Structure and process are focused on the health care provider and institution, whereas outcomes are focused on the patient. Donabedian emphasized that structure and process are important for providing quality health care; however, outcomes are the ultimate measure of quality. Outcomes determine the extent of benefit or harm to the patient.

Outcomes are the end results of care. They reflect the effectiveness of the health care services provided. They represent what happened to the patient. Traditionally, outcomes have been measured in clinical terms, such as the results of blood pressure readings or laboratory tests. Today, they are being measured in terms of curing diseases such as cancer or heart disease; preventing disabilities such as stroke, blindness, or amputation; and preventing death. Outcomes have also been expanded to include quality of life, patient satisfaction, patient preference, and mental and physical functioning. Favorable outcomes are the goal of health care, although occasional unintended effects occur as well. Outcomes-based therapy seeks to increase desired outcomes and decrease undesired outcomes. All health care services should be evaluated on the basis of outcomes as health care moves from just providing a service to determining the outcome of that service.

Donabedian's terms can be applied to the practice of pharmacy. Structure is related to the physical setting of the pharmacy, such as the drug and supply inventory, the computer system, the patient profiles, and pharmacy technician coverage. Process is related to activities that occur between the pharmacist and the patient, for example, taking a medication history, monitoring a patient's drug regimen, and counseling the patient. Outcomes are related to what happens to the patient as a result of drug therapy and can include the relief of symptoms, a change in the length of hospitalization, or adverse drug reactions. Pharmacists have a responsibility to ensure positive outcomes of drug therapy for their patients.

## PHARMACEUTICAL CARE

A discussion of pharmaceutical care is central to the discussion about pharmacists in the U.S. health care system. The profession of pharmacy is shifting from providing a *product* to providing a *service*. Pharmaceutical care involves the process in which a pharmacist cooperates with the patient and his other health care providers in designing, implementing, and monitoring a therapeutic plan that will produce specific outcomes for the patient. It is a type of patient care service that is unique to pharmacy.

Pharmaceutical care was defined in 1990 by two pharmacists who were professors at the University of Florida College of Pharmacy, C. D. Hepler and L. M. Strand. They defined **pharmaceutical care** as "the responsible provision of drug therapy for the purpose of achieving definite outcomes that improve a patient's quality of life." These outcomes are curing disease, reducing or eliminating symptoms, arresting or slowing disease progression, and preventing disease or symptoms. The pharmaceutical care process involves three major functions performed by the pharmacist on behalf of the patient. These functions are identifying potential and actual drug-related problems, resolving drug-related problems that do develop, and preventing potential drug-related problems (Hepler & Strand, 1990).

A **drug-related problem** is defined as an event or situation involving drug therapy that actually or potentially interferes with an optimum outcome for the patient. Drug-related problems include:

- *Untreated indication.* A patient has a medical problem that needs drug therapy but is not receiving a drug for that problem. An example would be a patient with congestive heart failure who does not receive an ACE inhibitor.

- *Improper drug selection.* A patient has a medical problem but is taking the wrong drug for that problem. An example would be a patient who is allergic to penicillin and is taking penicillin for an infection.

- *Subtherapeutic dosage.* A patient has a medical problem that is being treated with too little of the correct drug. An example would be a patient with epilepsy taking a seizure drug but still experiencing seizures.

- *Failure to receive a drug.* A patient has a medical problem that is the result of not receiving a drug. An example would be a patient with diabetes who does not receive his insulin injection and experiences hyperglycemia.

- *Overdosage.* A patient has a medical problem that is being treated with too much of the correct drug. An example would be a patient with asthma taking theophylline who has a high theophylline blood level.

- *Adverse drug reaction.* A patient has a medical problem that is the result of an adverse drug reaction. An example would be a patient taking an ACE inhibitor and experiencing a dry cough.

- *Drug interactions.* A patient has a medical problem that is the result of a drug's interacting with another drug, food, or laboratory test. An example would be a patient taking fluconazole for a fungal infection along with erythromycin for a bacterial infection and experiencing heart palpitations.

- *Drug use without an indication.* A patient is taking a drug for no medically valid reason. An example would be a patient taking an H2-receptor antagonist drug for vague symptoms of an upset stomach.

Drug-related problems are a major concern. They cause serious health problems, disability, and even death. Thousands of people are hospitalized yearly as a result of drug-related problems. Through the pharmaceutical care process, pharmacists work to achieve positive outcomes and prevent negative outcomes by identifying and managing drug-related problems.

Pharmaceutical care has been described as a philosophy of practice, and some pharmacists have been practicing pharmaceutical care for many years already. It can be applied in all pharmacy practice settings. Pharmaceutical care incorporates the three measures for assessing quality: structure, process, and outcomes. Again, although structure and process are important, it is the incorporation of outcomes into the daily practice of pharmacy that is unique to pharmaceutical care. What are some specific examples of pharmaceutical care services provided by pharmacists? They include performing drug regimen reviews, counseling patients, monitoring patient compliance, performing pharmacokinetic calculations to ensure correct dosing of critical medications, educating other health care professionals, and developing and managing formularies. Examples of the many outcomes that can occur as a result of pharmaceutical care are provided in Box 1–3.

---

### BOX 1–3    Outcomes That Occur As a Result of Pharmaceutical Care

Better disease control or cure
Fewer total medications
Less emergency room use
Better self-care by patients
Appropriate generic use
Fewer specialist referrals
Fewer drug-related home health visits
Fewer adverse drug reactions
Lower levels of nursing home care
Fewer hospitalizations
Less urgent care use
Increased patient satisfaction
Fewer unscheduled physician visits
Fewer phone calls to physicians
Better patient compliance
Increased quality of life

Pharmaceutical care is the pharmacy profession's opportunity to shift from providing a product to providing a true service. It complements the trend emerging in health care today, especially in managed care. Pharmacists are being called on to deliver cost-effective, accessible, quality pharmaceutical services. Pharmacy technicians are a big part of accomplishing this goal. Pharmaceutical care can help pharmacists and pharmacy technicians achieve it. It is clearly the wave of the future.

## KEY CONCEPTS

- Any health care system has three components: cost, access, and quality.
- There are many types of health care systems in place throughout the world, some under government control and some with limited government control.
- Many types of health care personnel provide health care services, including pharmacists and pharmacy technicians, physicians, nurses, physician assistants, and various allied health personnel.
- Health care institutions provide health care services on an outpatient or inpatient basis.
- Three types of health care services are provided in our health care system: primary care, secondary care, and tertiary care.
- Financing for the U.S. health care system comes from private and public sources and involves a three-party payment system.
- Problems relating to cost, access, and quality exist in the current U.S. health care system, examples being rising health care costs, the lack of health coverage for all citizens, the uneven distribution of services, and the lack of adequate quality control and safety systems.
- Various health care reforms, especially the use of managed care and the emphasis on outcomes of health care services, may bring solutions of some of our nation's health care problems.
- Managed care combines health care financing with health care delivery and is changing the way health care services are provided and paid for.
- Structure, process, and outcomes can be measured to ensure the quality of health care, but outcomes are the ultimate measure and apply to the practice of pharmacy.
- Pharmaceutical care is the provision of drug therapy to achieve definite outcomes that improve a patient's quality of life.

## SELF-ASSESSMENT QUESTIONS

### MULTIPLE CHOICE

1. By providing pharmaceutical care, pharmacists can:
   a. improve a patient's quality of life
   b. reduce drug costs
   c. prevent drug-related problems
   d. all of the above

2. Pharmaceutical care emphasizes the pharmacist's responsibility in regard to:
   a. drug dispensing
   b. patient outcomes
   c. diagnosing disease
   d. compounding

3. The drivers of any health care system are all of the following except:
   a. cost
   b. institutions
   c. access
   d. quality

4. All are examples of inpatient care institutions except:
   a. a patient's home
   b. nursing homes
   c. hospitals
   d. surgery centers

5. Hospitals are classified by:
   a. number of beds
   b. length of patient stays
   c. types of services provided
   d. all of the above

6. Outcomes can be described as:
   a. a change in the patient's health status as a result of a health care service
   b. the end result of care
   c. the ultimate measure of quality
   d. all of the above

7. The following statements about ambulatory care are all true except:
   a. it costs less than inpatient care
   b. it is provided to a patient in a bed
   c. it is provided on an outpatient basis
   d. it can be provided in a retail pharmacy

8. Which is not an outpatient care institution?
   a. outpatient pharmacy
   b. physician medical practice
   c. renal dialysis center
   d. nursing home

9. All of the following statements about the U.S. health care system are true except:
   a. the emphasis is on the diagnosis and treatment of disease
   b. the U.S. government has a limited role
   c. the United States spends a large amount of its GDP on health care
   d. health care is available to every American

10. A drug-related problem can be:
    a. an overdose of a drug
    b. an underdose of a drug
    c. the wrong drug
    d. all of the above

## TRUE/FALSE (CORRECT THE FALSE STATEMENTS.)

1. _____ The continuation of care from one health care setting to another is called continuity of care.
2. _____ The goal of managed care is to reduce health care costs while maintaining the quality of health care.
3. _____ The foundation of a managed care organization is the specialist physician.
4. _____ Most primary care services are provided in outpatient care institutions.
5. _____ Outcomes-based therapy is a change in the patient's health as a result of the health care system.
6. _____ Funding for the U.S. health care system comes from public sources.
7. _____ In a three-party payment system, a payment is made directly to a health care provider by the patient.
8. _____ Managed care provides both the financing and delivery of health care.
9. _____ A preferred provider organization provides health care services to members on a capitation basis.
10. _____ A drug-related problem can interfere with an optimum outcome.

## FILL-IN

1. Immediate care for serious or acute illness or injury is referred to as _____ _____.
2. Direct payment to a health care provider by a patient is referred to as an _____ _____ _____ payment.
3. A fee-for-service payment, where payment is made *after* a health care service is provided, is referred to as a _____ payment.
4. A capitation payment, where payment is made *before* a health care service is provided, is referred to as a _____ payment.
5. A group of health care providers linked through a contract to provide a range of health care services is called a _____.
6. A primary care physician is referred to as a _____.
7. A _____ _____ _____ is an event or situation involving drug therapy that actually or potentially interferes with an optimum outcome for the patient.
8. Basic general health care is referred to as _____ care.
9. _____ care is the most advanced and expensive type of health care.
10. Many different health care personnel working together and communicating for the good of the patients is described as _____ health care.

## CRITICAL THINKING

1. What are the consequences of managed care for patients, health care providers, and payers?
2. What are the problems associated with an undersupply of primary care physicians and an oversupply of specialist physicians?
3. Does health care spending demand too great a share of the gross domestic product in the United States?
4. Who are the uninsured in America, and how can health care coverage be extended to them?
5. Why is pharmaceutical care necessary in our health care system?

## BIBLIOGRAPHY

American Heart Association. (2005). *Managed health care plans.* [On-line] AHA. Available: www.americanheart.org.

American Hospital Association. (2006). *American Hospital Association guide, 2006 edition.* Chicago: Author.

American Hospital Association. (2006). *American Hospital Association statistics, 2006 edition.* Chicago: Author.

American Society of Consultant Pharmacists. (2005). *Statement on pharmaceutical care.* [On-line] ASCP. Available: www.ascp.com.

Centers for Medicare and Medicaid Services. (2005). *Highlights—National health expenditures, 2003.* [On-line] CMS. Office of the Actuary. National Health Statistics Group. Available: www.cms.gov.

Centers for Medicare and Medicaid Services. (2005). *National health care expenditures projections: 2004–2014.* [On-line] CMS. Office of the Actuary. National Health Statistics Group. Available: www.cms.gov.

Centers for Medicare and Medicaid Services. (2005). *The nation's health dollar: 2003.* [On-line] CMS. Office of the Actuary. National Health Statistics Group. Available: www.cms.gov.

Donabedian, A. (1978). The quality of medical care. *Science, 200,* 856–864.

Drug Store News Tech Ed Program. (2002). Health care overview for retail pharmacy technicians. *Drug Store News, 10,* 1–8.

Hepler, C. D., & Strand, L. M. (1990). Opportunities and responsibilities in pharmaceutical care. *American Journal of Hospital Pharmacy, 47,* 533–543.

Jonas, S. (2003). *An introduction to the U.S. health care system* (5th ed.). New York: Springer Publishing Company.

Kovner, A., & Jonas, S. (Eds.). (2005). *Jonas and Kovner's health care delivery in the United States* (8th ed.). New York: Springer Publishing Company.

Mayer, F. (2006). It's time for health care for everyone. *Drug Topics, 150*(15), 52.

McCarthy, R., & Schafermeyer, K. (2004). *Introduction to health care delivery: A primer for pharmacists.* Gaithersburg, MD: Aspen Publishers, Inc.

National Home Infusion Association. (2005). Health care spending growth steady, slowdown expected to level off. *Infusion, 11*(1), 9–10.

Navarro, R. (2005). *Managed care pharmacy practice* (2nd ed.). Gaithersburg, MD: Aspen Publishers, Inc.

Pal, S. (2005). Use of complementary and alternative medicines. *U.S. Pharmacist, 30*(12), 8.

Pennsylvania Pharmacists Association, Academy of Alternative Pharmacy Practice. (2005, May/June). Prescription drug trends: A focus on driving factors. *Pennsylvania Pharmacist, 17,* 22.

Pharmacy Technician Certification Board. (2005). *Your guide to PTCB certification 2005.* Washington, DC: Author.

Posey, M. (2006). Fixing what's wrong with American health care. *Pharmacy Today, 12*(8), 18.

Relman, A. S. (1988). Assessment and accountability: The third revolution in medical care. *New England Journal of Medicine, 319*(18), 1220–1222.

Sanofi Aventis Pharmaceuticals. (2006). *Managed care digest series: Hospitals/Integrated Health Systems Digest 2006.* Bridgewater, NJ: Author.

Smith, M., Wertheimer, A., & Fincham, J. (2005). *Pharmacy and the U.S. health care system* (3rd ed.). Binghamton, NY: Pharmaceutical Products Press.

U.S. Census Bureau. (2005a). *Current population survey health insurance definitions.* [On-line] U.S. Census Bureau. Available: www.census.gov.

U.S. Census Bureau. (2005b). *Health insurance coverage: 2004.* [On-line] U.S. Census Bureau. Available: www.census.gov.

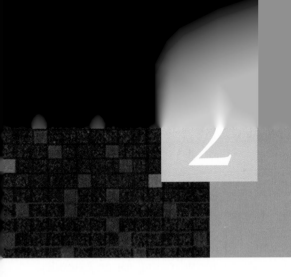

# Long-Term Care

## Learning Objectives

Upon completion of this chapter, the student should be able to:

- Describe the unique characteristics of long-term care.
- Explain the funding for long-term care.
- Discuss the three types of long-term settings and give examples of each.
- Discuss the elderly population.
- List the risk factors for the development of drug-related problems in the elderly.
- Describe an adverse drug reaction.
- Explain pharmacy's role in long-term care.

## Key Terms

| | | |
|---|---|---|
| activities of daily living (ADLs) | continuum of care | long-term care |
| adverse drug reaction | instrumental activities of daily living (IADLs) | resident |
| assisted living | | respite care |

## Introduction

Long-term care is a unique and growing part of the health care market. It is provided in many forms and in many settings. Although it is provided to patients of all ages when needed, the majority of long-term care is provided to the elderly. The elderly have many health problems and take multiple medications. They are at risk for many drug-related problems, especially adverse drug reactions. There is a need here for the pharmacist's expertise in solving drug-related problems and improving the outcomes of drug therapy. Pharmacists and pharmacy technicians must be knowledgeable about the long-term care environment in order to understand their roles in it. This chapter discusses long-term care and the elderly and provides the background for the discussion of pharmacy practice in long-term care. ■

## OVERVIEW OF LONG-TERM CARE

Long-term care is an important component of today's health care system. **Long-term care** is defined as care that is provided to an individual for an extended period of time. It includes a variety of health care, personal care, and social and housing services. It is care provided to sick individuals or individuals with disabilities who do not need acute hospital care but cannot carry out normal activities without assistance. A patient's need for long-term care is determined by many factors: marital status, poverty, gender, mental status, physical functioning, chronic medical problems, age, and family support. The goal of long-term care is to allow an individual to maintain the highest level of independent functioning and dignity. Long-term care is really the attempt to meet the physical, mental, social, and spiritual needs of the patient.

### CHARACTERISTICS OF LONG-TERM CARE

Long-term care has several unique characteristics. It is not age-specific. Long-term care is provided to any patient who has a chronic or long-term health problem that limits her ability to perform daily activities without assistance regardless of her age. Examples of patients who may need long-term care are the elderly, accident victims, children with birth defects, the mentally retarded, the physically disabled, and people with chronic illnesses such as Alzheimer's, AIDS, cancer, multiple sclerosis, and other diseases. The majority of patients needing long-term care, however, are the elderly.

Long-term care is flexible care that responds to the individual needs of the patient. Long-term care provides a continuum of care. A **continuum of care** refers to moving through continuous levels of care, from one level to the next, as the patient's needs change. These levels of care range from health care services provided at home, to services provided in the community, to services provided in long-term care institutions, up to acute hospital care. Patients move up and down the various levels of care, depending on the types of services they need. The continuum of long-term care is shown in Figure 2–1.

Long-term care is supportive and rehabilitative care rather than curative care. Most long-term care patients have health problems that cannot be cured but can be managed for the long term, such as diabetes, hypertension, depression, heart disease, and arthritis, to name a few. Other long-term care patients require some type of rehabilitation to help restore functioning, such as accident victims and the physically disabled.

Long-term care is interdisciplinary care. It is provided by a team of health care professionals. It involves the services of a wide variety of individuals: pharmacists, physicians, nurses, physical therapists, occupational therapists, speech therapists, dieticians, social workers, administrators, and others.

Finally, long-term care is cost-effective care. It is less expensive than acute hospital care. In fact, cost is the main force in the shift from acute hospital care

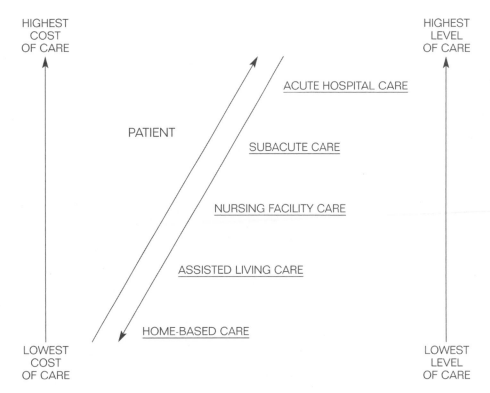

HIGHEST
COST
OF CARE

HIGHEST
LEVEL
OF CARE

ACUTE HOSPITAL CARE

PATIENT

SUBACUTE CARE

NURSING FACILITY CARE

ASSISTED LIVING CARE

HOME-BASED CARE

LOWEST
COST
OF CARE

LOWEST
LEVEL
OF CARE

**FIGURE 2–1**    The Continuum of Long-Term Care

to long-term care, although, as a consequence, patients are being discharged from hospitals sooner and being admitted to various types of long-term care settings when they are still quite ill. Cost is also sometimes a factor in determining which long-term care setting is selected, because some long-term care settings have lower costs of care than others.

## FUNDING FOR LONG-TERM CARE

There are several sources of funding for long-term care. The money comes primarily from three sources: public programs, private insurance, and out-of-pocket spending.

The bulk of long-term care is financed through the public programs of Medicaid and Medicare. Medicaid, the federal and state welfare program for the poor, pays for long-term care for the poor elderly and for those who have depleted their savings after entering a nursing facility and paying for their care. Medicaid is the primary source of publicly funded long-term care. Despite the growth in other long-term care settings, such as community-based and home-based care, the majority of Medicaid funds for long-term care go for institutional care.

Medicare, the federal health insurance program for the elderly, provides limited long-term care coverage. Medicare Part A covers a short-term stay in a nursing facility of up to 100 days if the resident is admitted within 30 days following a hospital stay of at least 3 days. A daily co-payment by the resident is required after 20 days of care in the nursing facility.

Private insurance, in the form of Medigap plans or private employer group health plans, may cover a small portion of long-term care services. However, most health insurance plans provide little or no coverage for long-term care.

Long-term care insurance is being promoted today by private insurance companies. Long-term care insurance is a type of private insurance that provides financial assistance for long-term care services in the event that a person needs to enter a nursing facility. The benefits and costs of these plans vary widely. Many are confusing and expensive and have limitations, such as no lifetime benefit, exclusions for high-risk patients, premium increases, and no adjustment for inflation.

If the patient does not have private insurance that covers long-term care or does not qualify for Medicaid, the patient or the patient's family pays the cost of care. About one-half of all long-term care costs are paid *out of pocket* by the patient or family (Medicare, 2005). Because nursing facility care is expensive, costing thousands of dollars per year, care for an extended period of time can be financially devastating.

## LONG-TERM CARE SETTINGS

Long-term care can be provided in a variety of settings. Although long-term care is commonly thought of in terms of a nursing home, the nursing home is only one of many long-term care settings. Long-term care is found in other environments, each with its own unique characteristics and challenges. Long-term care settings can be divided into three types: institutional settings, community settings, and the home-based setting. Surprisingly, the majority of people who receive long-term care are in the community and home-based settings. The remainder of people needing long-term care are admitted to some type of institutional long-term care setting. There are many factors that determine the long-term care setting for an individual. These include the type and severity of medical problems, how well the patient can function physically and mentally, the availability of a caregiver, and finances, among others. New long-term care settings are continually emerging.

### INSTITUTIONAL SETTINGS

A long-term care institution provides inpatient care, usually with a patient assigned to a bed. Institutional-based care provides care over a longer period of time than would be possible or permitted in an acute care hospital. It also provides less expensive care than in a hospital setting. It is designed to accommodate patients who do not require hospital care but who do need a wide range of medical, nursing, and personal care and social services. Licensed and trained health care professionals provide these services. These long-term care institutions are regulated by law. Examples of institutional long-term care settings include subacute care units, nursing facilities, psychiatric hospitals and other specialty hospitals (such as chronic disease hospitals and long-term acute care hospitals), and correctional facilities.

#### Subacute Care Units

Subacute care is defined as inpatient care that lies between acute hospital care and nursing facility care. It is the first step in the continuous series of long-term care settings. Subacute care is less complex care than in a hospital. However, it is more complex or at a higher level than in a nursing facility. Patients are quite ill, suffering from a serious illness or injury or worsening of a chronic disease, yet they do not need the intensive services of a hospital. Subacute care is interdisciplinary, and the staff is licensed and highly trained as in a hospital. This type of care is usually provided immediately after a hospitalization or even instead of a hospital stay. One example would be an elderly individual who sustains a hip fracture and is transferred to a subacute care unit for rehabilitation after hospitalization for surgery. Another example would be an individual admitted directly to a subacute care unit rather than to a hospital for complex intravenous antibiotic therapy. Most subacute care units are based in hospitals, in nursing facilities, or in freestanding subacute care facilities, that is, facilities dedicated only to subacute care. Subacute care is less expensive than acute hospital care. With managed care today, the trend is to move from acute care to lower-cost subacute care for the patients who can be treated in this setting. Subacute care is intended to be more short-term and transitional in nature than other long-term care settings. The goal is to improve the patient's condition so that she can be moved down the continuum of care to a less-intensive long-term care setting. Therefore, although the patient is sicker in this type of setting, less time is spent in this setting than in other long-term care settings.

## Nursing Facilities

The nursing facility is only one type of long-term care facility, but it is the one most people think of in relation to long-term care. It was previously referred to as a nursing home. Nursing facilities provide a level of care between acute hospital care and community-based long-term care. Nursing facility care offers a lower level of care than in an acute care hospital or subacute care setting. However, nursing facilities still care for patients with complicated medical problems. In addition to basic medical and nursing care, they also offer intravenous therapy, nutritional therapy, chemotherapy, respiratory therapy, cardiac rehabilitation, and specialized care, for example, for Alzheimer's and AIDS. The staff in nursing facilities is also licensed and highly trained but at a lower ratio to patients than in a hospital or subacute care unit.

The cost of care in a nursing facility is less than the cost of care in a hospital or subacute care unit. There is also a shift today from nursing facility care to community-based and home-based long-term care as a result of mounting financial pressure to lower the cost of long-term care. Nursing facility costs represent the majority of the nation's expenditures for long-term care.

There are three types of ownership for nursing facilities. The majority of nursing facilities are for-profit; some are not-for-profit; and a small percentage are government-owned. Some nursing facilities operate independently or as part of a chain, with the numbers of chain nursing facilities increasing. The majority of funding for nursing facility care comes from Medicaid and Medicare; a small percentage comes from HMOs and private insurance; the remainder is paid out of pocket by the patient.

A nursing facility patient is referred to as a **resident.** Most residents are elderly, women, white, and widowed. Almost all residents have one or more chronic conditions, with more than half having three or more conditions. The most common chronic conditions found in nursing facility residents are heart disease, hypertension, arthritis, diabetes, dementia, arteriosclerosis, and stroke. Many residents use wheelchairs, have difficulty controlling their bladder and bowel functions, and have a visual or hearing impairment. Most residents need a complete range of services, including nursing, drug therapy, personal care, and nutrition therapy.

The length of stay in a nursing facility can vary greatly. Nursing facility residents can be grouped into two types, based on their length of stay. A short-term resident remains in the nursing facility less than 6 months. These are patients who are recovering from an illness or accident and who expect to be discharged to home, or they are extremely ill patients who have a short life expectancy, such as patients with cancer or patients with end-stage congestive heart failure. Many people believe that once patients are admitted to a nursing facility they are never discharged. However, short-term residents disprove that belief. A long-term resident resides in a nursing facility more than 6 months, with the average length of stay being 2 years. These are patients who are chronically ill or who are physically or mentally impaired.

Alzheimer's disease is an example of a chronic disease that requires a long-term stay in a nursing facility. People with this disease begin with a gradual decline in memory. As the disease progresses, they do not remember family and friends, and they forget how to dress, eat, bathe, or go to the bathroom. When they leave their rooms, they become disoriented and cannot remember how to return. They need help with medications, daily activities, and health care. Alzheimer's units in nursing facilities are specially designed for safety and security. They allow the patients to walk around in a protected environment. These units are staffed by specially trained personnel and offer special programs to address the particular needs of patients with Alzheimer's disease.

### Psychiatric Hospitals and Other Specialty Hospitals

Psychiatric hospitals and other specialty hospitals are also considered to be long-term care institutions because patients reside in these facilities for long periods of time. As mentioned previously, psychiatric hospitals treat mentally ill patients as well as those addicted to drugs and alcohol. Specialty hospitals provide services for specific medical conditions and include rehabilitation hospitals, chronic disease hospitals such as cancer hospitals, and long-term acute care hospitals.

### Correctional Facilities

Correctional facilities provide long-term care to their residents. Although they have features that distinguish them from nursing facilities and other long-term care institutions, correctional facilities are indeed long-term care facilities. They include jails and prisons. County and local jails are usually short-term holding centers, with prisoners constantly entering and leaving. Because the average stay in jail is only a few weeks, health care services focus on disease prevention and healthier living.

Federal and state prisons, on the other hand, are where sentenced criminals reside for the long term. Inmates in prison tend to be older and have chronic health conditions. Every inmate is entitled to health care, and this health care focuses on chronic health problems. A major problem is infection—tuberculosis, AIDS, HIV, and hepatitis. Another is dental care problems due to neglect or drug abuse. Other chronic health problems are hypertension, heart disease, and diabetes.

## COMMUNITY SETTINGS

Community settings provide long-term care but not in an institution or in a traditional long-term care facility. Community-based care is care that falls between institutional-based care and home-based care. It has more of a social focus than a medical focus. This type of long-term care provides assistance with activities that are essential to daily living, such as bathing, dressing, walking, eating, and toileting. These are referred to as **activities of daily living,** or ADLs, and are related to personal care functions. This type of long-term care also provides assistance with other activities that are important for personal independence, such as cooking, shopping, banking, housekeeping, taking medications, and transportation. These are referred to as **instrumental activities of daily living,** or IADLs, and are related to household and social functions. The type of assistance that an individual needs to perform ADLs and IADLs determines the type of community-based long-term care setting needed, because the type of assistance varies with each setting. Community-based long-term care allows an individual to remain in the community and to maintain her independence as much as possible.

The majority of people in community-based settings are elderly. The remainder are mentally retarded or physically disabled. Care is usually provided by non-licensed and medically untrained personnel, who may have an inadequate understanding of drug therapy. Community-based long-term care services are paid for by a combination of funds from Medicaid, Medicare, and other federal, state, and local social programs. Community-based settings are not federally regulated.

Community-based care is the area of long-term care that is growing the fastest. Individuals who would have once received long-term care services in an institution are now receiving these services in the community. This trend is due to the need to control health care costs. As can be expected, community-based long-term care is less expensive than institutional-based long-term care.

Community-based care is offered in a number of ways and in many different types of community settings. Examples are given in Box 2–1. The most important settings are discussed.

---

### BOX 2–1    Community-Based Long-Term Care Settings

Assisted living facilities
Board and care homes
Home health care
Adult day care
Hospice
Respite care
Continuous care retirement communities
Retirement housing
Group homes
Senior centers
Adult foster care
Personal care homes
Subsidized apartments
Community mental health centers

### Assisted Living Facilities

**Assisted living** is defined as a combination of housing, personalized support services, and health care for individuals who require help with activities of daily living (Assisted Living Federation of America, 2005). It is an important residential option in the long-term care environment. Assisted living provides a homelike setting to individuals who need some support but do not require nursing care. This type of care provides personal care services (ADLs such as bathing, dressing, eating, toileting), medication management, limited health care services, meals, housekeeping, laundry service, activities, and transportation. It is less intensive care than that provided in a nursing facility but more intensive care than that provided in a board and care home. Assisted living provides *assistance with living* while giving the individual as much independence as possible. Table 2–1 lists other characteristics of assisted living and compares them with nursing facility characteristics.

There are many reasons for the need for assisted living. The most important reason is the need for assistance with activities of daily living. Other reasons are frailty, safety and security, nutritional needs, companionship, decreasing mental function, and the need for medication management. Assisted living is a booming sector of the long-term care market. The number of assisted living facilities is growing owing to the increase in the elderly population, the fact that assisted living is less expensive than other long-term care options, and the shift from nursing facility care to this type of community-based care. If the individual is physically able to live in this type of a setting, it is one of the most cost-effective living options.

Assisted living care can be found in many settings. It can be found in a free-standing assisted living facility, in a continuous care retirement community, or along with or within a nursing facility. Usually the individual resides in a room, apartment, or other type of arrangement. Specialized Alzheimer's care is also available in some assisted living settings. Assisted living facilities may be owned on a not-for-profit or for-profit basis, and as part of a chain. Assisted living care or an assisted living setting does not guarantee future nursing care

**TABLE 2–1    Assisted Living vs. Nursing Facility Characteristics**

| ASSISTED LIVING FACILITY | NURSING FACILITY |
| --- | --- |
| Homelike setting | Hospital-like setting |
| Less licensed staff | More licensed staff |
| Lower staff-to-patient ratio | Higher staff-to-patient ratio |
| Personal care | Nursing care and personal care |
| Less stringent federal regulations | Stringent federal regulations |
| Promotes independence | Promotes dependence |
| Focus on wellness | Focus on illness |
| Less expensive care | More expensive care |
| Lack of regulations for pharmacy | Federal regulations for pharmacy |

(unless it is in a continuous care retirement center). In most cases, there is no entrance fee, a lump-sum charge paid before entry, but there is a monthly fee. Assisted living is not covered by Medicare or private health care insurance. In some states, Medicaid will reimburse for assisted living services. A growing number of private long-term care insurance policies are starting to cover the costs. In reality, about two-thirds of assisted living costs are paid for by the assisted living resident or by the resident's family (NCAL, 2005).

There are no federal regulations for assisted living facilities. Assisted living facilities are regulated by the individual states, and state legislation and regulations vary as to the licensing, staffing, design, and quality of services offered. However, two organizations, the Joint Commission and the Commission for Accreditation of Rehabilitation Facilities, have accreditation standards for assisted living. These standards are important in establishing national guidelines for assisted living, since there are no federal regulations at this time.

### Board and Care Homes

Board and care homes are another type of community-based long-term care setting. A board and care home is a nonmedical living arrangement for the elderly, mentally retarded, or physically disabled. By definition, it is two or more people who live together but are not related to the owner or operator of the home. Services provided are housekeeping and meals (room and *board*), supervision, and some personal care services, but no medical or nursing care. Many board and care residents have multiple chronic medical problems and take multiple medications. Care is usually delivered by unlicensed and medically untrained staff. There is no Medicare funding for this type of care. In some cases, Medicaid or private long-term care insurance will pay for this type of living arrangement. Currently, the regulation and licensing of these facilities are the responsibility of each individual state.

### Home Health Care

Home health care is defined as health care services provided to patients in their homes. The emphasis is on medical and nursing care as well as other services, but not on housing. Home health care involves a team of licensed and trained health care professionals, not medically untrained personnel. Home health care is another cost-effective alternative to institutional long-term care and is experiencing tremendous growth. Medicaid and Medicare cover many home health care services, as do many health insurance programs. Because home health care is an advanced practice area for pharmacists and presents an opportunity for pharmacists to provide a unique type of pharmaceutical care, it is covered in depth in Chapters 6 and 7.

### Adult Day Care

Adult day care is a range of personal care services and social services provided to adults who need supervision while their caregiver works. It is provided outside of the home in a group setting at a central location. Adult day care centers usually operate during normal working hours 5 days a week, and some may offer services in the evenings or on weekends. This type of long-term care setting allows a family caregiver to continue to work. It is an alternative to full-time institutional long-term care for families caring for elderly relatives who are not able to supervise them during the day. Adult day care fills this gap in care. It is reimbursable by Medicaid up to a certain dollar limit. There are no federal regulations for these centers, but there are some national standards of care.

### Hospice

Hospice is an organized program of services to meet the special needs of terminally ill patients. It is a special philosophy for caring for individuals at the end of life that focuses on their comfort rather than on a cure for disease. Hospice services include health care services, nursing services, spiritual support services, and other services in a variety of settings but most often in the home. Hospice has gained acceptance as an alternative to hospital care for the terminally ill. Hospice patients often have special medication needs. Because hospice is also an advanced practice area for pharmacists and presents an opportunity for pharmacists to provide a unique type of pharmaceutical care, it is covered in depth in Chapter 11.

### Respite Care

**Respite care** is defined as short-term, temporary care provided to an individual so that a family caregiver can take a break from the daily routine of caregiving. It provides a *respite,* or a rest, for the caregiver of an elderly or chronically ill person. It can be a few hours, overnight, or several days of care. It can be provided in the patient's home or outside of the patient's home, such as a temporary stay in a nursing facility or other setting.

### Continuous Care Retirement Communities

A continuous care retirement community, or CCRC, sometimes referred to as a life care community, is a property that provides complete residential services and future health care services. It offers all the benefits of living independently combined with the peace of mind in knowing that personal care services and nursing care are available should they ever be needed. There are usually three levels of living available in a CCRC corresponding to the different levels of long-term care: independent living in a house or apartment, assisted living in a room or apartment, and nursing care in the nursing facility part of the retirement community. This type of setting allows the individual to move into the retirement community while she is relatively healthy and independent and to move through the continuum of long-term care, that is, move from one level of care to another, when needed. The distinguishing feature of a continuous care retirement community is that *guarantee* of lifelong access to long-term care. Continuous care retirement communities offer not only housing and future nursing and personal care but also social services, recreational programs, sports facilities, transportation, and social events.

A continuous care community usually requires a substantial monthly fee that includes services such as utilities, maintenance, housekeeping, meals, transportation, and other needs. Many communities also require a large up-front entrance fee that functions as a form of insurance toward future long-term care costs. The high cost of these communities makes them inaccessible to many elderly.

**Retirement Housing**

Retirement housing, often referred to as a naturally occurring retirement community, or NORC, is defined as rental units for healthy, mostly retired elderly. It provides the elderly with an alternative to living in and maintaining a home. Essentially, it is housing without medical, nursing, or personal care services. The elderly residing in these units are relatively healthy and independent. They do not need help with activities of daily living or instrumental activities of daily living. They are responsible for their own medications. Through this type of living arrangement, they enjoy social contact, security, and usually some planned social, fitness, and health programs. Residents with low to moderate incomes may qualify for federal and state programs that will help pay for this type of housing.

## THE HOME-BASED SETTING

It is difficult to consider an individual's home as a long-term care setting. However, home-based care is a major but largely unrecognized source of long-term care. Home-based care includes a wide variety of personal care and social services provided to individuals in their homes. Home is where the majority of the elderly live, alone or with a spouse, family, or friends. It is the most desirable living environment, not only for them but also for other types of long-term care patients, such as the mentally retarded or children and adults with physical disabilities. A large number of long-term care patients are taken care of at home by *family caregivers*. The National Family Caregivers Association (NFCA) estimates that over a quarter of the adult population are family caregivers; that is, they are involved in providing care for an elderly, disabled, or chronically ill individual at home. A family caregiver can be a spouse, adult child, parent, other relative, friend, or neighbor. Traditionally, most of these family caregivers were women, but today almost as many men as women provide this type of care (NFCA, 2005). These caregivers are unpaid and usually medically untrained. They often have other responsibilities such as work or caring for their own families. They sacrifice time, energy, and money in taking care of the individual. Home-based care plays an important role in long-term care. In fact, most people who need personal care services receive them outside the formal long-term care system, that is, outside of institutional and community settings. For some people, there are no other options for long-term care than home-based care.

Many services are provided in home-based care. Caregivers provide assistance with activities of daily living and instrumental activities of daily living. One critical task is helping to manage and administer medications, for example, taking medications on time, taking the medications as directed, and obtaining medications. In fact, being able to manage medications is what enables many individuals to remain at home. The inability to manage medications is one of the top reasons for admission to a nursing facility or an assisted living facility. The quality of care is difficult to measure in this setting because most of the time it cannot be observed; services occur in the home, with only the individual and caregiver present. Nonetheless, this type of long-term care allows an individual to remain relatively independent and in her own home.

## THE ELDERLY POPULATION

The elderly population is defined as persons 65 years of age or older. They can be divided into three age groups. The elderly aged 65 to 74 years are referred to as the young-old. They are relatively healthy and may still be employed. Most are active, are financially independent, and have a positive outlook on life. When long-term care is needed, it is usually received in a community or home-based setting. Elderly aged 75 to 84 years are referred to as the middle-old. They are able to live independently or with some assistance. They are still relatively healthy but are at a greater risk of illness or problems owing to their age. The need for long-term care increases in this age group. Finally, persons 85 years of age and older are referred to as the old-old. They are often widowed and alone. They are frequently frail and have several chronic illnesses. They often need long-term care services. The elderly population has been increasing over the years. However, the old-old age group is the fastest growing segment of the elderly population.

In general, today's elderly population is healthier and is living longer than in the past. This trend is due to many factors. There are new and better treatments for chronic diseases. Advances in new technology and surgical techniques, such as cataract surgery, hip replacements, and pacemakers, enable the elderly to continue to function independently. Today's elderly are more educated and have a higher level of experience and a higher income level, all of which are associated with better health. They are maintaining healthier lifestyles by eating well, exercising, and generally staying active. The healthy elderly are the least likely to need long-term care.

There are many in the elderly population, however, who are not healthy and have several chronic medical problems. Many elderly Americans have at least one chronic health problem. The most common chronic conditions in the elderly are listed in Box 2–2.

As people age, they become more likely to develop chronic health problems. In general, elderly with chronic health problems are frail and are likely to need long-term care.

---

### BOX 2–2    Chronic Conditions in the Elderly Population

Alzheimer's disease
Depression
Parkinson's disease
Arthritis
Hypertension
Hearing impairment
Cataracts
Heart disease
Diabetes
Tinnitus
Visual impairment

## DRUG-RELATED PROBLEMS IN THE ELDERLY

The elderly make up approximately 13 percent of the U.S. population, yet they consume a disproportionate amount, about one-third, of the nation's health care costs (ASCP, 2005). As already stated, the elderly have many chronic health problems. They visit physicians more often than younger individuals. They are more likely to be admitted to a hospital and have longer hospital stays than younger patients. Because of their chronic health problems and the increased use of physicians and hospitals, the elderly have a high rate of medication use.

Most Americans over 65 years of age take at least one medication. Some take several medications. Nursing facility residents take multiple medications. In 2006, a national survey showed that nursing facility residents received an average of seven regularly scheduled medications per day. With the increased use of drugs comes the increased risk of experiencing a drug-related problem. The most important risk factor for the development of a drug-related problem in the elderly is the use of many or multiple medications. It has been demonstrated that the more medications an elderly patient takes, the greater the chance of drug-related problems. The elderly have the potential for drug-related problems based on the *number* of medications they take alone.

As discussed in Chapter 1, a drug-related problem is an undesirable experience involving drug therapy that can actually or potentially interfere with a desired outcome. Drug-related problems include underdosing, overdosing, improper drug selection, drug therapy needed but not given, drug interactions, using drugs without a reason, and adverse drug reactions. Drug-related problems are a major cause of negative outcomes that occur in the elderly. These negative outcomes include hospitalization, falls, decreased physical and mental functioning, changes in thinking, worsening of the health condition, and even death. The cost of drug-related problems is also staggering. In nursing facilities, it is estimated that approximately $2 is spent to treat drug-related problems for every $1 spent on prescribed medications (ASCP, 2005).

In addition to multiple medications, there are other risk factors for the development of drug-related problems in the elderly. These risk factors are multiple health problems, decreased kidney and liver function, other age-related changes in the body, low body weight, advanced age, and the types of medications being taken. Multiple health problems may require that the patient take several different types of medications. Decreased kidney and liver functions make it more difficult to eliminate medications from the body. Age-related changes in the body can cause a difference in the way the elderly react to medications. Low body weight and advanced age make the elderly more sensitive to medications in the usual adult dosages. Finally, there are many medications in different therapeutic classes that are commonly involved in drug-related problems. These medications may be safe and effective in younger people but can often cause adverse reactions in the elderly. They are considered by medical experts to be potentially inappropriate for use in the elderly unless the potential benefits outweigh the risks. In 1991, researchers led by Dr. Mark Beers identified potentially inappropriate medications in elderly nursing home residents. The list became known as the "Beers criteria" and is the most widely used tool to examine medication use in the elderly. The Beers criteria were updated in 1997, to identify medications that are inappropriate for use in *all* seniors, and again in 2003.  The Beers criteria have been used over the years as guidelines by pharmacists and physicians to improve the use of medications in the elderly.  Based on this information, the Centers for Medicare and Medicaid Services has released "drug therapy surveyor guidelines" to help nursing home surveyors monitor the use of medications that are potentially inappropriate for use in residents. More recently, these criteria have been used to develop formularies as part of the Medicare Prescription Drug Benefit. Table 2–2 lists medications that are considered potentially inappropriate and that should be avoided in the elderly (Fick et al., 2003).

Adverse drug reactions are the most serious drug-related problem in the elderly. An **adverse drug reaction** is defined as any response to a drug that is unexpected, unintended, undesired, or excessive when used in appropriate doses. Almost any drug, prescription or nonprescription, can cause some type of adverse drug reaction, depending on that drug and the patient's health. These adverse drug reactions present themselves as a wide variety of signs and symptoms that can range from mild to severe. Examples of adverse drug reactions are confusion, depression, loss of appetite, weakness, drowsiness, tremor,

**TABLE 2–2   Medications Considered Inappropriate For Use In The Elderly**

| | |
|---|---|
| Anticholinergics | Dry mouth, urinary retention, dizziness |
| Antihistamines | Sedation, anticholinergic side effects |
| Barbiturates | Sedation, addiction |
| Chlorpropamide | Excessive lowering of blood sugar |
| Dipyridamole, short acting | Low blood pressure in an upright position |
| GI antispasmodics (ex. dicyclomine, hyoscyamine) | Sedation, anticholinergic side effects |
| Long-acting benzodiazepines (ex. chlordiazepoxide, diazepam) | Excessive sedation |
| Meprobamate | Excessive sedation, addiction |
| Methyldopa | Decreased heart rate, worsens depression |
| Muscle relaxants (ex. carisoprodol, cyclobenzaprine) | Excessive sedation, weakness |
| Nonsteroidal anti-inflammatory drugs (ex. ibuprofen, naproxen) | Nausea, GI bleeding, sedation |
| Older tricyclic antidepressants (ex. amitriptyline, imipramine) | Sedation, tremor |
| Propoxyphene | Sedation, psychosis, confusion |
| Ticlodipine | More toxic than aspirin but no better |
| Thioridazine | Sedation, tremor |

Adapted from "Updating the Beers Criteria for Potentially Inappropriate Medication Use in Older Adults," by D. Fick, J. Cooper, W. Wade, et al., 2003, Archives of Internal Medicine, 163(22), 2716–2724.

**TABLE 2–3    Examples of Adverse Drug Reactions**

| INITIAL PROBLEM | DRUG THERAPY | ADVERSE DRUG REACTION | ADDITIONAL DRUG THERAPY |
|---|---|---|---|
| Arthritis | NSAID | GI upset | H2-receptor antagonist |
| Depression | Older tricyclic antidepressant | Constipation | Laxative |
| Pain | Codeine | Constipation | Laxative |
| Agitation | Older antipsychotic | Tremor, stiffness | Parkinson's medication |

constipation, diarrhea, blurred vision, and urinary retention. Sometimes an adverse drug reaction is misinterpreted as a new medical condition. This error can lead to the prescribing of additional medications to treat the adverse drug reaction, further increasing the risk of a patient's experiencing a drug-related problem. Examples of adverse drug reactions are given in Table 2–3.

The risk of drug-related problems in the elderly, especially adverse drug reactions, calls for close and continuous monitoring of their medications. Although some drug-related problems are unpredictable, most can be anticipated and prevented. Prevention is accomplished through better education of health care patients and providers and the careful review of a patient's drug regimen by a pharmacist in what is referred to as a drug regimen review. The drug regimen review is discussed in Chapter 5.

## THE ROLE OF PHARMACY IN LONG-TERM CARE

Pharmacy practice in long-term care began in the mid-1960s. Before Medicare and Medicaid were enacted in the mid-1960s, conditions in nursing facilities were poor. There was no accounting for medication use in the facility, and there was little or no involvement on the part of the pharmacist. Medicare and Medicaid first addressed the issue of drug-related problems in nursing facilities by requiring a monthly review of the patient's medications, first by a nurse and physician, then, after 1974, by a pharmacist. The rationale for having pharmacists perform the drug regimen review was that they have unique expertise in the use of medications and could solve drug-related problems when others could not. Since that time, pharmacy practice in long-term care has evolved into a well-defined specialty that is referred to as consultant pharmacy practice. The long-term care pharmacist, referred to as a consultant pharmacist, has been recognized as a drug therapy expert and an important member of the interdisciplinary long-term care team.

Long-term care presents an opportunity for pharmacists to help improve the outcomes of drug therapy in the elderly and to reduce the cost of drug-related problems. It has been demonstrated that drug regimen review and other pharmaceutical care services in long-term care settings increase the effectiveness of drug therapy and decrease drug-related problems, thereby also reducing costs. According to an ASCP-funded study called the Fleetwood Project, consultant pharmacists in nursing facilities save approximately $3.6 billion annually in costs associated with drug-related problems such as hospital costs, physician costs, laboratory tests, and other ancillary services, while improving outcomes by 43 percent (ASCP, 2005). Thus, pharmacists play an important role in long-term care. What is consultant pharmacy practice, and what are the many pharmaceutical care services that consultant pharmacists provide in the long-term care setting? These are two very important topics that have far-reaching effects. Because of their importance, Chapter 5 is devoted entirely to the role of the pharmacist and the accompanying role of the pharmacy technician in long-term care.

There are many challenges and opportunities ahead for long-term care. The long-term care industry is changing because of changes in regulation and payment. Long-term care is striving for better outcomes of care. It is expanding because of an increase in the elderly population and the shift from expensive hospital care. Several trends are emerging, such as a decrease in the number of nursing facility beds; an increase in the number of assisted living beds; an increase in the number of beds in hospitals becoming long-term care beds, as hospitals try to get more into the long-term care market; and an increase in the number of beds in hospitals becoming subacute care beds (Sanofi Aventis Pharmaceuticals, 2006).

Current issues in long-term care are related to the three components of our health care system: cost, access, and quality.

- *Cost.* Long-term care is expensive. Who should pay for it? Can long-term care insurance be made more affordable? Can long-term care be delivered in less expensive settings?

- *Access.* Who should be eligible for long-term care services? Will long-term care be available to those who need it? Can long-term care services keep pace with the increase in the elderly population?

- *Quality.* Donabedian's concepts of structure, process, and outcome are being applied to long-term care. Nursing facility structures and processes are being related to the outcomes experienced by residents, and these outcomes are being used to determine the quality of that care. Pharmacists are involved in ensuring quality, cost-effective drug therapy in this health care setting.

## KEY CONCEPTS

- Long-term care is care provided over an extended period of time and includes health care, personal care, and social and housing services; it is not age-specific but is flexible, supportive and rehabilitative, interdisciplinary, and cost-effective.

- The majority of funding for long-term care is through public programs.

- Long-term care can be provided in a variety of settings, such as institutional, community, and home-based settings.

- The elderly population is composed of three age groups with different characteristics and needs.
- The elderly are at risk for drug-related problems, especially adverse drug reactions due to multiple medications and multiple health problems.
- An adverse drug reaction is any response to a drug that is unexpected, unintended, undesired, or excessive when used in appropriate doses.
- Pharmacists can help improve the outcomes of drug therapy in the elderly and decrease costs through drug regimen review and other pharmaceutical care services.

## SELF-ASSESSMENT QUESTIONS

### MULTIPLE CHOICE

1. Funding for long-term care comes from the following sources except:
   a. public programs
   b. donations
   c. private insurance
   d. out-of-pocket spending

2. Which is not a long-term care setting?
   a. acute care facility
   b. correctional facility
   c. mental institution
   d. life care community

3. Patients who need long-term care can be:
   a. accident victims
   b. children with birth defects
   c. the mentally retarded
   d. all of the above

4. Community-based long-term care can be provided in:
   a. board and care homes
   b. senior centers
   c. retirement housing
   d. all of the above

5. All are true statements about continuous care retirement communities except:
   a. they allow movement through levels of care
   b. they offer complete residential services and future health care services
   c. they guarantee lifetime access to long-term care
   d. they do not require a good income

6. Retirement housing provides:
   a. personal care services and housing but not medical or nursing care
   b. housing but not medical, nursing, or personal care services
   c. medical, nursing, and personal care services but not housing
   d. housing and future medical, nursing, and personal care services

7. All of the following statements concerning home-based long-term care are true except:

   a. it involves medically untrained caregivers
   b. it is a major source of long-term care
   c. it is the same as home health care
   d. it involves medication management

8. Active, healthy, sometimes employed elderly under 75 years of age are referred to as:

   a. young-old
   b. middle-old
   c. old-old
   d. retired

9. The most important risk factor for the development of drug-related problems in the elderly is:

   a. multiple health problems
   b. the use of inappropriate drugs
   c. changes in kidney and liver function
   d. multiple medications

10. Which it not a characteristic of assisted living facilities?

    a. focus on wellness
    b. less stringent federal regulations
    c. homelike setting
    d. nursing care

## TRUE/FALSE (CORRECT THE FALSE STATEMENTS.)

1. _____ Long-term care is defined as care provided for acute illness.
2. _____ Community-based long-term care has a social emphasis rather than a medical emphasis.
3. _____ The inability to manage medications is a major factor contributing to an elderly patient's need for long-term care.
4. _____ Medicare is the primary source of publicly funded long-term care.
5. _____ The majority of patients needing long-term care are the elderly.
6. _____ The elderly consume a smaller percentage of drugs than younger people.
7. _____ Long-term care settings can be institutional-based, community-based, or home-based, each with its own characteristics and challenges.
8. _____ The majority of people who receive long-term care are in the institutional setting.
9. _____ Most nursing facility patients are white, women, and widowed.
10. _____ Activities of daily living are related to personal care functions.

**FILL-IN**

1. The average number of routine medications taken by a nursing facility patient is _____.
2. A long-term care facility is generically called a _____.
3. A nonmedical living arrangement consisting of two or more elderly people unrelated to the owner or operator is a _____.
4. _____ is short-term, temporary long-term care provided by one caregiver on behalf of another caregiver.
5. The fastest growing age group of the elderly population is the _____.
6. The most serious drug-related problem in the elderly is _____.
7. The long-term care setting that is growing the fastest is _____.
8. A nursing facility patient is often referred to as a _____.
9. The first step in the continuum of long-term care settings is _____.
10. Activities that are related to household and social functions are called _____.

**CRITICAL THINKING**

1. Identify examples of the different types of long-term care settings, institutional-, community-, and home-based, in your area.
2. Identify elderly relatives and friends in terms of the three age groups of the elderly.
3. Select three types of drug-related problems and give an example of each.
4. What are the results of the movement away from institutional long-term care settings to community long-term care settings?
5. Why are community and home-based long-term care settings important to the continuum of care?

## BIBLIOGRAPHY

American Correctional Association. (2005). *Standards for health services.* [On-line] ACA. Available: www.aca.org.

American Medical Directors Association. (2004). *AMDA and ASCP joint position statement on the Beers list of potentially inappropriate medications in older adults.* [On-line] AMDA. Available: www.amda.com.

American Society of Consultant Pharmacists. (2005). *ASHP guidelines on pharmaceutical services in correctional facilities.* [On-line] ASHP. Available: www.ascp.com.

American Society of Consultant Pharmacists. (2005). *The Fleetwood Project Research Initiative.* [On-line] ASHP. Available: www.ascpfoundation.org.

American Society of Consultant Pharmacists. (2005). *Senior care pharmacy facts.* [On-line] ASHP. Available: www.ascp.com.

Assisted Living Federation of America. (2005). *What is assisted living?* [On-line] ALPHA. Available: www.alpha.org.

Barlas, S. (2004). Federal regulatory assistance for assisted living? *Geriatric Times, 5*(5), 3.

Calis. K., & Young, L. (2004). Clinical analysis of adverse drug reactions: A primer for clinicians. *Hospital Pharmacy, 39*(7), 697–712.

Clark, T. (2002). Medication management in assisted living: Assuring the accuracy of medication administration. *The Consultant Pharmacist, 17*(9), 761–764.

Crownover, B. (2005). Implementation of the Beers criteria: Sticks and stones—or throw me a bone. *Journal of Managed Care Pharmacy, 11*(5), 416.

Crutchfield, D. (2004). Potentially inappropriate drugs. *Geriatric Times, 5*(4), 31–32.

Fick, D., Cooper, J., Wade, W., et al. (2003). Updating the Beers criteria for potentially inappropriate medication use in older adults—Results of a U.S. consensus panel of experts. *Archives of Internal Medicine, 163*(22), 2716–2724.

Gebhart, F. (2005). Inappropriate meds linked to adverse nursing home events. *Drug Topics, 149*(3), 81.

Guay, D. (2004). Beers 2003 update: An advance or more of the same? *The Consultant Pharmacist, 19*(4), 364–370.

Health Alliance Plan. (2005). *Are you at risk for polypharmacy?* [On-line] HAP. Available: www.hap.org.

Kaldy, J. (2004). The evolution of criteria for inappropriate drugs. *Caring for the Ages, 5*(8), 131–132.

Kaldy, J. (2005). Multidisciplinary medication management. *Caring for the Ages, 6*(6), 8–9.

McCarthy, R., & Schafermeyer, K. (2004). *Introduction to health care delivery: A primer for pharmacists.* Gaithersburg, MD: Aspen Publishers, Inc.

Medicare. (2005). *Alternatives to nursing home care: Other options.* [On-line] Medicare. Available: www.medicare.gov.

Medicare. (2005). *Paying for care.* [On-line] Medicare. Available: www.medicare.gov.

National Center for Assisted Living. (2005). *Assisted living state regulatory review 2005.* [On-line] NCAL. Available: www.ncal.org.

National Family Caregivers Association. (2005). *Caregiving statistics.* [On-line] NFCA. Available: www.nfcacares.org.

Posey, M. (2006). Fixing what's wrong with American health care. *Pharmacy Today, 12*(8), 18–19.

Resnick, B. (2005). Is home always best? *Caring for the Ages, 6*(9), 3–4.

Sanofi Aventis Pharmaceuticals. (2006). *Managed care digest series: Senior care digest 2006.* Bridgewater, NJ: Author.

Terrie, Y. (2004). Understanding and managing polypharmacy in the elderly. *Pharmacy Times, 70*(12), 84–85.

Wick, J. (2005). 10 risky drugs for elders. *Pharmacy Times, 71*(1), 80–82.

Wick, J. (2006). The Beers criteria: Red flags for elders. *Pharmacy Times, 72*(6), 56.

Zangaria, M. A. (2005). The effects of aging on drug efficacy. *U.S. Pharmacist, 30*(5), 54–57.

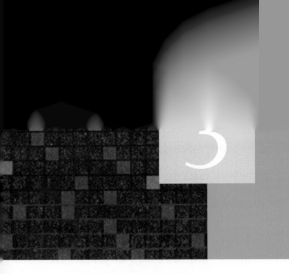

# 3 Care Pharmacy

## Learning Objectives

Upon completion of this chapter, the student should be able to:

- Define a long-term care pharmacy.
- Understand the difference between an open-shop and a closed-shop pharmacy.
- Describe the elements of a long-term care pharmacy.
- Describe the types of drug distribution systems and the differences between them.
- Explain the unique prescription-dispensing process and delivery services of a long-term care pharmacy.
- Describe an emergency medication supply and its use in the long-term care facility.
- Discuss the types of medication storage used in the long-term care facility.
- List and explain the various forms and reports provided to the long-term care facility.

## Key Terms

behavior monitoring form

blended unit-dose system

closed-shop pharmacy

cycle fill

drug distribution system

e-prescribing

electronic medical record

emergency drug

long-term care pharmacy

medication administration record

modified unit-dose system

modular cassette

multiple medication package

open-shop pharmacy

physician order form

treatment administration record

turn-around system

unit-dose system

## Introduction

The long-term care pharmacy is the primary source of medications for long-term care or nursing home residents. Over the years, many retail pharmacies have expanded and concentrated their services in long-term care. Other large long-term care pharmacies have emerged. The long-term care pharmacy is unique and complex and requires special knowledge and skills. It also involves special equipment and supplies.

A long-term care pharmacy provides not only medications but also other services that help to promote the safe and effective use of medications in the long-term care facility. These services involve the use of sophisticated drug distribution systems as well as computer and automated technology. This chapter examines these systems and services and provides an overview of the day-to-day operations in a long-term care pharmacy. The legislation and regulations pertaining to a long-term care pharmacy and the roles of the pharmacist and pharmacy technician in this area are covered in the chapters that follow. ■

## OVERVIEW OF A LONG-TERM CARE PHARMACY

A **long-term care pharmacy** is defined as a pharmacy that dispenses medications to residents in a long-term care facility. Long-term care pharmacies are found in a variety of styles and settings. They can range from small independent community pharmacies to large-volume long-term care pharmacies that are part of long-term care pharmacy corporations and resemble mail-order pharmacies. Long-term care can be the majority or the only type of pharmacy business for a particular pharmacy, or it can be just a small percentage of its business. There are two types of long-term care pharmacies: an open-shop pharmacy and a closed-shop pharmacy.

An **open-shop pharmacy**, also referred to as an open-door pharmacy, is defined as a pharmacy that dispenses medications for both long-term care facility residents and regular retail or "walk-in" patients. It is usually a community retail pharmacy, either an independent or a chain pharmacy.

A **closed-shop pharmacy**, also referred to as a closed-door pharmacy, is defined as a pharmacy that dispenses medications for only long-term care facility residents. It does not dispense prescriptions to retail or walk-in patients, that is, to patients who do not reside in a long-term care facility. A closed-shop pharmacy can be *in-house* or *out-of-house*. An in-house pharmacy is a closed-shop pharmacy that is located inside the long-term care facility, usually as a separate department of the facility. It is usually found in facilities that are large enough or have enough residents to support a pharmacy of their own. An out-of-house pharmacy is a closed-shop pharmacy that is not located inside a long-term care facility but is located outside and independent of it. A long-term care facility that is too small to support its own in-house pharmacy will negotiate and contract with a specific out-of-house pharmacy to provide its pharmaceutical services. An out-of-house closed-shop pharmacy can be a community retail pharmacy. However, most are large, high-volume pharmacies that are part of long-term pharmacy corporations, such as NCS Healthcare, Inc., Omnicare, and PharMerica, that service several long-term care facilities.

## ELEMENTS OF A LONG-TERM CARE PHARMACY

There are many elements that make up a long-term care pharmacy. Some of these elements are the same as those found in a traditional retail pharmacy. Some of these elements, however, are unique. The two most important elements of a long-term care pharmacy are personnel and equipment and supplies.

### PERSONNEL

A variety of personnel is needed in a long-term care pharmacy to ensure its efficient operation and to provide the many services offered. A pharmacist who works in a long-term care pharmacy is referred to as a long-term care pharmacist. The long-term care pharmacist ensures that long-term care residents receive medications on a timely basis according to the physician's orders. He has special knowledge in the areas of geriatrics, psychotropic medications, and other specialties, such as Alzheimer's care, intravenous infusion therapy, or AIDS therapies. The pharmacy technician is an important member of the long-term care pharmacy team. The technician assists the pharmacist in all areas of drug distribution as well as in purchasing, clerical duties, and quality control. A driver or delivery person is needed to deliver the medications to the long-term care facility in a timely, courteous manner. Finally, a billing clerk or bookkeeper handles the various accounting tasks. The appropriate number of pharmacists and pharmacy technicians will depend on the number and types of long-term care facilities served by the pharmacy, the number of residents in the facility, the drug distribution system used by the facility, and the types of services provided by the pharmacy.

### INVENTORY

The drug inventory in a long-term care pharmacy is generally the same as the drug inventory in a retail pharmacy. However, the long-term care pharmacy may stock more dosage forms of medications for long-term care residents who are unable to take oral medications, such as injectable, suppository, and liquid forms. It may also stock many special over-the-counter products that are used by the elderly, such as dermal ulcer products, incontinence products, dry skin products, and nutritional supplements. Long-term care pharmacies that provide intravenous infusion therapies will have a drug inventory similar to the inventory in a hospital pharmacy. In all cases, the inventory in a long-term care pharmacy will be customized to meet the needs of the residents of the long-term care facilities served by the pharmacy.

### PHARMACY DESIGN

Because a long-term care pharmacy can be found in a variety of styles and settings, there is no one type of design for this type of pharmacy. In general, a community long-term care pharmacy resembles a community retail pharmacy. A large, high-volume long-term care pharmacy that is part of a long-term care pharmacy corporation resembles a mail-order pharmacy. Mail-order pharmacy is discussed in Chapter 9.

## EQUIPMENT AND SUPPLIES

A variety of equipment and supplies is found in the long-term care pharmacy. Some equipment and supplies are unique to this type of pharmacy operation. The computer is essential for prescription processing, as well as for billing, purchasing, record keeping, and clinical functions. In the long-term care pharmacy, specialized computer software specific to long-term care pharmacy operations is required. This software enables the pharmacy to provide the various forms and reports that are required by the facility. A long-term care pharmacy may also use a variety of printers to accommodate the different labeling requirements of various drug distribution systems. In addition to computers and printers, facsimile machines, copiers, and paging devices for drivers are used. Finally, some type of automated drug repackaging equipment will be found in a long-term care pharmacy, such as a unit-dose machine, punch card sealing machine, or strip packaging machine, depending on the drug distribution system used by the long-term care facility.

Traditional pharmacy supplies, such as prescription vials, labels, auxiliary labels, prescription pads, prescription files, and bags, are found in a long-term care pharmacy. In addition, specialized pharmacy supplies that accompany each type of drug distribution system will also be found. These include special boxes, labels, and blister materials. Again, the variety of supplies will depend on the drug distribution system used by the long-term care facility.

Finally, there are special forms and reports that are used in the long-term care facility for a variety of purposes. These forms and reports are provided to the nursing facility by the provider pharmacy.

## DELIVERY SERVICE

The safe and timely delivery of medications to the nursing facility is one of the most important elements of a long-term care pharmacy operation. Timely delivery is necessary to avoid delaying the start of or interrupting drug therapy for a nursing facility resident. Routine deliveries are usually made to the facility at a predetermined time each day. They can also be made on a "stat" or emergency basis as needed. Delivery service after pharmacy hours is usually available with a pharmacist and a driver on call. The delivery service also includes the pickup of medication reorder forms and unused noncontrolled substance medications from the facility.

# DRUG DISTRIBUTION SYSTEMS FOR LONG-TERM CARE

A **drug distribution system** is defined as a safe and economical method of distributing a drug. It refers to the packaging or container that holds and stores the drug during its transfer from the pharmacy to the patient. Any drug package must meet USP/NF standards for light and moisture resistance. The goals of any drug distribution system are safety and efficiency. The drug distribution system chosen for use by the long-term care facility should maximize patient safety by minimizing the chance of errors. It should be easy to use and should provide accountability for drugs. It is important that pharmacy technicians become familiar with the various drug distribution systems available for use in the long-term care setting in order to use them in drug distribution activities.

## UNIT-DOSE SYSTEM

A **unit-dose system** is defined as a drug distribution system that provides a medication in its final "unit-of-use" form. It is a drug distribution system that was originally developed and designed for use in acute settings such as hospitals. A unit-dose system is a safe and efficient system for use in the long-term care facility. It increases nursing productivity and provides error-resistant drug ordering, distribution, storage, and administration. There are many types of unit-dose systems, but they all share the same feature: a single-unit package of a drug that is dispensed just before it is administered to the patient. The drug is contained in a small packet. One side of the packet is made of a thermal paper and foil laminate; the other side is made of a poly film material, which may be transparent or colored (for light-sensitive drugs). In compliance with USP labeling requirements, as discussed in Chapter 4, medication information is printed on the paper backing by means of a stencil and ink system or by a computer-generated thermal printing system that interfaces with the unit-dose packaging machine (Figure 3–1). The unit-dose system is a product of automation. Separate and sophisticated machinery is required to package and label unit-dose medications.

There are manual, semiautomatic, and automatic loading unit-dose packaging machines. All of these machines produce unit-dose packages in strips separated by perforations. A single-drop unit-dose machine can package up to 60 packages per minute, whereas a double-drop machine can package up to 120 packages per minute. The machine "drops" the drug into a package, seals the package, and prints the medication information, all in one operation (Figure 3–2).

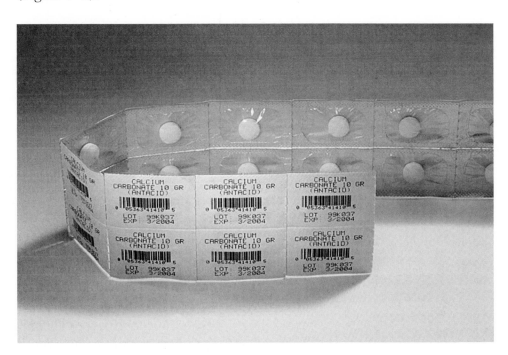

**FIGURE 3–1**    Individual Unit-Dose Packages. (Courtesy of AutoMed Technologies, Inc.)

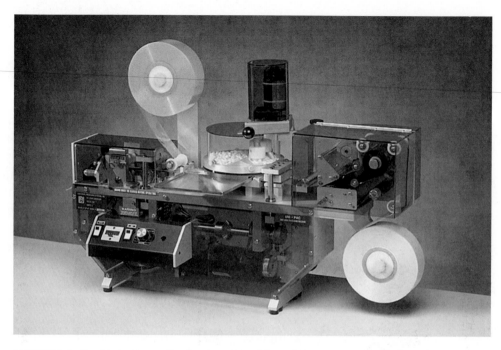

**FIGURE 3–2**   Unit-Dose Packaging Machine. (Courtesy of AutoMed Technologies, Inc.)

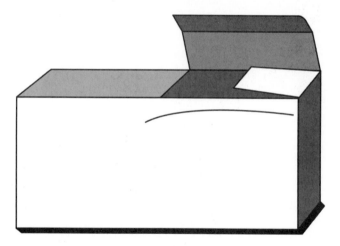

**FIGURE 3–3**   Unit-Dose Box.

Special supplies are used with a unit-dose drug distribution system. Unit-dose boxes made of paper or cardboard hold the unit-dose packaged medications in strips. Usually a 30-day supply of unit-dose medication is contained in these boxes. Thirty-day supplies are common because the drug therapy of most long-term care residents is relatively constant and there are few day-to-day changes. However, some long-term care facilities prefer a 7- or 14-day supply of medications (Figure 3–3).

The prescription label is compatible with the unit-dose box and is usually a two-part label for ease of reordering. One part of the label is removed, usually by peeling it off, and this is affixed to a compatible medication reorder form (Figure 3–4). The other part of the label remains on the box as the legal prescription label. A reorder reminder, also compatible with the unit-dose box, appears near the bottom of the current supply to prompt the nurse to reorder

# MEDICATION REORDERS

**Refills Only**

☐ Check here if you need additional forms

Form # MP5222 (Rev. 03/07)  Reorder From: MED-PASS, INC.  XFM 072796P

**DIRECTIONS:** If completing form by hand, enter one medication per reorder field; or attach reorder label below and indicate any new directions/label changes. "X" out unused areas and provide form to pharmacy. If faxed, attach activity report after faxing. *Please phone the pharmacy if you need a medication prior to routine delivery.* Put initials in box when received and retain according to facility policy.

| Facility Name | Wing/Station | Faxed By | Date | Time Faxed ☐AM ☐PM | Page ___ of ___ |
|---|---|---|---|---|---|

Resident ___ RM # ___
Drug/Strength ___ Qty. ___
Directions ___ Indication ___
Rx # ___ Dr. ___
Comments/Direction change: | Initial If Phoned in | Received By Qty.

*(reorder fields repeat 8 times)*

| PHARMACY USE ONLY | Order Taken By | Computer Technician | Picked By | Packed By | Checked By | Checked By | Delivered By | Received By | Date/Time |

**FIGURE 3–4** Medication Reorder Form. (Courtesy of MED-PASS, Inc.)

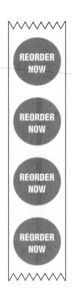

**FIGURE 3–5**    Reorder Reminder. (Courtesy of MED-PASS, Inc.)

the medication (Figure 3–5). In the long-term care facility, unit-dose packages of medication in boxes are stored in mobile medication carts with separate drawers or sections for each patient's medications.

## MODIFIED UNIT-DOSE SYSTEM

A **modified unit-dose system** is a drug distribution system that combines unit-dose medications blister-packaged onto a multiple-dose card instead of being placed into a box. These cards are known as *punch cards, bingo cards,* or *blister cards*. A single medication of 30, 60, or even 90 units can be packaged on one card. The medication is dispensed by pushing it through the foil on the back of the card. The "blisters" are available in different formats and sizes to accommodate the particular drug (Figure 3–6).

The complete system is composed of the lidding stock, perforated blisters, and a punch card. The lidding stock is the thermal paper and foil laminate perforated to match the particular number of blisters on the card. The medication information is printed on the paper side of the lidding stock to comply with the labeling requirements for unit dose. The perforated blisters are made of plastic material formed by heat to create a certain number of blisters. They may be clear, amber, or light-resistant. The punch card is made of cardboard and has an adhesive along the edge. There is a space for the prescription label, and the

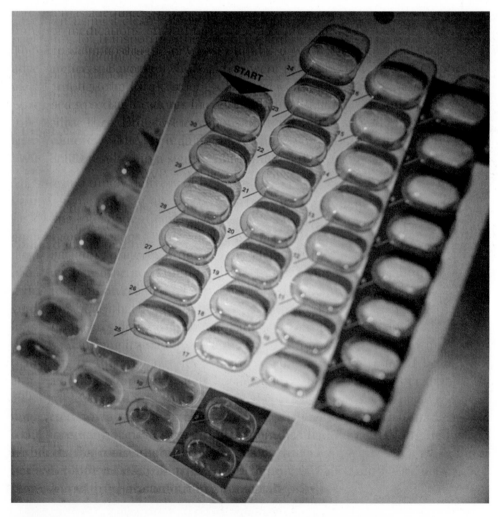

**FIGURE 3–6**    Punch Cards. (Courtesy of AutoMed Technologies, Inc.)

blisters are numbered for instant drug counts. There also is a reorder reminder by way of a colored ribbon with the last few doses.

The cards are assembled by printing the medication on the paper side of the lidding stock on each perforated square, filling the perforated blisters either by hand or by machine, and then sealing. There are two methods of sealing: heat sealing and cold sealing. In the first method, a heat-sealing machine uses heat at a minimum setting to produce a seal. Cold sealing can be accomplished either manually or by the use of a cold-sealing machine. The manual method uses a handheld roller to apply pressure and obtain a seal. A cold-sealing machine uses an automatic roller to apply the correct pressure over the entire card.

No other special supplies are needed to complete the modified unit-dose system. Punch cards are also stored in mobile medication carts in the facility.

## BLENDED UNIT-DOSE SYSTEM

A **blended unit-dose system** is a drug distribution system that combines a "unit-of-use" medication package with a non-unit-dose drug distribution system. There are two types of blended systems: the multiple medication package system and the modular cassette system.

A **multiple medication package**, also called a pouch package or a compliance package, is a medication package in which all medications for a specific administration time are packaged together; for example, all medications to be administered at 8 A.M. (Figure 3–7). Packages are produced in a continuous

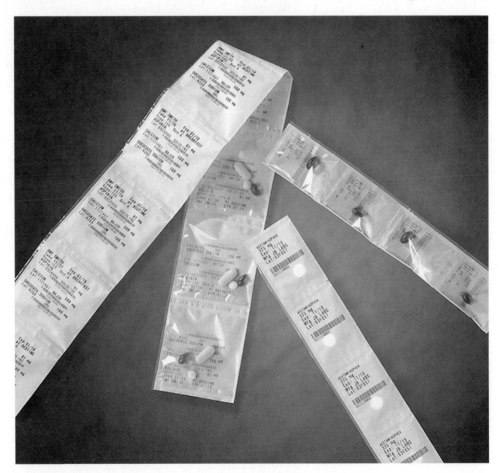

**FIGURE 3–7** Multiple Medication Package. (Courtesy of AutoMed Technologies, Inc.)

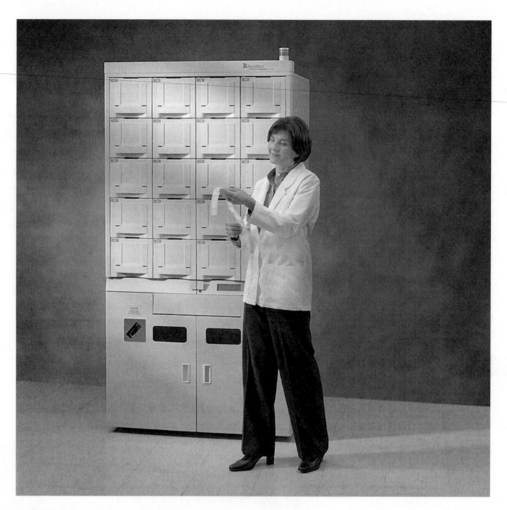

**FIGURE 3–8    Strip Packaging Machine. (Courtesy of AutoMed Technologies, Inc.)**

strip sequenced according to their time of administration; for example, 8 A.M., followed by 12 noon, followed by 4 P.M., followed by 8 P.M., followed by 8 A.M., and so on. This method expands the benefits of unit dose by allowing medications to be packaged more "patient ready" for administration. Multiple medication packages are produced by automated strip packaging machines, which are much more expensive than traditional unit-dose packaging machines (Figure 3–8). Multiple medication packages are stored in the facility in mobile medication carts in accessories that accommodate the strips of packages in a roll.

A **modular cassette** is a combination of a cassette or drawer exchange system (as used in hospitals) with unit-dose or blister-packaged medications. It is available as a 7-day system or a 14-day system. It incorporates a 7-day or 14-day strip of medication with a "reserve" or backup dose inside a narrow type of cassette, often referred to as a "slide tray." Unlike a paper or cardboard unit-dose box, this cassette is constructed of heavy plastic and is reusable. Modular cassettes are stored in specially designed mobile medication carts in the facility (Figure 3–9).

There are many advantages to using a type of unit-dose drug distribution system in the long-term care setting, mostly enjoyed by the long-term care facility. These systems save nursing time because there is no need to prepare or

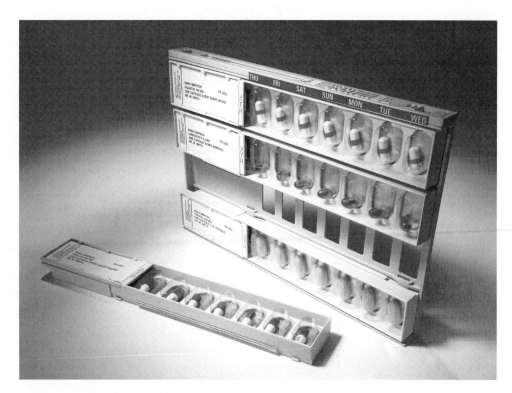

**FIGURE 3–9**   Modular Cassette. (Courtesy of Artromick International, Inc.)

"pour" medications at the time of administration to the patient, and the chance of medication errors is decreased. There are built-in reordering procedures. These systems provide better accountability of medications, discourage drug diversion and abuse, and simplify bookkeeping. Finally, unit-dose systems minimize waste.

There are several disadvantages of unit-dose drug distribution systems that are mostly related to the long-term care pharmacy. The pharmacy must stock additional inventory of medications in unit-dose form, needing additional space for their storage. Specialized equipment is required to prepare these forms, such as unit-dose packaging machines, punch card sealing machines, or strip packaging machines, as well as the space in which to operate the machines. Preparing unit-dose medications is time- and labor-intensive and requires additional personnel, and, although it is more expensive to package medications in unit-dose form, there is usually no additional reimbursement for it. Finally, nurses in the long-term care facility sometimes complain that it is difficult to open some types of unit-dose packages.

## TRADITIONAL VIAL SYSTEM

A traditional vial system is a drug distribution system in which medications are packaged in traditional multiple-dose prescription vials. There are several advantages to this system for the long-term care pharmacy. This system does not require any specialized equipment, supplies, time, or expense to package these medications. There is no need to stock extra inventory. It also does not disrupt the traditional day-to-day operations of the pharmacy. However, there are several disadvantages to this system that relate to the long-term care facility. There is little control of the medication once it leaves the pharmacy. It is more difficult to keep an accurate inventory. To account for a medication, the nurse must empty the prescription vial and count the contents individually. There is no built-in reordering system. Additional nursing time is needed for medication administration. Medications must be poured into small cups, which can be confused or spilled, increasing the chance of medication errors. Finally, discontinued medications that are not in unit-dose form cannot be returned to the pharmacy to be reused but must be destroyed.

## AUTOMATED DISPENSING SYSTEMS

An automated dispensing system is a drug distribution system in which medications are stored and dispensed in a unit outside of the long-term care pharmacy. This unit is electronically linked with the pharmacy's computer, which controls the process, and all medication orders are reviewed by the pharmacist prior to dispensing. It features an "automated teller machine–like" dispensing cabinet that holds the medications and computer-controlled access. A nurse obtains access to medication through the use of a password or fingerprint scan. Documentation, reordering, and billing are done automatically. The advantages of an automated dispensing system include reduced medication errors, improved documentation, and enhanced security. The disadvantages include cost, space requirements for the unit, and computer problems. Automated dispensing systems are usually found in large long-term care facilities. An example is the Pyxisstation by Pyxis Corporation.

## SPECIALIZED MEDICATION DISPENSERS

There are specialized containers for medications, such as controlled substances, that require greater accountability in the nursing facility. They are often referred to as *security containers,* and examples of these include slide cases, narcotic cubes, and narcotic dispensers. These containers are usually constructed of hard plastic and have numbered compartments to hold the medication. The top or covering over each compartment is clear or opaque plastic, which allows visibility. Thus the number of doses of medication remaining in inventory can be quickly counted. Tampering is prevented by the tops, which are designed to be broken away when the medication is removed from the compartment for dispensing to the patient (Figure 3–10).

There are also specialized medication containers that have been developed for residents who administer their own medications, to improve patient compliance. They are referred to as *reminder boxes, medication dispensers, pill tenders,* or *medication planners.* These containers are also made of plastic and are sturdy, lightweight, dishwasher safe, and reusable. They are available in many types and styles. Most are weekly containers with four compartments for the different administration time periods—morning, noon, evening, and bedtime for each day of the week—a total of 28 compartments. There are large-capacity containers for patients with multiple medications in each compartment or for large-sized medications. They can be made child-resistant. There are also containers that use Braille or raised strips for visually impaired residents (Figure 3–11).

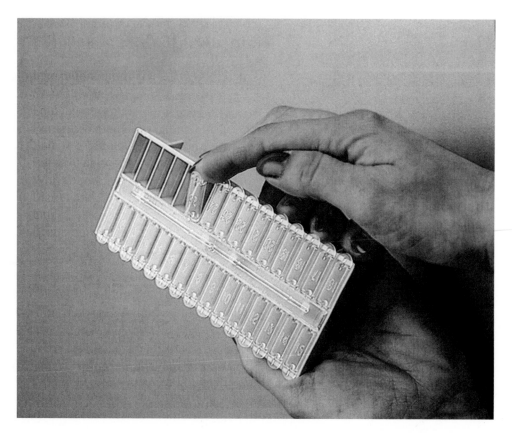

**FIGURE 3–10**    Narcotic Dispenser. (Courtesy of Health Care Logistics, Inc.)

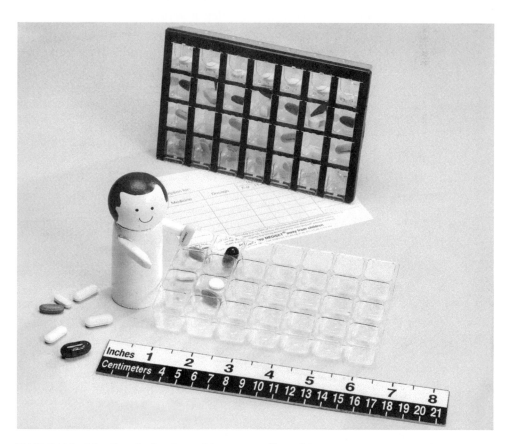

**FIGURE 3–11**    Reminder Box. (Courtesy of Health Care Logistics, Inc.)

## THE PRESCRIPTION-FILLING PROCESS IN A LONG-TERM CARE PHARMACY

The process of dispensing a prescription for a resident in a long-term care facility differs from the process used to dispense a prescription for a regular retail patient or customer in several ways. The process in the long-term care setting involves three parties—the long-term care nurse, the long-term care pharmacist, and the prescribing physician—as opposed to two parties—the retail pharmacist and the prescribing physician—in a traditional community retail setting. The process begins when a nurse makes an assessment of a resident's condition or problem and contacts the physician. The physician reviews the problem and information from the patient's chart and then gives a prescription order to the nurse, verbally by phone, by facsimile, or electronically. The nurse enters the order into the resident's chart and then communicates the new prescription to the pharmacy by phone, facsimile, or electronically. The order received from the long-term care facility must be clear, unambiguous, and complete.

The prescription order is received in the pharmacy and screened through the use of the computerized patient medication profile for the appropriate dose, route of administration, drug or food interactions, allergies, contraindications, and therapeutic duplications. Computer entry leads to the generation of a computerized prescription label. The prescription is then packaged, using the appropriate drug distribution system for the facility, and labeled to comply with applicable federal and state regulations. After the pharmacist checks the completed order, it is delivered to the nursing facility.

Requests for refills are received by phone, facsimile, medication reorder form, or electronically. The refill-dispensing service to a long-term care facility is based on a **turn-around system.** This is a system for obtaining refills that requires a nurse to reorder a medication at a predetermined time before the medication runs out. This time can be anywhere from 3 to 7 days; thus the system is called a "3-day turn-around" or "7-day turn-around" system. Medication order reminders, placed near the end of the medication supply, alert the nurse to start the order process. Reordering involves removing one part of the two-part prescription label on the medication package and placing it on a reorder form. This form is sent to the pharmacy by facsimile or with the driver. Refills can also be phoned in to the pharmacy or transmitted electronically. The medication is refilled at the pharmacy and delivered to the facility, and the cycle begins again.

Another dispensing service provided to the long-term care facility is called **cycle fill.** It is a system for obtaining refill medications automatically from the pharmacy without involving the nursing staff. A resident's medication is identified for refill at the appropriate scheduled time by the use of a pharmacy computer program. This frees the nursing staff from the responsibility of reordering medications. Both refill systems ensure the safe, efficient, and timely delivery of medications to the nursing facility resident.

### ELECTRONIC MEDICAL RECORDS AND E-PRESCRIBING IN THE PRESCRIPTION-FILLING PROCESS

For long-term care facilities, long-term care pharmacies, and prescribing physicians who have implemented electronic technology into their practices, the three-way communication among nurses, pharmacists, and physicians and the process of ordering and filling prescriptions for long-term care residents are simplified. This technology involves the use of electronic medical records and e-prescribing.

An **electronic medical record** is defined as an electronic patient chart that is stored in a computer. It has the same elements as a paper chart, including a problem list, vital signs, allergies, physician orders and progress notes, current medication orders, lab results, consults, and referrals. The electronic medical record requires the use of a laptop personal computer and a dial-up connection (to a server on the network). It allows different health care providers in different locations to access, add to, or edit a patient's information. Electronic medical records minimize errors, reduce costs, and improve patient care. The security of electronic medical records is mandated by the Health Insurance Portability and Accountability Act (HIPAA) and is provided through the use of access privileges to ensure the protection of a patient's medical information.

In the long-term care setting, a compatible computer system is required within the nursing facility. The electronic medical record replaces the paper, handwritten chart located on-site and saves valuable time spent manually searching the large chart that a nursing facility resident typically has due to longer stays. It makes the information in the chart available at any time to nurses, pharmacists, and physicians, wherever they may be. It is especially important because it allows the pharmacist to easily and effectively communicate medication-related concerns to other health care providers. In addition, it enables the pharmacist to communicate through e-prescribing.

**E-prescribing** is defined as the transmission of a prescription, called an e-prescription, between a physician and a pharmacist by way of an electronic medium, with the Internet, dial-up lines, or e-prescribing networks as examples of these mediums. It is essentially computer-to-computer prescribing. E-prescriptions are different from written prescriptions and facsimile prescriptions, which are *images* of a written prescription. However, an e-prescription may be formatted to be electronically received by a facsimile machine. Technology is built into the system to have the prescription validated by way of an electronic signature and to maintain patient confidentiality. E-prescribing allows a physician, at the time of prescribing, to review patient information, such as age, weight, and allergies; drug information, such as interactions and side effects; and a patient's prescription drug benefit and its drug formulary, to determine excluded drugs or drugs that may need an approval. E-prescribing requires a small investment in technology and handheld computers. In return, it reduces medication errors that result from poor handwriting or transcribing errors from verbal orders, and it increases the efficiency of the prescribing process.

In the long-term care setting, like the requirement for electronic medical records, e-prescribing requires a compatible computer system within the facility. This allows three-way communication, not only between the physician and the pharmacist but also with the nurse in the facility, and it creates a secure, closed system. It decreases the time required to get a medication to a long-term care resident by eliminating phone calls involving medication-related problems or formulary problems among the three parties. Although many nursing facilities still use manual handwritten charts and traditional ordering systems, electronic technology is becoming more widely used. Electronic technology continues to improve, and new standards are being developed for the use of electronic medical records and e-prescribing as these tools are rapidly adopted in the long-term care setting.

## THE PRESCRIPTION PACKAGING PROCESS

The prescription packaging process involves the transfer of a medication from a manufacturer's original stock container to a drug distribution system. The actual process may be done manually, as in the case of a cold-sealed punch card, or by an automated system, such as a unit-dose or strip packaging machine. Regardless of the process, certain steps must be taken to assure the safety and quality of the medication in its final form.

A separate work area should be dedicated to packaging operations. It should be separate from other pharmacy activities, such as traditional vial dispensing, compounding, shipping, billing, or returns. Only one medication should be packaged at a time, and no other medications should be present in the work area. Prior to starting, the manufacturer's stock container should be examined to verify the correct drug and strength and to assess the integrity of the drug, that is, to determine whether there is contamination or damage from heat, light, or moisture. The machine to be used should be cleaned and inspected and should be operated safely according to the manufacturer's instructions. Drug labeling materials should be assembled in the work area, and the resulting drug packages should be labeled immediately upon completion according to USP labeling standards (see Chapter 4). Finished drug packages should then be removed from the packaging area and brought to the area of the pharmacy designated for their storage. A control record must be maintained according to state and federal guidelines and should include the drug name, strength, dosage form and manufacturer, the manufacturer's lot number and expiration date, the lot number and the expiration date assigned to the drug package, the date and amount of drug packaged, and the initials of the packager.

At the end of the packaging operation, any unused drug remaining in the manufacturer's original container should be returned to stock. Machines should again be cleaned and inspected. Any remaining unused medication labels should be destroyed to prevent them from inadvertently being placed on the wrong drug package. Finally, the control record should be filed. The entire process may then be repeated for another drug.

## THE USE OF BAR CODING IN THE PRESCRIPTION PACKAGING PROCESS

The packaging of medications into safe and efficient drug distribution systems is the mainstay of the long-term care pharmacy. There are several automated technologies and systems in use in the long-term care pharmacy today, for example, high-speed unit-dose packaging machines and strip packaging machines. However, a new technology has emerged that holds promise for safer medication use in the long-term care setting: the bar coding of medication packages. Individual bar codes are being added to the labels of packaged medications in the long-term care pharmacy through the use of specialized computer programs. The bar code contains information about the medication and may also contain information about the patient and the administration time. In the nursing facility, the nurse scans the bar code on the resident's identification wristband at the bedside using a handheld bar code scanning device. She then scans the bar code on the medication package before opening it to assure that the correct medication is being administered to the correct patient. The use of bar codes in this way ensures patient safety by preventing medication administration errors.

The bar code scanner can also be used by the nursing staff to reorder medications from the pharmacy, eliminating phone calls, label peeling, and facsimile orders. It can also be used to track medication deliveries. Although bar code technology is relatively new in the long-term care setting, a growing number of long-term care pharmacies and facilities are using this technology.

## SERVICES OF A LONG-TERM CARE PHARMACY

A long-term care pharmacy dispenses medications to residents in a long-term care facility in the appropriate drug distribution system for the facility. Just as important, the long-term care pharmacy provides various services to the long-term care facility to ensure the safe ordering, distribution, storage, administration, accountability, and record keeping of medications in the facility.

### AUDITING SYSTEM FOR CONTROLLED SUBSTANCES

The long-term care pharmacy assists the long-term care facility in tracking controlled substances prescribed for its residents. Owing to the nature of these drugs and the potential for abuse and diversion, it is important that the facility have systems in place for their receipt, administration, and disposal. One method of tracking these medications is to use a type of security container as the drug distribution system for controlled substances. Another method is for the long-term care pharmacy to provide a delivery record to be used by the nursing staff to verify the receipt of the controlled substances. Finally, the pharmacy can provide the facility with specialized forms for record keeping and tracking of controlled substances within the facility.

### EMERGENCY MEDICATION SUPPLY

An emergency supply of medications in limited quantities is kept in the long-term care facility. These medications are supplied and maintained by the long-term care pharmacy. An **emergency drug** is defined as a drug that can result in discomfort, distress, or an acute or life-threatening condition if not administered to a resident within a reasonable length of time, usually a few hours. These medications should be used only for a medical emergency and not as a routine source of medications for the resident.

The emergency drugs to be kept in the long-term care facility are determined by the long-term care pharmacist, representatives from the medical and nursing staff, and state regulations. The drugs should meet the specific needs of the resident population of the long-term care facility, and they should be periodically reviewed. The categories of medications that may be included in the emergency medication supply are listed in Box 3–1.

Emergency medications are stored in a portable, sealed container in the long-term care facility. The container is kept in a secured area of the facility, such as in a locked cabinet or medication room, to prevent unauthorized access and to ensure the proper storage environment for the medications. Commercially available emergency boxes, as well as ordinary fishing tackle boxes and plastic sewing boxes, can be used (Figure 3–12). The box is sealed or locked in such a way that the seal is visibly altered when the box is opened. Plastic, cut-away locks are used for this purpose.

An inventory list must be attached to the emergency box. It must include the name of the medication (brand or generic), its dosage strength, and the quantity. The medications in the box must be labeled with the name, dosage

## BOX 3–1    Categories of Emergency Supply Medications

Analgesics
Antibiotics
Anticoagulants and vitamin K
Antidiarrheals
Antihistamines
Antinauseants
Antipsychotics
Diuretics
Hypergylcemics and hypoglycemics
IV additives
Large-volume parenterals
Narcotic antagonists
Seizure control medications
Steroids

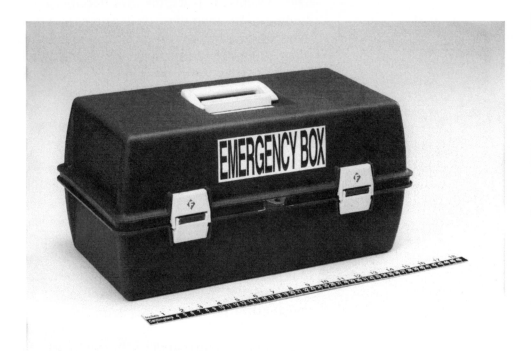

**FIGURE 3–12**    Emergency Box. (Courtesy of Health Care Logistics, Inc.)

strength, quantity, expiration date, and name of the provider pharmacy. A sample inventory list is provided in Table 3–1.

The long-term facility is required to record medication use from the emergency box. The patient's name, drug name, strength, quantity, date and time, and the name of the individual removing the medication must be recorded. The facility should have a policy and procedure for the use of the emergency box. A nurse receives an order for an emergency medication from a physician. The emergency box is opened by breaking the seal or lock, and enough medication is removed to last until delivery of medication from the pharmacy. Use of the medication is recorded, and the provider pharmacy is notified. There are two methods of

**TABLE 3–1 Sample Emergency Medication Inventory List**

| MEDICATION | QUANTITY |
|---|---|
| Acetaminophen 325 mg tablet | 6 |
| Acetaminophen 650 mg suppository | 4 |
| Adrenalin 1:1000 – 1 mL | 2 |
| Amoxicillin 250 mg capsule | 6 |
| Atropine sulfate 0.4 mg/mL – 1 mL | 2 |
| Cefazolin 1 gram vial | 2 |
| Cephalexin 250 mg capsule | 6 |
| Ciprofloxacin 250 mg tablet | 6 |
| Dexamethasone 0.4 mg/mL – 1 mL | 2 |
| Diazepam 5 mg/mL – 2 mL | 2 |
| Digoxin 0.125 mg tablet | 4 |
| Diphenhydramine 50 mg/mL – 1 mL | 2 |
| Erythromycin 250 mg tablet | 6 |
| Furosemide 40 mg tablet | 2 |
| Furosemide 40 mg/4 mL – 4 mL | 2 |
| Glucagon 1 mg/mL – 1 mL | 1 |
| Glipizide 5 mg tablet | 2 |
| Haloperidol 5 mg/mL – 1 mL | 1 |
| Heparin 5,000 Units/mL – 1 mL | 1 |
| Hydrocodone/APAP 5/500 | 6 |
| Hydroxyzine 50 mg/mL – 1 mL | 1 |
| Insulin, Humulin Regular 100 Units/mL – 10 mL | 1 |
| Loperamide 2 mg capsule | 4 |
| Morphine sulfate 10 mg/mL – 1 mL | 2 |
| Morphine sulfate concentrate 20 mg/mL – 30 mL | 1 |
| Nitroglycerin 1/150 gr (0.4 mg) – 25-tablet bottle | 1 |
| Phytonadione 10 mg/mL – 1 mL | 1 |
| Prednisone 5 mg tablet | 4 |
| Promethazine 50 mg/ml injection | 2 |
| Promethazine 25 mg suppository | 2 |
| Promethazine 25 mg tablet | 4 |
| Sulfamethoxazole/Trimethoprim DS tablet | 4 |
| Warfarin 5 mg tablet | 4 |
| Water for injection – 30 mL | 1 |

replacement. In the first method, only the emergency medication that was used is delivered to the facility. A nurse is responsible for restocking the emergency box and resealing it. In the second method, the opened and used emergency box is replaced by a new, complete, and sealed box delivered to the facility. The used box is then returned to the pharmacy for inventory and restocking. The emergency box is inventoried by the provider pharmacy periodically to ensure that it is complete and there are no expired medications. A helpful way to monitor the expiration dates of the contents is to list the date that corresponds to the earliest expiration date of a medication in the box on the outside of the emergency box.

The use of an automated dispensing machine is another method of obtaining emergency medications in the long-term care facility. In addition to immediate access to emergency medications, automation has the advantages of automatic record keeping, billing, and reordering.

## MEDICATION STORAGE IN THE LONG-TERM CARE FACILITY

Medications for nursing home residents, once received from the provider pharmacy, must be correctly and securely stored in the long-term care facility. Mobile medication carts are used for this purpose. There are many types of carts as well as numerous manufacturers. There are differences in materials and construction, but the most important difference is in configuration. The configuration of the cart describes the arrangement of the drawers and compartments in the cart. The configuration will depend on the drug distribution system being used in the facility. Carts can be configured or arranged to accommodate unit-dose boxes, punch cards, slide trays, multiple medication packages, and traditional prescription vials (Figures 3–13 and 3–14). Usually a resident will have an individual drawer or section in the cart for his medications. There are also separate drawers or storage areas for liquids, ophthalmic and otic bottles,

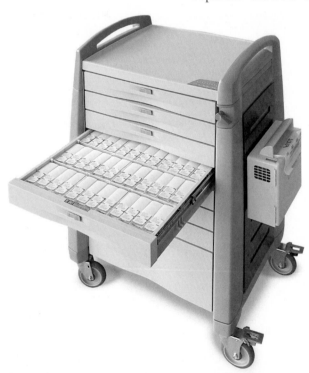

**FIGURE 3–13** Unit-Dose Box Medication Cart. (Courtesy of Artromick International, Inc.)

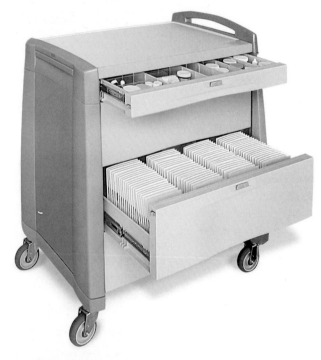

**FIGURE 3–14** Punch Card Medication Cart. (Courtesy of Artromick International, Inc.)

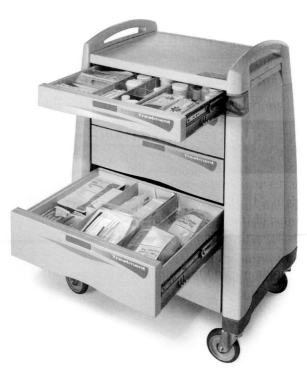

**FIGURE 3–15** Treatment Cart. (Courtesy of Artromick International, Inc.)

inhalers, transdermal medications, and opened bottles of insulin. There is a separate, locked compartment for storing Schedule II controlled substances, providing storage under double locks. Carts are locked when not in use for medication administration and are kept in the medication room or at the nursing station. The carts are usually provided to the facility by the provider pharmacy, with the cost of the carts being calculated into the price of the pharmaceutical services. The pharmacy then is responsible for maintaining the carts.

External medications must be stored separately from internal medications. There are specialized mobile carts for storing external medications, bandages, and other first aid–type supplies. These carts are referred to as treatment carts (Figure 3–15).

A refrigerator must be available in the long-term care facility for the storage of insulin, vaccines, other refrigerated injectables, sterile intravenous infusions, suppositories, and liquid antibiotics. It is preferably found in the medication room or at the nursing station. A locked compartment or box within the refrigerator is required for the secure storage of refrigerated Schedule II controlled substances, such as Dilaudid (hydromorphone) suppositories (Figure 3–16).

Some long-term care facilities provide a locked cabinet or drawer, usually in the medication room or at the nursing station, for the storage of overflow medications, excluding refrigerated medications, external medications, and Schedule II controlled substances. Discontinued medications are usually stored in a locked or secure area until disposal or pickup by the provider pharmacy.

## FORMS AND REPORTS

A long-term care pharmacy provides various forms and reports to the long-term care facility as part of its comprehensive service. Forms and reports are used for two purposes in the facility: record keeping and communication. Forms and reports are tools for complying with federal and state laws and regulations for

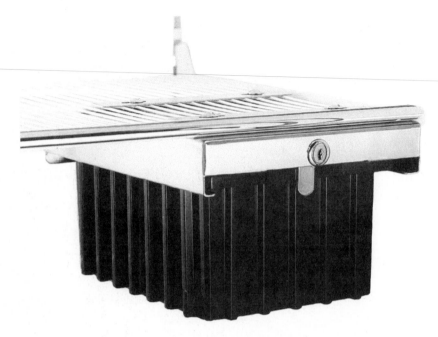

**FIGURE 3–16** Locking Refrigerator Box. (Courtesy of Health Care Logistics, Inc.)

long-term care. Certain forms allow for the proper documentation of drug and other therapies, medication administration, and medication accountability and are referred to as charting forms. Forms and reports are also tools for improving communication between the interdisciplinary team members in the long-term care facility. Each facility uses forms and reports specific for its needs. The choice of forms is made using input from the long-term care pharmacist and the nursing staff. Forms should be easy to use in order to be used effectively. The forms and reports are compatible with most major computer software systems and are usually printed on durable paper to withstand repeated handling. There are many types of forms provided to the long-term care facility by the provider pharmacy.

### Physician Order Form

The **physician order form,** also called a physician order sheet, or POS, is a complete list of all of the physician's orders for a long-term care resident. It contains both drug orders and nondrug orders. The drug orders are based on the patient's medication profile. The nondrug orders are varied and include allergies, diagnoses, diet orders, directives, laboratory orders, oxygen orders, and orders for ancillary services such as physical therapy, occupational therapy, respiratory therapy, or speech therapy. Resident activities, special resident preferences (for food or grooming), and specialist physician or dental consults are also included as nondrug orders. The physician order form is a communication tool and is essential to the resident's overall care in the facility. It is updated and printed monthly and is part of the patient's chart. An example of a physician order form is shown in Figure 3–17. A set of physician orders can also be computer generated without the use of a specific commercially available form.

### Medication Administration Record

The **medication administration record,** or MAR, is a form used to document medication administration to a patient. It is an important component of a good

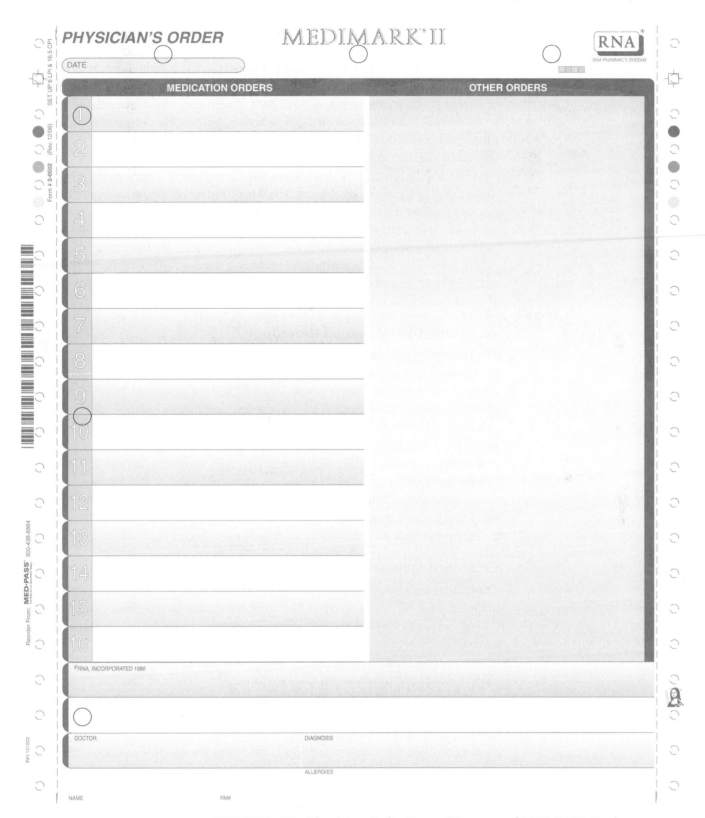

**FIGURE 3–17** Physician Order Form. (Courtesy of MED-PASS, Inc.)

drug distribution system. Proper medication administration is required to protect the health and safety of the nursing facility resident. The medication administration record includes all the information needed for the proper administration of medication. It includes the drug, dose, route of administration, frequency of administration, and administration times. It also includes the resident's drug allergies and diagnoses. It may include nondrug treatments or monitoring requirements, such as monitoring the pulse of a patient receiving digoxin or monitoring the blood pressure of a patient receiving antihypertensive medications.

The medication administration record is used every time a medication is administered to a patient and is usually kept on the medication cart. The nurse documents the administration of a dose by placing his initials in the proper space on the form corresponding to the medication and the administration time. Documentation must be done immediately after the administration of the medication. The MAR is a monthly form used to document medication administration over an entire month. It is also part of the resident's chart. An example of a medication administration record is shown in Figure 3–18.

### Treatment Administration Record

The **treatment administration record,** or TAR, is a form used to document external treatments administered to a patient. It is similar in format to the medication administration record, but it is used specifically for documenting external treatments. Treatment medications such as creams, ointments, enemas, and suppositories are usually found on the treatment administration record rather than on the medication administration record. Examples of treatments include wound care treatments, decubitus ulcer treatments, dry skin treatments, scalp and shampoo treatments, foot care treatments, and incontinence treatments. Documentation is in the form of the nurse's initials in the proper space corresponding to the treatment and the administration time. It is also a monthly form and part of the patient's chart. An example of a treatment administration record is shown in Figure 3–19.

### Controlled Substance Forms

Controlled substances are subject to special ordering, storage, administration, disposal, and record keeping in the long-term care facility in accordance with federal and state laws and regulations. There are several forms that assist in the accountability of controlled substances in this setting.

A controlled substance count form allows for nursing shift count verification of controlled substance medications. This refers to the counting of an individual controlled substance medication at each change of nursing shift, witnessed and signed by the outgoing and incoming nurses. The incoming nurse then assumes responsibility for the medication while on duty (Figure 3–20).

A controlled substance usage form monitors the receipt, administration, and disposal of an individual controlled substance medication for an individual resident. It documents the delivery of the controlled substance medication to the facility, the use of the medication, and, finally, the disposal of the medication once it is no longer being taken by the resident. A separate form is used to account for each controlled substance medication that a resident may be taking (Figure 3–21).

### Resident Monitoring Forms

There are many different forms that are used in the long-term care facility to monitor medication regimens, patient behaviors, and medical conditions. One

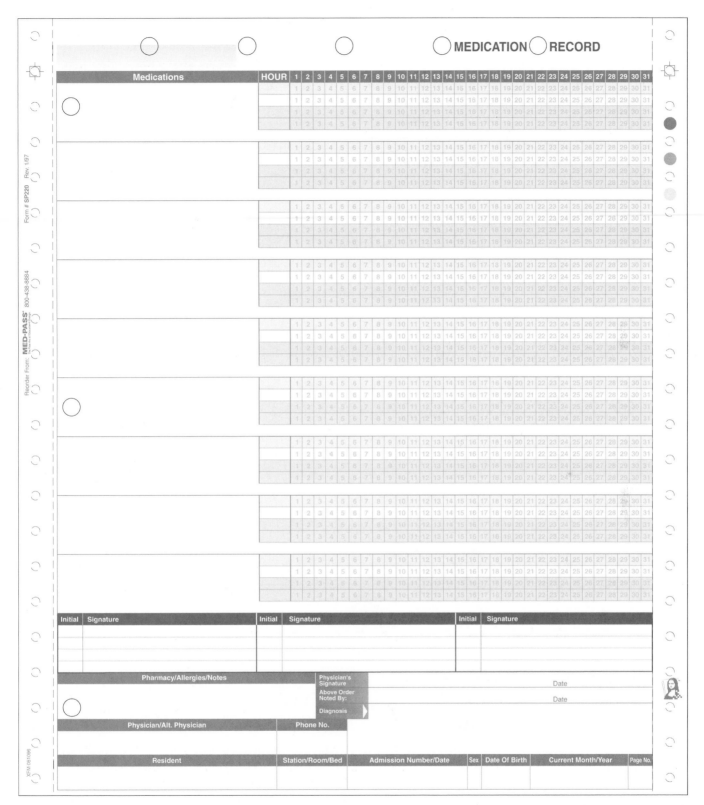

**FIGURE 3–18** Medication Administration Record. (Courtesy of MED-PASS, Inc.)

of the most useful types of forms is a behavior monitoring form. A **behavior monitoring form** is a form used to document a patient's behaviors and information relevant to them. It is a monthly form that allows documentation of a resident's behaviors, any precipitating factors, drug and nondrug interventions,

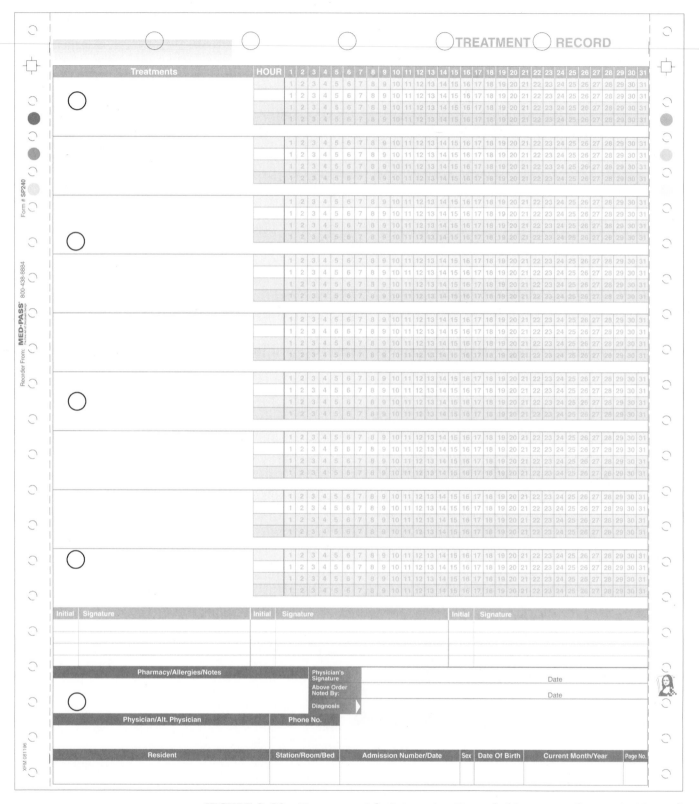

**FIGURE 3–19**   Treatment Administration Record. (Courtesy of MED-PASS, Inc.)

outcomes, and adverse drug reactions. This form will be used any time a resident is taking a psychotropic medication, such as an antipsychotic, antianxiety, antidepressant, or sedative-hypnotic medication. It is a method for preventing the overuse of these types of medications while encouraging nondrug interventions in residents who display certain types of behaviors (Figure 3–22).

Healthcare Center

## EIGHT HOUR/SHIFT VERIFICATION
## OF CONTROLLED SUBSTANCES COUNT

**DIRECTIONS:** Use this form to verify that the Controlled Drugs on hand have been counted and that each medication count is in agreement with quantity stated on Controlled Drug Record(s). Use the comment section to note discrepancies and notify appropriate facility staff according to facility policy.

| DATE | SHIFT | SIGNATURE ON-COMING NURSE | SIGNATURE OFF-GOING NURSE | COMMENTS/DOCUMENTATION |
|------|-------|---------------------------|---------------------------|------------------------|
| / / | | | | |
| / / | | | | |
| / / | | | | |
| / / | | | | |
| / / | | | | |
| / / | | | | |
| / / | | | | |
| / / | | | | |
| / / | | | | |
| / / | | | | |
| / / | | | | |
| / / | | | | |
| / / | | | | |
| / / | | | | |
| / / | | | | |
| / / | | | | |
| / / | | | | |
| / / | | | | |
| / / | | | | |
| / / | | | | |
| / / | | | | |
| / / | | | | |
| / / | | | | |
| / / | | | | |
| / / | | | | |
| / / | | | | |
| / / | | | | |
| / / | | | | |
| / / | | | | |

Form # MP5212   Rev. 01/02

Reorder From: **MED-PASS** 800-438-8884

© 1993 MED-PASS, INC.

INH-102000

**FIGURE 3–20**   Controlled Substance Count Form. (Courtesy of MED-PASS, Inc.)

## INDIVIDUAL RESIDENT'S CONTROLLED SUBSTANCE RECORD

| Medication Name | | Medication # | Dosage | Method of Administration | Pharmacist Name |
|---|---|---|---|---|---|
| Amount Ordered | Amount Received | Signature of Nurse Receiving Medication | | | Date |

### DISPOSITION OF REMAINING DOSES - Per Facility Policy

☐ Doses transferred to a medical waste container — Quantity / Date

☐ Doses flushed — Nurse Signature

☐ Doses Incinerated — Witness Signature / Title

☐ Doses Transferred to other Disposal Record — Date / Signature / Title

☐ Doses Discharged with Resident (See Record on Chart) — Quantity / Date / ☐ Party Receiving (*See Discharge Note) / Nurse Signature

OPTIONAL BOX
FOR LABEL

| NAME OF PERSON GIVING | DATE | TIME | AMT. ON HAND | AMT. RECEIVED | AMT. GIVEN | AMT. REMAINING |
|---|---|---|---|---|---|---|
| | | | | | | |
| | | | | | | |
| | | | | | | |
| | | | | | | |
| | | | | | | |
| | | | | | | |
| | | | | | | |
| | | | | | | |
| | | | | | | |
| | | | | | | |
| | | | | | | |
| | | | | | | |
| | | | | | | |
| | | | | | | |
| | | | | | | |
| | | | | | | |
| | | | | | | |
| | | | | | | |
| | | | | | | |
| | | | | | | |

| Resident Name | ID # | Room # | Physician |
|---|---|---|---|

Form # MP5211   (Rev. 08/06)

Reorder From: MED-PASS® 800-438-8884

© 1993 MED-PASS, Inc.

INH 120200

These colors (Teal and Pink) are a trademark of Med-Pass, Inc.

**FIGURE 3–21** Controlled Substance Usage Form. (Courtesy of MED-PASS, Inc.)

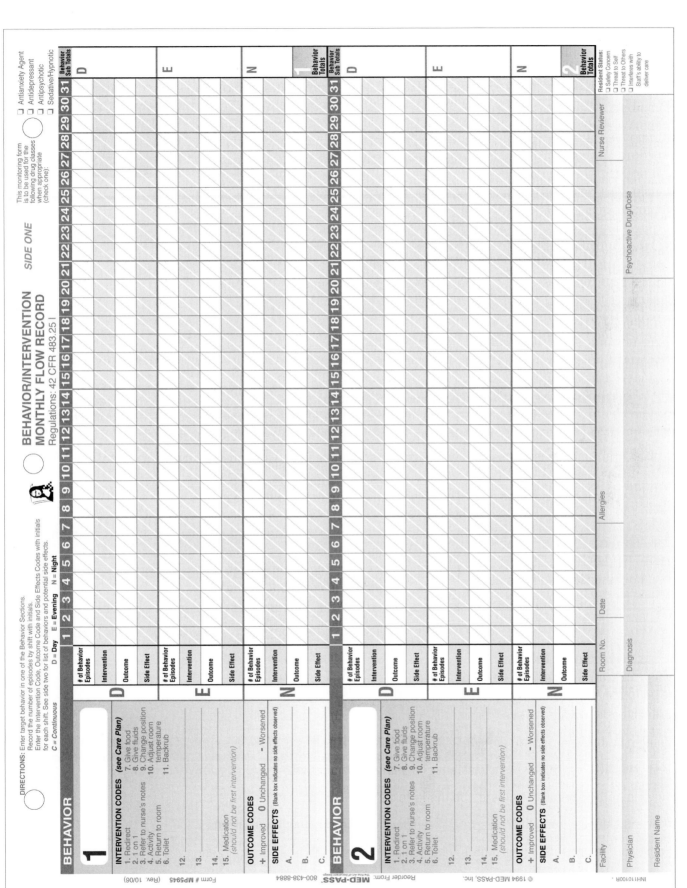

**FIGURE 3–22** Behavior Monitoring Form. (Courtesy of MED-PASS, Inc.)

**Medication Delivery Record**

There are reports that provide accountability and quality control for medication distribution between the long-term care pharmacy and the long-term care facility. A medication delivery record is a computer-generated report that accompanies the delivery of medications to the facility. It is the list of medications that is found in a particular delivery. The medications to be delivered are checked against the delivery record in the pharmacy. They are checked against the delivery record again when they are delivered to the facility. Any discrepancies are immediately reported to the provider pharmacy.

## KEY CONCEPTS

- A long-term pharmacy is a pharmacy that dispenses medications to residents in a long-term care facility.
- The two types of long-term care pharmacies are the open-shop and closed-shop pharmacies.
- A long-term care pharmacy has many unique elements, including special equipment, supplies, and refill systems.
- The different types of drug distribution systems used in long-term care are the unit-dose system, modified unit-dose system, blended unit-dose system, traditional vial system, and automated dispensing system.
- The unique prescription-dispensing process in the long-term care pharmacy features three parties—the nurse, pharmacist, and physician—an appropriate drug distribution system, and delivery to the long-term care facility, as well as unique refill reordering systems.
- Emergency medications supplied and maintained by the long-term care pharmacy are found in the long-term care facility.
- Medications are stored in the long-term care facility in specially designed mobile medication carts.
- The long-term care pharmacy supplies many forms and reports to the long-term care facility, including physician order forms, medication and treatment administration forms, controlled substance forms, behavior monitoring forms, and medication delivery records.

## SELF-ASSESSMENT QUESTIONS

### MULTIPLE CHOICE

1. Which is not an emergency medication?
   a. antidiarrheal
   b. multiple vitamin
   c. analgesic
   d. antihistamine

2. The drug distribution system that is not used in long-term care is:
   a. bingo cards
   b. multiple medication packages
   c. 7-day modular cassettes
   d. 24-hour cassettes

3. All of the following are advantages of a unit-dose drug distribution system except:
   a. decreased inventory of medications in the pharmacy
   b. decreased chance of medication errors
   c. decreased nursing time
   d. decreased drug abuse

4. A long-term care pharmacy provides all of the following forms to a long-term care facility except:
   a. a medication administration record
   b. a behavior monitoring form
   c. a physician order form
   d. an intravenous compounding record

5. A long-term care pharmacy can be:
   a. an independent pharmacy
   b. an open-shop pharmacy
   c. a long-term care pharmacy corporation
   d. all of the above

6. A punch card is an example of a:
   a. blended unit-dose system
   b. unit-dose system
   c. modified unit-dose system
   d. traditional vial system

7. All of the following are accurate statements concerning emergency medications except:
   a. the nursing facility administrator decides the contents of the emergency box
   b. the emergency medication supply must be periodically inventoried
   c. an emergency medication can be dispensed only on a physician's order
   d. record keeping is involved in the use of emergency medications

8. All of the following are accurate statements concerning a medication cart except:
   a. each patient has his own drawer in the cart
   b. there are special areas for storing liquids
   c. there is a separate locked compartment for Schedule II controlled substances
   d. it is not necessary to lock a medication cart

9. Which is not a component of the delivery service of a long-term care pharmacy?
   a. a routine daily delivery time
   b. hourly delivery

c. stat or emergency delivery

d. after-hours delivery

10. Medication used in the long-term care facility cannot be stored in:

a. a refrigerator

b. treatment carts

c. the resident's nightstand

d. medication carts

## TRUE/FALSE (CORRECT THE FALSE STATEMENTS)

1. _____ A closed-shop pharmacy can fill prescriptions for any patient, including long-term care residents.

2. _____ Automation plays a role in the long-term care pharmacy.

3. _____ The cycle fill system frees the nursing staff from the responsibility of reordering medications.

4. _____ The emergency medication supply can be used as a routine source of medications for long-term care residents.

5. _____ The storage unit for medications in the long-term care facility is the mobile medication cart.

6. _____ The medication administration record must be used every time a medication is administered.

7. _____ The physician order form contains nondrug orders as well as drug orders.

8. _____ External medications must be stored separately from internal medications in the long-term care facility.

9. _____ The goals of any drug distribution system are economy and simplicity.

10. _____ The use of automated dispensing machines in the long-term care facility is a method of obtaining emergency medications.

## FILL-IN

1. The drug distribution system used in long-term care that involves individual medication packages is called _____.

2. A drug that can result in discomfort, distress, or an acute or life-threatening condition if not administered quickly is referred to as an _____ _____.

3. A long-term care pharmacy that is found inside a long-term care facility is referred to as _____.

4. The refill dispensing service to a long-term care facility is based on a _____ system.

5. The method of distributing a drug is called the _____ _____ _____.

6. The system that combines unit-dose medication packaging with non-unit-dose distribution is called a _____ unit-dose system.

7. A medication packet in a continuous strip sequenced according to administration time is a _____ _____ _____.

8. A _____ _____ is a specialized medication container designed to provide accountability for controlled substances.

9. The _____ describes the arrangement of drawers and compartments in a medication cart.
10. The form similar in format to the medication administration record for documenting the use of external treatments is the _____ _____ _____.

## CRITICAL THINKING

1. Compare and contrast pharmacy operations in a long-term care pharmacy with those in a traditional community retail pharmacy.
2. Identify examples of the different types of long-term care pharmacies in your community.
3. What are some examples of nondrug orders found on a physician order form?
4. Apply *structure, process,* and *outcomes* to a long-term care pharmacy.
5. Provide examples of situations in which an emergency medication would be used.

## BIBLIOGRAPHY

American Society of Consultant Pharmacists. (2005). *White paper prepared for the Long-Term Care Health Information Technology Summit.* [On-line] ASCP. Available: www.ascp.com

Barry, D. (2006). Entering the e-prescribing era. *Pharmacy Today, 12*(1), 16.

Erickson, A. (2004). Zipping from physician to pharmacist. *Pharmacy Today, 10*(3), 19.

Hurdle, J. (2004). Can electronic medical records improve geriatric care? *Geriatric Times, 5*(2), 25–26.

Institute of Medicine. (2005). *Key capabilities of an electronic health record system.* [On-line] IOM. Available: www.iom.edu.

Kaldy, J. (2005). Multidisciplinary medication management. *Caring for the Ages, 6*(6), 8–9.

Schuerenberg, B. (2005). Electronic records find long-term use. *Health Data Management, 4*(2), 30–34.

University of the Sciences in Philadelphia. (2005). *Remington: The Science and Practice of Pharmacy* (21st ed.). Easton, PA: Mack Publishing Company.

Zwillich, T. (2004). Feds issue bar-code rules but clash with lawmakers. *Drug Topics, 148*(6), 70.

# 4 Regulations for Long-Term Care Pharmacy

## Learning Objectives

Upon completion of this chapter, the student should be able to:

- List the organizations that regulate long-term care pharmacy.
- Describe the history of federal pharmacy legislation and regulations.
- Discuss the drug regimen review and the purpose of indicators used in its performance.
- Understand the scope of Omnibus Budget Reconciliation Act regulations.
- Explain freedom of choice as it relates to pharmacy services in the long-term care facility.
- Discuss the Anti-Kickback Act as it relates to long-term care pharmacy, and identify "safe harbors."
- Discuss Drug Enforcement Agency regulations that pertain to long-term care pharmacy.
- Explain the expiration date labeling of medications packaged for use in the long-term care facility.
- Understand the issues concerning the return and reuse of medications from the long-term care facility.
- Discuss the provision of material safety data sheets by a long-term care pharmacy to the long-term care facility.
- Explain the Medicare Prescription Drug Benefit.
- Describe the state's role in long-term care pharmacy regulation.
- Understand the role of the Joint Commission in long-term care pharmacy.

## Key Terms

| | | |
|---|---|---|
| apparent irregularity | indicator | remuneration |
| bundling | kickback | safe harbor |
| drug regimen review | material safety data sheet | unnecessary drug |
| hazardous chemical | | |

## Introduction

The evolution of pharmacy practice into long-term care has resulted in the enactment of legislation and regulations that pertain specifically to long-term care pharmacy practice. These regulations pertaining to long-term care pharmacy are extensive. They present a challenge in that they reflect issues from both institutional and retail pharmacy practice and include new and very different types of legislation and regulations that pertain only to long-term care. It is important that pharmacists and pharmacy technicians be familiar with the legislation and regulations that govern the practice of long-term care pharmacy and that affect the entire long-term care industry. This chapter discusses the current pharmacy legislation and regulations for long-term care pharmacy. ∎

## OVERVIEW OF LEGISLATION AND REGULATIONS FOR LONG-TERM CARE PHARMACY

The long-term care industry is heavily regulated. It is one of the two most highly regulated industries in the United States, the other being the nuclear industry. There are many laws, or legislation, and regulations that pertain to long-term care facilities and long-term care pharmacies. In the legislative process, a law is passed by the legislature and establishes required, permissible, or prohibited conduct. Violation of the law can lead to civil or criminal penalties. A regulation also establishes rules of conduct, but it is issued by a federal agency rather than by the legislature. Regulations are intended to help carry out laws by providing guidelines to those governed by the laws, for example, long-term care facilities and long-term care pharmacies, as well as to those responsible for enforcing the laws, for example, long-term care surveyors.

There are many organizations that regulate long-term care facilities and long-term care pharmacies. These include the Centers for Medicare and Medicaid Services (CMS), Department of Health and Human Services (DHHS), Occupational Safety and Health Administration (OSHA), Drug Enforcement Administration (DEA), Joint Commission, state-licensing agencies for long-term care facilities, and state boards of pharmacy.

Medication management in the long-term care facility is an important part of the regulations pertaining to long-term care pharmacy. The long-term care pharmacist has several roles within the facility pertaining to medication management, which is discussed in Chapter 5. In order to understand current legislation and regulations that pertain to long-term care, one must understand their history.

## HISTORY AND EVOLUTION OF LEGISLATION AND REGULATIONS FOR LONG-TERM CARE PHARMACY

Before the mid-1960s, conditions in long-term care facilities were very poor. The facilities were unsanitary and physically unsafe. Social services were not available. Medications were misused, and there was no accountability for them. There were few government regulations, and there was little or no pharmacy involvement.

In 1965, the federal government became involved in long-term care for the first time with the enactment of Medicare and Medicaid. CMS, which oversees Medicare and Medicaid, established requirements in order for a long-term care facility to participate in and be reimbursed by the Medicare and Medicaid programs. These requirements were called Conditions of Participation. One of these conditions was a monthly drug regimen review for each resident. A **drug regimen review** was defined then and still is defined as the process of reviewing all of a resident's medications and corresponding medical information, formulating a clinical recommendation, and communicating that recommendation. (The drug regimen review is discussed in detail in Chapter 5.) At that time, the requirement specified that a charge nurse and prescribing physician together review each resident's medications monthly. The pharmacist was not mentioned. Drug therapy problems continued, although they were starting to be recognized and addressed.

The Conditions of Participation were revised in 1974. The requirement now called for the drug regimen review to be performed by a pharmacist. This change was based on the assumption that the pharmacist is a drug therapy expert and can solve drug-related problems. The revision further added that the pharmacist must report any "irregularities" to the director of nursing, the attending physician, or both, and that this report must be acted on. The pharmacist's involvement in the long-term care facility was also strengthened by the formation of a pharmaceutical services committee within the facility, with the pharmacist as a member. This committee met at least monthly to oversee pharmaceutical services in the facility and to develop written policies and procedures for safe and effective medication use, administration, and control. A survey process was also established to help promote good patient care, to identify inappropriate patient care, and to correct patient care problems. This process consisted of periodic visits to the nursing facility by a surveyor.

There were problems and challenges for the pharmacists performing drug regimen reviews. Most of the pharmacists were not familiar with the drug regimen review because it was not included in pharmacy education at that time. There were no standards for performing the drug regimen review that pharmacists could refer to, so the drug regimen reviews were individual and inconsistent. Long-term care surveyors were also unfamiliar with the drug regimen review, and there was no way for them to determine if it was being performed properly. But this was the beginning of consultant pharmacy practice.

In 1980, standards were developed by CMS to help surveyors assess the performance of the drug regimen review. These standards are referred to as indicators. An **indicator** is described as a tool used by a surveyor to assess the performance of a pharmacist in performing a drug regimen review. The indicators are considered to be *minimal* standards for performing the drug regimen review. They were developed to decrease the subjectiveness of the long-term care surveyor. The following is the list of indicators for assessing the performance of the drug regimen review.

- *Excessive reviews performed on the same day.* No more than 100 reviews should be performed in one day. Drug regimens are complex. In order to perform adequate reviews, the pharmacist should devote more than a few minutes to each one.

- *The location of the reviews.* The reviews should be performed in the long-term care facility, where the pharmacist has access to sources of data such as nurse's notes, physician progress notes, laboratory results, the medication administration record, and even interviews with the patient.

- *The average number of medications per resident.* The average number of medications per resident in the long-term care facility should conform to the national average. In 2006, the national average was seven medications. Drug regimen review should reduce drug use in long-term care facilities.

- *The number of reviews performed vs. the average census.* The number of reviews performed monthly should correspond to the average monthly census, or number of residents, in the long-term care facility. For example, if the average census is 100, the number of reviews performed should be approximately 100.

- *Apparent irregularities.* An irregularity is a potential drug therapy problem. An **apparent irregularity** is a drug therapy circumstance that *may* constitute an irregularity. The pharmacist is responsible for identifying an irregularity and reporting it. A complete list of apparent irregularities is found in Appendix A. Some common examples are the use of duplicate medications, inappropriate doses, and inappropriate monitoring.

These indicators have since been revised and expanded. Individual indicators do not signal a poor drug regimen review. Taken together, however, they provide evidence of whether an adequate drug regimen review is being performed by the pharmacist.

## OMNIBUS BUDGET RECONCILIATION ACT OF 1987

The Omnibus Budget Reconciliation Act of 1987, referred to as OBRA 87, was a piece of federal legislation that made extensive revisions to the Medicare and Medicaid Conditions of Participation for long-term care facilities. It contained numerous revisions to protect the residents' rights and to promote quality care in the long-term care facility. It prompted extensive regulations by CMS that set the standards for resident care. These regulations were so specific that CMS published *interpretive guidelines* to help nursing facilities follow the law and to help long-term care surveyors enforce the law. Further revisions were made in 1990 in OBRA 90. Many of these regulations and guidelines address issues that are related to drug therapy in the long-term care facility and for which pharmacists have a major responsibility. These issues deal with unnecessary drugs, antipsychotic drugs and antipsychotic dose reductions, medication errors, pharmacy services, consultant pharmacist services, and the labeling and storage of drugs.

## UNNECESSARY DRUGS

According to CMS regulations, *each resident's drug regimen must be free of unnecessary drugs*. An **unnecessary drug** is defined as a drug whose use should be reduced or discontinued based on monitoring data or an adverse drug reaction. The interpretive guidelines state that unnecessary drugs are drugs given:

- In excessive dose
- For excessive or insufficient duration
- Without adequate monitoring
- Without a reason for use
- In the presence of adverse drug reactions
- Any combination of these reasons

## ANTIPSYCHOTIC DRUGS

According to CMS regulations, *the long-term care facility must ensure that residents who have not used antipsychotic drugs are not given these drugs unless they are necessary to treat a specific condition, which must be diagnosed and documented in the resident's chart*. The interpretive guidelines state that these drugs should be used only if the resident has a specific condition that warrants the use of these drugs. These conditions are found in Box 4–1.

The guidelines further state that these drugs should not be used if certain behaviors are the only reasons for their use. These behaviors are found in Box 4–2.

The final guideline is that "as needed," or *p.r.n.*, antipsychotic drug orders should not be used more than five times in a 7-day period without a physician's reviewing the resident's condition.

---

**BOX 4–1     Conditions That Warrant the Use of Antipsychotic Drugs**

Schizophrenia
Schizo-affective disorder
Delusional disorder
Psychotropic mood disorders
Acute psychotic disorders
Brief reactive disorders
Schizophreniform disorder
Atypical psychosis
Tourette's disorder
Huntington's disease
Organic mental syndromes

From "Interpretive Guidelines: Skilled Nursing Facilities and Intermediate Care Facilities," CMS, 1992, www.cms.gov, accessed 1/2006.

> ## BOX 4–2    Behaviors That Do Not Warrant the Use of Antipsychotic Drugs
>
> Pacing
> Wandering
> Poor self-care
> Restlessness
> Crying out, yelling, or screaming
> Impaired memory
> Anxiety
> Depression
> Insomnia
> Unsociability
> Indifference to surroundings
> Fighting
> Nervousness
> Uncooperativeness
> Unspecified agitation
>
> From "Interpretive Guidelines: Skilled Nursing Facilities and Intermediate Care Facilities," CMS, 1992, www.cms.gov, accessed 1/2006.

Antipsychotic drugs are powerful drugs with the potential for serious adverse effects. Before OBRA 87, they were prescribed freely and inappropriately for long-term care residents. They were used as *chemical restraints*. They were used to sedate residents in order to reduce staffing needs in the long-term care facility. These drugs were responsible for debilitating and often irreversible adverse effects. OBRA 87 regulations specified when antipsychotic drugs could be used and resulted in a significant decline in their use.

## ANTIPSYCHOTIC DOSE REDUCTIONS

According to CMS regulations, *residents who use antipsychotic drugs must receive gradual dose reductions, drug holidays, or behavioral programming in an effort to discontinue these drugs.* A drug holiday refers to the temporary discontinuation of a drug to test the need for its continued use. Behavioral programming means trying to change a resident's behavior or environment or both. The interpretive guidelines state that a gradual dose reduction consists of tapering the dose to see if the resident's symptoms can be controlled by a lower dose or if the dose can be eliminated altogether. At the minimum, after no more than 6 months of therapy, a resident with a stable condition should be tapered at a maximum of approximately 25 percent of the initial dose per month. As an example, a resident taking 2 mg of Risperdal (risperidone) per day would be tapered down to 1.5 mg per day. The guidelines do state that gradual dose reductions are not necessary if the resident has had a gradual dose reduction within the last 6 months and is taking the lowest possible dose that will control her symptoms. Dose reductions are important. Studies have documented that adverse drug reactions and patient falls increase with higher dosages of antipsychotics.

## MEDICATION ERRORS

According to CMS regulations, *the long-term care facility must ensure that it is free of significant medication error rates. The facility must ensure that residents are free of any significant medication errors.* According to the interpretive guidelines, a medication error is the difference between what the physician orders and what is administered to the resident. A significant medication error is one that causes the resident discomfort or puts her health or safety at risk. Medication error rates for the facility must be calculated. The rate should not be greater than 5 percent. Examples of significant medication errors in the long-term facility include the following:

- Omission—the drug is ordered but not administered
- Unauthorized drug—the drug is administered but not ordered
- Wrong dose
- Wrong route of administration
- Wrong dosage form
- Wrong drug ordered
- Wrong time

It is important to examine medication errors. Errors can be a symptom of a faulty drug administration system or inadequate long-term care facility staff training. Most important, medication errors can result in harm to residents.

## PHARMACY SERVICES

According to CMS regulations, *the long-term care facility must provide routine and emergency drugs to its residents or obtain them under an agreement with a pharmacy.* The interpretive guidelines state that a facility must provide pharmaceutical services to meet the needs of each resident. This provision includes procedures for accurate ordering, receiving, dispensing, and administering medications. The facility can enter an agreement with a long-term care pharmacy to provide pharmacy services. However, it is the responsibility of the facility to ensure that those services are provided in a timely manner so that the resident does not experience any discomfort and that her health or safety is not in danger.

## CONSULTANT SERVICES

According to CMS regulations, *the facility must employ or obtain the services of a licensed pharmacist who provides consultation on all aspects of pharmacy services in the facility.* Also, *the drug regimen of each resident must be reviewed at least once a month by a licensed pharmacist (or at least quarterly in an intermediate-care facility for the mentally retarded). The pharmacist must report any irregularities to the director of nursing or the attending physician, or both, and these reports must be acted upon.* According to the interpretive guidelines, the director of nursing and the physician must act on the pharmacist's recommendations; that is, they must investigate the irregularity identified by the pharmacist and consider the pharmacist's recommendations, but they do not have to agree with or accept those recommendations. Nurses and physicians must document their actions concerning the recommendations made by pharmacists.

## LABELING OF DRUGS

According to CMS regulations, *the facility must label drugs according to currently accepted professional principles, including the expiration date.* According to the interpretive guidelines, the critical elements of the drug label are the name of the drug and its strength. The names of the resident and the physician do not have to be on the label of the drug package. The drug package must be associated with the resident in some way, however, so that the drug is administered to the correct resident. All medications must be labeled with an appropriate expiration date regardless of the drug distribution system used by the facility.

## STORAGE OF DRUGS

According to CMS regulations, *the facility must store all drugs in locked compartments at the proper temperatures according to state and federal laws and can permit only authorized personnel to have access to the keys.* The interpretive guidelines state that compartments can be drawers, cabinets, rooms, refrigerators, mobile carts, and boxes.

## OBRA REVISIONS

Later revisions to OBRA have resulted in additional requirements for long-term care pharmacy. These include:

- Infection control. *The facility must establish and maintain an infection control program designed to provide a safe, sanitary, and comfortable environment for residents and help prevent the spread of disease and infection.* This requirement has resulted in the formation of infection control committees, with pharmacists as members, and policies and procedures for infection control within the facility.

- Self-administration of drugs. *A nursing home resident may administer his own medications if the interdisciplinary team determines that this practice is safe.* The pharmacist, as an important member of the long-term care interdisciplinary team, helps with this decision.

- Restraints. *The resident has the right to be free from any physical or chemical restraints used for discipline or the convenience of the staff.* Antipsychotic drugs are considered to be chemical restraints.

- Resident assessment. *The facility must perform a comprehensive assessment of a resident's needs, examine each resident no less than once every 3 months, and revise the resident's assessment as appropriate.* This requirement has led to the process of care planning.

- Storage of controlled substances. *The facility must provide a separately locked compartment for the storage of Schedule II controlled substances and any other drugs subject to abuse, except when the facility uses a unit-dose drug distribution system in which the quantity of controlled substances stored is minimal and a missing dose can be readily detected.* According to the interpretive guidelines, "separately locked" means that the key to the separately locked Schedule II controlled substances is not the same key that is used to gain access to the non–Schedule II controlled substances.

There have been many benefits and far-reaching effects of OBRA 87 for long-term care pharmacy. With federal regulations defining the duties of a consultant pharmacist in the nursing facility, the pharmacist has become an important member of the long-term care interdisciplinary team. Through drug regimen review, the pharmacist helps improve the outcomes of medication for the long-term care resident. Long-term care pharmacists also help the long-term care facility comply with federal regulations, as well as help control the costs related to drug therapy in the facility. The importance of pharmacy in long-term care has been recognized.

## FREEDOM OF CHOICE

According to CMS regulations, a long-term care facility must provide routine and emergency drugs to its residents or obtain them under an agreement. This agreement is made between the facility and a specific long-term care pharmacy. The provider pharmacy, or contract pharmacy, supplies the drugs in the drug distribution system selected for use by the facility. The selection of a specific drug distribution system that meets the needs of the facility is part of the facility's medication use policy. It should be mentioned here that there is no law that prohibits this "exclusive" arrangement between a long-term care facility and a long-term care pharmacy.

One of a long-term care resident's rights is freedom of choice. A resident has the right to choose a pharmacy other than the contract pharmacy to provide her medications. Oftentimes, this other pharmacy, referred to as an outside pharmacy, may not be able to provide the resident's medication in the drug distribution system used by the facility. The Department of Health and Human Services (DHHS) states that freedom of choice applies to any service that is *not* included in the package of services provided in a long-term care facility. Most facilities include medications as part of their package of services; therefore, a resident of that facility has no further choice regarding her medications. The patient can exercise freedom of choice *before* entering the facility by deciding whether to enter that facility. Furthermore, a facility can deny admission to a resident if she does not agree to obtain her medications from the contract pharmacy and use the drug distribution system selected by the facility. Of course, a long-term care facility should explain this situation clearly to a resident before admission.

The CMS has further expanded on this issue by stating that a long-term care facility has the right to develop medication use policies to protect the health and safety of its residents and that it can prohibit the use of an outside pharmacy that does not meet with its policies. An outside pharmacy that does not or cannot provide medications to a long-term care resident in the drug distribution system in use in the facility does *not* meet with the facility's policies. Multiple drug distribution systems can lead to confusion and error in all aspects of medication use in the facility.

Therefore, freedom of choice as it pertains to long-term care pharmacy means that:

1. A long-term care resident can choose an outside pharmacy to supply her medications if medications are *not* included in the facility's package of services.

2. A long-term care facility may refuse admission to a resident who refuses to use the drug distribution system in place in the facility.

3. A long-term care facility has the right to establish medication use policies to protect its residents and may require all outside pharmacies to comply with its policies.

## ANTI-KICKBACK LEGISLATION

The Federal Health Care Program Anti-Kickback Act, formerly known as the Medicare and Medicaid Anti-Kickback Statute, is a fraud and abuse law relevant to long-term care pharmacy practice. The Anti-Kickback Act *imposes criminal penalties for the knowing and willful payment, solicitation, or receipt of remuneration in return for referring an individual to a person for, or in return for, purchasing, leasing, ordering, or for arranging or recommending the purchase, lease, or order of items or services reimbursable by a federal health care program.* Stated simply, the Anti-Kickback Act prohibits the payment of anything of value to influence the referral of goods or services covered under the Medicare and Medicaid programs. **Remuneration** refers to a payment made directly or indirectly in the form of cash or free or discounted goods or services and includes kick-backs, bribes, and rebates. A **kickback** is defined as a portion of a payment returned to another party according to a secret agreement. This act imposes a criminal penalty (a fine of up to $25,000 and imprisonment for up to 5 years) for the individual (e.g., a pharmacist) or the organization (e.g., the long-term care pharmacy) that offers, pays, solicits, or receives a kickback in order to induce business that is paid for by the government, that is, Medicare and Medicaid. In addition, the act excludes the individual or organization from further participation in the Medicare and Medicaid programs.

This act has been expanded several times. In 1996, under the Health Insurance Portability and Accountability Act (HIPAA), it was broadened to include all federal health care payers. Additionally, the Balanced Budget Act of 1997 imposes a $50,000 penalty for each violation of the Anti-Kickback Act and damages up to three times the amount of the kickback. The Department of Health and Human Services' Office of the Inspector General (OIG) is responsible for prosecuting Medicare and Medicaid fraud.

There are several reasons for the Anti-Kickback Act. Kickbacks and other types of payment result in increased health care costs and increased use of goods and services. These types of activities compromise the integrity of legitimate referrals and therapy decisions. The OIG stresses that the most important aspect of a kickback is that it attempts to induce referrals. Because this act is very broad and unclear at times, the OIG has issued a number of practices that are not considered unlawful under the Anti-Kickback Act. These practices are known as "safe harbors."

### SAFE HARBOR REGULATIONS

**Safe harbor** regulations were adopted by the Department of Health and Human Services to protect legitimate business arrangements and relationships, that is, arrangements and relationships in which there is no danger of patient

## BOX 4–3    Safe Harbor Areas

Investment interests
Space rental
Equipment rental
Personal services
Sale of a practice
Referral services
Warranties
Discounts
Employee compensation
Group purchasing organizations
Waiving coinsurance or deductibles

From "Medicare and State Health Care Programs: Federal Abuse: OIG Anti-Kickback Provisions," DHHS, Office of the Inspector General, 1991, www.dhhs.gov, accessed 1/2006.

or program abuse. These regulations describe what can be done without fear of prosecution. An activity that falls outside of a safe harbor is not necessarily illegal. The regulations only mean that the legality of the activity needs to be determined. This determination is done by examining the activities and relationships and comparing them with the provisions set forth in the Anti-Kickback Act. Sometimes there is a fine line between a legitimate practice and a violation of the law. There are 23 broad areas of safe harbors. Several of these areas that pertain to long-term care pharmacy are listed in Box 4–3.

The following are several examples of safe harbors that apply to long-term care pharmacy practice:

- The long-term care pharmacy provides a free facsimile machine or computer to the long-term care facility. It is a safe harbor *if* it is used only for pharmacy-related purposes. This restriction requires a dedicated or separate phone line and auditing the use of the equipment.

- The long-term care pharmacy pays the long-term care facility to handle the billing for its prescription business. It is a safe harbor *if* the amount paid for this service does not exceed the fair market value.

- The long-term care pharmacy provides consultant pharmacist services to the long-term care facility. It is a safe harbor *if* the pharmacy charges the facility the fair market value for these services. It is *not* a safe harbor if the pharmacy performs these services at no cost or charges below fair market value.

- The long-term care pharmacy provides mobile medication carts or other equipment to the long-term care facility. It is a safe harbor *if* the equipment is rented to the facility at fair market value, or the fair market value of the equipment is incorporated into the pharmacy's overall charge to the facility for pharmacy services.

- The long-term care pharmacy rents space in the long-term care facility for performing consulting services. It is a safe harbor *if* there is a specific rental agreement and the rent paid does not exceed fair market value.

An example of a long-term pharmacy business arrangement that is an abuse of the safe harbor regulations is bundling. **Bundling** refers to the practice of providing a group of goods and services together at no charge or below fair market value in order to obtain or keep business. As an example, a long-term care pharmacy could bundle valuable goods and services, such as consultant pharmacist services, facsimile machines or computers, mobile medication carts, forms and reports, and in-service training to facility staff, with providing medications to the facility.

Enforcement of the Anti-Kickback Act has increased over the years, because many questionable business practices do not fall within safe harbors. Long-term care pharmacy agreements with long-term care facilities can expect to come under scrutiny for several reasons. Long-term care residents by their very nature are a vulnerable group. A consultant pharmacist can influence the drug regimens of long-term care residents. A consultant pharmacist who also dispenses drugs to the facility can have a conflict of interest. There exists the potential for increased drug use and costs. In order to comply with fraud and abuse laws, long-term care pharmacists must examine their own business arrangements with long-term care facilities. Payments and charges should always be at fair market value and should not be tied to any other activity. Pharmacists must continue to serve the best needs of the residents.

## DRUG ENFORCEMENT AGENCY REGULATIONS

The Drug Enforcement Agency (DEA) is the federal agency responsible for combating controlled substance abuse through enforcement and prevention. There are several specific DEA regulations that pertain to long-term pharmacy practice.

### TRANSMISSION OF SCHEDULE II PRESCRIPTIONS BY FACSIMILE

In general, prescriptions for Schedule II controlled substances must be in writing and cannot be refilled. DEA regulations allow for the transmission of a Schedule II prescription between the physician and the pharmacy via a facsimile machine. However, the original written prescription must be presented to the pharmacist and verified against the facsimile copy before the drug is actually dispensed.

There is an exception to this written prescription requirement for Schedule II prescriptions for residents in a long-term care facility. For these patients, the facsimile copy is considered a written prescription, and it is not necessary for the original written prescription to be delivered to the long-term care pharmacy, either before or after the delivery of the drug to the facility. The facsimile copy, of course, must contain all of the data required for a normal written Schedule II prescription, including the physician's signature. The pharmacy is required to retain the facsimile copy in the same manner as a normally written Schedule II prescription.

All types of Schedule II drugs in all dosage forms, including oral medications, injectables, suppositories, transdermal patches, and intravenous infusions, can be dispensed on the basis of the facsimile copy. This exception helps to eliminate the need to treat these prescriptions as "emergency prescriptions," which limit the amount of drug that can be dispensed. It also speeds the delivery of these medications to the long-term care resident, when medication needs change quickly and the physician's orders need to be communicated rapidly.

## ELECTRONIC PRESCRIPTIONS FOR SCHEDULE II CONTROLLED SUBSTANCES

The DEA does not have a regulation for the electronic prescribing of Schedule II controlled substances. It is currently gathering information in order to revise federal regulations to allow electronic prescriptions for these drugs. This is necessary to meet and keep up with the technological advances in pharmacy practice, including long-term care pharmacy practice. The new regulations will include a way to certify the authenticity of the prescribing physician as well as of the receiving pharmacy, and to provide confidentiality.

## PARTIAL FILLING OF SCHEDULE II PRESCRIPTIONS

The DEA permits partial filling of a Schedule II prescription when a pharmacy is unable to supply the full quantity called for in the prescription. The remaining portion must be filled within 72 hours of the initial partial filling.

There is an exception to the conditions for partial filling of Schedule II prescriptions for residents in a long-term care facility or for patients diagnosed with a terminal illness. Schedule II prescriptions for these patients can be filled in partial quantities under certain conditions. Partial prescriptions may be filled for up to 60 days from the date of issue of the prescription, unless the medication is discontinued sooner. The total quantity of medication dispensed through partial filling cannot exceed the original quantity prescribed. The pharmacist must also note in some way on the written prescription that the patient is a "long-term facility patient" or "terminally ill patient." A Schedule II prescription that is partially filled and does not contain this notation is considered to have been filled in violation of the Controlled Substances Act.

For each partial filling, the pharmacist must record the following information: date of the partial filling, quantity dispensed, remaining quantity allowed to be dispensed, and the dispensing pharmacist. This information must be recorded on the back of the written prescription or on any other appropriate record, including a computerized record, that can be maintained and retrieved.

## DESTRUCTION OF CONTROLLED SUBSTANCES IN THE LONG-TERM CARE FACILITY

The destruction or disposal of unused controlled substances is a problem for most long-term care facilities. Unused controlled substances result when the controlled medication is discontinued or the patient dies. These unused medications cannot be redispensed to other long-term care facility patients and must be destroyed. Under the federal Controlled Substances Act, controlled substances may be returned only between DEA registrants, that is, organizations that are registered with the DEA. Pharmacies are DEA registrants. Most long-term care facilities do not have their own pharmacies and are not DEA registrants; therefore, they are not permitted to return controlled substances to their contract pharmacy. This means that the long-term care facility must deal with the problem of unused controlled substances and their disposal in accordance with state and federal laws.

The DEA has no authority over the destruction or disposal of controlled substances in the long-term care facility because most long-term care facilities are not DEA registrants. It can only make recommendations. The first line of authority is the states. State regulations usually mandate who can conduct the disposal, who can witness the disposal, and what type of documentation is required. However, most states do not mandate how to perform the actual disposal. Traditionally, the destruction of controlled substances has been accomplished by flushing them into the sewer system. This method poses a threat to the environment. The Environmental Protection Agency (EPA) has enacted federal guidelines for the disposal of hazardous waste, which includes controlled substances, under the Resource Conservation and Recovery Act. State and local authorities have followed by implementing similar guidelines, and several states have enacted more stringent regulations. As a result, the flushing of controlled substances is no longer acceptable in most states. Furthermore, some controlled substances are classified as hazardous chemicals under the federal Occupational Safety and Health Administration's (OSHA) Hazard Communication Standard (HCS). These medications require special handling during their destruction to protect the employee and prevent accidental absorption (through the skin), inhalation, or ingestion. An alternative method of disposal for the long-term care facility is incineration. Incineration, either on-site at the facility or off-site at a commercial incinerator, is approved in most states.

It is easy to see that there is no simple answer to the problem of what a long-term care facility should do with unused controlled substances. Long-term care pharmacists often assist the long-term care facility in the destruction process as a service to the facility. However, long-term care pharmacists should consult federal DEA regulations; state environmental, occupational, and safety regulations; and state board of pharmacy regulations before getting involved in the destruction of controlled substances in the facility.

## USE OF AUTOMATED DISPENSING SYSTEMS IN LONG-TERM CARE FACILITIES

In 2005, the DEA amended regulations to allow a long-term care pharmacy to install and operate an automatic dispensing system or machine in a long-term care facility where state law permits. In states that do allow this practice, the pharmacy must register with the DEA to operate an automated dispensing system at the facility, along with proof of a state-issued permit for this activity. Currently, many states do not allow a long-term care pharmacy to operate an automated dispensing system in a long-term care facility. These states may in the future amend their pharmacy practice acts to allow this activity.

A long-term care pharmacy that services several long-term care facilities must have a separate registration for each facility in which it operates an automated dispensing system. Drugs stored in the automated dispensing system are considered to be part of the inventory of the long-term care pharmacy, and drugs dispensed from the system are considered to have been dispensed by the pharmacy. The operation of the automated dispensing system must be under the supervision of a licensed pharmacist. The pharmacist does not need to be physically present in the long-term care facility, but regulations require that the drug utilization review must be performed electronically by the pharmacist before the drug is dispensed.

This change in DEA regulations has the greatest impact on the dispensing of controlled substances to long-term care facility residents. It facilitates record keeping, decreases the ordering time, improves security, and reduces waste. The use of an automated dispensing system in the long-term care facility provides an alternative to address the problem of unused controlled substances and their disposal at the long-term care facility.

## EXPIRATION DATE LABELING OF MEDICATIONS

OBRA regulations require that medications that are packaged for use in the long-term care facility be labeled with an appropriate expiration date based on current accepted professional principles. According to CMS, this date is based on United States Pharmacopeial Convention (USP) standards for expiration dating (as well as packaging and temperature monitoring). For nonsterile solid and liquid dosage forms that are repackaged in unit-dose containers, the requirement is 1 year or the manufacturer's expiration date, whichever is sooner. According to CMS and the USP, modified unit-dose systems, such as punch cards, are considered to be unit-dose packages for the purpose of expiration dating. For multiple-dose containers, that is, traditional prescription vials, the requirement is 1 year from the date that the drug is dispensed or the manufacturer's expiration date, whichever is less. For multiple medication packages, which consist of two or more different solid oral dosage forms in the same package, the requirement is no longer than 60 days from the date of repackaging or the shortest manufacturer's expiration date of any of the medications in the package or the shortest recommended expiration date for any of the medications in the package. In addition, the long-term care pharmacist and the pharmacy technician must be aware of individual state laws concerning the expiration dating of medications.

New terminology is also being used. The term *beyond-use date* is being used rather than the term *expiration date*. The beyond-use date is considered to be a shorter date than an expiration date. It reflects the fact that the medication is no longer in the manufacturer's original package and therefore can be affected by factors such as temperature, humidity, and the type of medication packaging being used.

## RETURN AND REUSE OF MEDICATIONS FROM THE LONG-TERM CARE FACILITY

Millions of dollars of medications that are dispensed to residents in long-term care facilities are unused. Unused medications result from a change in therapy, the medication becoming outdated, or the resident's death or discharge from the facility. Under the appropriate circumstances, long-term care pharmacists can help to reduce waste and decrease health care costs through the return and reuse of medications.

In 2000, the FDA reversed a 20-year-old policy that prohibited the return and reuse of medications from hospitals and long-term care facilities and set standards for this practice. These standards include proper storage and handling, record keeping, and the integrity of returned medications. Since then, several states have passed laws that allow medications to be recovered from long-term facilities and to be dispensed again. Many of these regulations, however, do not clearly instruct the long-term care pharmacy on how to credit or adjust a claim for medications that have been returned.

In 2003, the American Society of Consultant Pharmacists (ASCP) updated its *Statement on the Return and Reuse of Medications in the Long-Term Care Facility*. This statement supports the return and reuse of medications under certain conditions. The American Medical Association (AMA) adopted an almost identical policy, and the two organizations have presented a united effort in developing and implementing solutions to this problem of medication waste.

The ASCP statement addresses the legitimate return and reuse of medications from the long-term care facility when federal and state laws and regulations (DEA regulations, EPA guidelines, OSHA standards, and USP standards) and the policies and procedures of the long-term care facility are met. In addition, specific safeguards for the medications and appropriate billing practices must be in place. ASCP supports the return and reuse of medications if:

- The returned medications are not controlled substances. Under the Controlled Substances Act, controlled substances can be returned only between DEA registrants. Long-term care facilities are not DEA registrants, and the long-term care pharmacy may not accept controlled substances from the facility.

- The medications are dispensed in tamper-evident packaging and returned with this packaging intact. Unit-dose and other types of packaging are acceptable for reuse as long as the seal is intact.

- The medications must meet all federal and state requirements for product integrity. This determination is made by the professional judgment of the long-term care pharmacist.

- Policies and procedures for the appropriate storage, transport, receipt, and security of the medications from the long-term care facility to the pharmacy are in place and are followed.

- A system is in place to track the reuse of medications. Tracking allows medications to be recalled if necessary. This system can take the form of a log of the returned medications, including the lot numbers and expiration dates.

- An electronic system is in place for billing a resident for only the number of doses used or for crediting the number of doses returned, regardless of the payer. The amount of credit issued should be the ingredient cost of the medication less pharmacy processing costs that reflect delivery and pickup of medications, repackaging, labor, record keeping, and overhead expenses.

Current USP regulations prohibit the return and reuse of medications in multiple medication packages. According to this regulation, once medications are packaged together, they may not be returned to stock and reused.

# PROVISION OF MATERIAL SAFETY DATA SHEETS TO THE LONG-TERM CARE FACILITY

The Occupational Safety and Health Administration (OSHA), through its Hazard Communication Standard (HCS), requires that a long-term care pharmacy provide a material safety data sheet (MSDS) for every hazardous chemical it delivers to the long-term care facility. The purpose is to protect the employees of the long-term care facility from exposure to these chemicals. The **material safety data sheet** is a document that provides detailed information on the hazards associated with a particular chemical substance. A **hazardous chemical** is a chemical substance that poses a threat to health or safety. There are two types of hazardous chemicals: chemicals that are physical hazards and chemicals that are health hazards. A physical hazard is a chemical that is combustible, flammable, explosive, or corrosive. A health hazard is a chemical that may cause acute or chronic health effects in an individual who has been exposed to it. A hazardous chemical can be a nondrug chemical, a compounding agent, or a drug. There are several nondrug chemicals and compounding agents that are considered hazardous and are found in the long-term care facility. These include camphor, iodine, isopropyl alcohol, menthol, and tincture of benzoin. They require an MSDS to be provided to the long-term care facility.

Many drugs are considered to be hazardous chemicals in their final, solid dosage forms (tablets, capsules, caplets, or gel caps) and especially when crushed or broken. They can cause sensitivities, irritation, cancer, malformations of a fetus, mutations, and other harmful effects. Examples of these are antibiotics, chemotherapy, potassium iodide, Propecia and Proscar (finasteride), Cytotec (misoprostol), and Zyrtec (cetirizine). Hazardous drugs can be identified from information provided on the package insert, *Physician's Desk Reference*, *American Hospital Formulary Service Drug Information*, and other references. These drugs require an MSDS to be provided to the long-term care facility. An example of an MSDS for a hazardous drug (Nolvadex [tamoxifen]) is found in Appendix B.

An MSDS is not required for nonhazardous drugs that are meant to be administered to the patient in a final solid dosage form. These are in a form that is not likely to result in exposure, even if they are crushed or broken just before administration. However, an MSDS is required for drugs that are meant to be crushed or broken before administration. These drugs are *not* in their final form and can result in exposure from inhalation. The long-term care pharmacy should provide an MSDS if it is aware that a drug will be used in this way.

Some drugs are hazardous only as a result of excessive handling, such as repackaging, in the long-term care pharmacy. They present a hazard only in the pharmacy, not in the long-term care facility. Therefore, an MSDS does not have to be sent to the facility. Pharmacy employees should take precautions, however, to minimize their exposure, such as using gloves, gowns, and masks when repackaging.

The source of the MSDS is the manufacturer of the chemical, who is responsible for developing the individual MSDS. The pharmacy receives the MSDS along with the chemical from the manufacturer or drug wholesaler. The pharmacy's legal responsibility is to deliver the MSDS to the long-term care facility. Many long-term care pharmacies, as a service, assist the long-term care facility by providing drug and hazardous chemical information, by helping to keep material safety data sheets filed and readily retrievable, and by providing overall assistance and education in case of an exposure.

## MEDICARE PRESCRIPTION DRUG BENEFIT

The Medicare Prescription Drug Benefit, or Medicare Part D, went into effect in 2006 as part of the Medicare Modernization Act (MMA) of 2003. It was the largest change in the Medicare program since it was created in 1965. Medicare Part D extends a prescription drug benefit to Medicare beneficiaries and is a voluntary program. Medicare Part D has presented a challenge to the Medicare beneficiary who resides in a long-term care facility, that is, the long-term care facility resident.

The long-term care facility resident is often sensitive to and intolerant of certain medications or has special medication needs and therefore requires access to a wide variety of medications. The limited formularies of some Medicare Part D prescription drug plans, with several excluded drug categories under these plans, such as weight loss and weight gain drugs, benzodiazepines, and over-the-counter drugs, offer less effective medications or medications with more side effects in the elderly. The appeals process for medications that are not covered is also a cause of concern, since the long-term care resident often needs immediate access to the medication and the appeals process may be lengthy. The CMS is addressing these specific long-term care issues.

The Medicare Prescription Drug Benefit also has several implications for the long-term care pharmacy. Any long-term care pharmacy may join any Medicare Part D plan as a provider if it meets certain criteria set forth by the CMS. The pharmacy must have a comprehensive inventory that includes drugs and dosage forms that are commonly used in a long-term care facility. It must be able to provide special drug distribution systems or packaging. The long-term care pharmacy must have a pharmacist on call 24 hours per day, 7 days per week. Finally, it must provide a delivery service, an emergency box, and forms and reports to the long-term care facility. As a result of these additional and distinct services provided by a long-term care pharmacy, the pharmacy will receive higher dispensing fees than a traditional community retail pharmacy under the Medicare Part D plans.

In addition to payment for prescription drugs, the Medicare Prescription Drug Benefit requires the creation and implementation of a medication therapy management (MTM) program for Medicare beneficiaries who meet certain criteria: they take multiple medications, have multiple chronic diseases, and have prescription drug costs that exceed a certain level. The purpose of MTM is to ensure positive outcomes of drug therapy. MTM is a pharmaceutical care service.

Medication therapy management as of this writing is in its formative stage. There are several models for MTM but no specific requirements. For example, pharmacists are the most effective health care professionals to provide MTM, but the law also allows other health care professionals to provide MTM services. The CMS is analyzing the early results of MTM and will release guidelines and additional requirements over the next several years.

In relation to long-term care pharmacy, medication therapy management is not meant to replace the OBRA-mandated drug regimen review as performed by a pharmacist. It is meant to be an additional set of clinical services. Again, final MTM regulations for long-term care pharmacy have yet to be finalized.

## STATE REGULATION OF LONG-TERM CARE PHARMACY

The dispensing and consulting services of a long-term care pharmacy are also regulated by the individual states. A long-term care pharmacy is licensed by its respective state board of pharmacy. It is usually licensed as a "retail" pharmacy because most states do not have a separate license category for long-term care pharmacies. The long-term care pharmacy must comply with all state as well as federal regulations. Some states require that a consultant pharmacist hold a special license to consult in addition to the traditional pharmacy license. Some states also have anti-kickback regulations of their own that parallel the federal anti-kickback regulations.

## JOINT COMMISSION STANDARDS FOR LONG-TERM CARE PHARMACY

The Joint Commission is an independent, not-for-profit organization dedicated to improving the quality of care in health care organizations. Originally formed to accredit hospitals, the Joint Commission has been accrediting long-term care pharmacies since 1996. The Joint Commission is currently the only organization that accredits these pharmacies.

The Joint Commission accreditation for the long-term care pharmacy is voluntary and not legally required. Therefore, the Joint Commission standards are considered to be quasi-legal standards. Accreditation is sought by the long-term care pharmacy itself, the long-term care facilities that it serves, managed care plans, and third-party prescription plans as a sign of the pharmacy's dedication to quality service. The Joint Commission accredits long-term care pharmacies because it considers them to be a critical field in health care, and it has recognized the importance of pharmaceutical care as well as dispensing services in long-term care.

Long-term care pharmacy accreditation is not intended for individual pharmacists. It applies to any organization that provides pharmaceutical care and pharmacy services to residents in a long-term care facility. The pharmacy organization is visited by surveyors who are themselves pharmacists with at least 5 years of long-term care pharmacy experience and who have specialized training in accrediting long-term care pharmacies. The survey includes a tour of the pharmacy, interviews with the pharmacy staff, examination of the pharmacy's records, interviews with the staff and residents of the long-term care facilities that the pharmacy serves, and briefings. The goals of the survey are to identify and correct problems and to improve the quality of services.

The basis for the survey is standards, which are the criteria for judging performance. These standards are customized to long-term care pharmacies and can be divided into patient-centered functions and pharmacy organization functions. Patient-centered functions are related to the provision of pharmaceutical care and pharmacy services to the long-term care resident and staff: for example, the drug regimen review or pharmacy education for staff members. Pharmacy organization standards are related to activities that are necessary for the long-term care pharmacy to be able to provide quality pharmaceutical care and pharmacy services: for example, adequate staff training or infection control procedures in the pharmacy. In short, the long-term care pharmacy is judged in areas that prove its commitment to providing the best service and achieving improved outcomes for its long-term care facility residents.

The Joint Commission has mandated new standards for pain assessment and management in long-term care. These standards discuss the multidisciplinary aspect of pain assessment and management and specifically discuss the role of the pharmacist in pain management. The long-term care pharmacy must be aware of these standards and attempt to improve pain management in the long-term care facility through its consultant services.

## KEY CONCEPTS

- Several organizations such as the Centers for Medicare and Medicaid Services, the Occupational Safety and Health Administration, the Drug Enforcement Administration, and the Joint Commission regulate long-term care pharmacy through extensive legislation, regulations, and standards.

- The federally required drug regimen review performed by a pharmacist was the beginning of consultant pharmacy practice.

- Standards called indicators have been developed to ensure the performance of an adequate drug regimen review.

- OBRA 87 regulations have made pharmacists responsible for all aspects of medication use in the long-term care facility.

- Freedom of choice legislation as it pertains to long-term care pharmacy includes both the patient's right to choose an outside pharmacy and the nursing facility's right to establish medication use policies and to enforce their compliance.

- Anti-kickback legislation and the development of safe harbors protect legitimate long-term care pharmacy practices.

- Current DEA regulations that pertain to long-term care pharmacy deal with the transmission of Schedule II prescriptions by facsimile, the partial filling of Schedule II prescriptions, the destruction of controlled substances in the long-term care facility, and the use of automated dispensing systems in the long-term care facility.

- Drugs packaged for use in a long-term care facility must bear an expiration date based on current accepted professional principles.

- Unused medications in a long-term care facility can be returned to the long-term care pharmacy and reused under certain conditions.
- A long-term care pharmacy must provide an MSDS for any hazardous chemical that it delivers to a long-term care facility.
- The Medicare Prescription Drug Benefit has several implications for long-term care pharmacy.
- Long-term care pharmacies are licensed and regulated by state boards of pharmacy.
- The Joint Commission accreditation is available for long-term care pharmacies; it is voluntary but sought by long-term care pharmacies as a sign of quality service.

## SELF-ASSESSMENT QUESTIONS

### MULTIPLE CHOICE

1. The regulatory organizations that affect long-term care pharmacy include all of the following except:
   a. OBRA
   b. OSHA
   c. the Joint Commission
   d. CMS

2. Which statement is correct concerning the consultant pharmacist's performance of the drug regimen review?
   a. the pharmacist must report any irregularities
   b. the pharmacist must perform the drug regimen review monthly
   c. no more than 100 reviews should be performed in a day
   d. all of the above

3. An unnecessary drug is a drug given:
   a. in an excessive dose
   b. for an excessive period of time
   c. without reason
   d. all of the above

4. All of the following are examples of medication errors in the long-term care facility except:
   a. omitted dose
   b. wrong drug
   c. wrong dose
   d. wrong place

5. An example of a nonhazardous chemical found in a long-term care facility is:
   a. iodine
   b. isopropyl alcohol
   c. tincture of benzoin
   d. normal saline irrigation

6. An area of responsibility for the pharmacist that is not required under OBRA is:

   a. the administration of drugs
   b. the use of antipsychotic drugs
   c. dose reductions for antipsychotic drugs
   d. the provision of consultant services

7. Long-term care pharmacy accreditation by the Joint Commission involves all of the following except:

   a. interviews with long-term care facility residents and staff
   b. a tour of the pharmacy
   c. interviews with the long-term care pharmacy staff
   d. an optional survey

8. An example of a safe harbor in a long-term care pharmacy practice is:

   a. a facsimile machine supplied to the facility for any use
   b. consultant pharmacist services at no cost to the facility
   c. renting medication carts to the facility at fair market value
   d. using space in the facility for pharmacy activities at no charge

9. All of the following statements regarding the facsimile transmission of Schedule II prescriptions in the long-term care pharmacy are true except:

   a. the fascimile copy does not have to be retained
   b. the fascimile copy is considered to be the original prescription
   c. the fascimile copy must include the physician's signature
   d. a prescription for any type of Schedule II medication can be transmitted through a facsimile machine

10. Conditions for the partial filling of a Schedule II prescription for a long-term care resident include:

    a. the notation of "long-term care facility patient" on the prescription
    b. the total quantity of medication cannot exceed the original quantity
    c. the date of each refill and the quantity must be recorded
    d. all of the above

## TRUE/FALSE (CORRECT THE FALSE STATEMENTS)

1. _____ The Joint Commission will accredit a long-term care pharmacist.
2. _____ Antipsychotic drugs should be used only if a long-term care resident has a specific condition that justifies the use of these drugs.
3. _____ A long-term care resident may administer her own drugs if it is determined that it is safe.
4. _____ Current DEA regulations permit controlled substances to be returned to a pharmacy by a long-term care facility.
5. _____ A MSDS must be provided to the long-term care facility by the pharmacy for any hazardous chemicals sent.
6. _____ A kickback is an attempt to induce referral business.
7. _____ A medication error is a discrepancy between what the physician ordered and what was administered to the resident.

8. _____ A long-term care resident has the right to be free of physical and chemical restraints.
9. _____ OBRA regulations made extensive revisions to the Medicare and Medicaid Conditions of Participation for long-term care facilities.
10. _____ All medications in the long-term care facility must be stored in locked compartments.

## FILL-IN

1. The drug regimen review is mandated under _____ regulations.
2. A _____ _____ is a long-term care pharmacy practice that can be done without fear of prosecution.
3. Partial prescriptions for Schedule II medications for long-term care residents can be refilled for up to _____ days.
4. A _____ _____ refers to discontinuing a drug to test the need for its continued use.
5. The _____ sets standards for expiration dating of medications.
6. The average number of medications per resident in a long-term care facility is _____.
7. A potential drug therapy problem is referred to as an _____.
8. P.R.N. antipsychotic medications should not be used more than _____ times per week.
9. The Joint Commission's basis for the survey and assessment of a long-term care pharmacy is _____.
10. Antipsychotic drugs are referred to as _____ restraints.

## CRITICAL THINKING

1. Compare and contrast the DEA final rule for the transmission of a Schedule II controlled substance prescription by facsimile in a long-term care pharmacy with that in a traditional community retail pharmacy.
2. What legal and ethical responsibility does a pharmacy technician have in regard to the safe harbor regulations? What should a pharmacy technician do if he observes questionable pharmacy practices that may violate these regulations?
3. Select six *apparent irregularities* as found in Appendix A, and give a specific example of each.
4. Select three cases in which an *unnecessary drug* may be given, and give a specific example of each.
5. Select three types of medication errors that may be found in a long-term care facility, and give a specific example of each.

## BIBLIOGRAPHY

Abood, R., & Brushwood, D. (2004). *Pharmacy practice and the law* (3rd ed.). Gaithersburg, MD: Aspen Publishers, Inc.

American Society of Consultant Pharmacists. (2003). *ASCP statement on the return and reuse of medications in long-term care facilities.* [On-line] ASCP. Available: www.ascp.com.

American Society of Consultant Pharmacists. (2004). *The consultant pharmacist guide to nursing facility regulations and the survey process.* Arlington, VA: Author.

Barry, D. (2006). Entering the e-prescribing era. *Pharmacy Today, 12*(1), 16.

Bishop, S. (2005). E-prescribing standards: First set proposed. *Pharmacy Today, 11*(4), 23–24.

Centers for Medicare and Medicaid Services. (2006). *Conditions of participation and conditions for coverage: Skilled nursing facilities.* [On-line] CMS. Available: www.cms.gov.

Centers for Medicare and Medicaid Services. (2006). *Prescription drug coverage.* [On-line] CMS. Available: www.cms.gov.

Clark, T. (Ed.). (2004). *ASCP policies, standards and guidelines—2004* (5th ed.). Arlington, VA: ASCP.

Coster, J. (2005). The Medicare Modernization Act, Part 1. *U.S. Pharmacist, 30*(7), 39–46.

Coster, J. (2005). The Medicare Modernization Act, Part 2. *U.S. Pharmacist, 30*(8), 47–50.

Crutchfield, D. (2004). Potentially inappropriate drugs. *Geriatric Times, 5*(4), 31–32.

Department of Health and Human Services. (2005). *Safe harbor regulations and preambles.* [On-line] Department of Health and Human Services, Office of the Inspector General. Available: www.dhhs.gov.

Foxhall, K. (2005). CMS warns that MTM will take time to set up. *Drug Topics, 149*(23), 12.

Gebhart, F. (2005). Long-term care pharmacies unhappy with Part D limits. *Drug Topics, 149*(22), 12.

Gebhart, F. (2005). Medication recycling: New patients for old pills. *Drug Topics, 149*(18), 37.

Goldfarb, N., & Maio, V. (2004). Ensure appropriate pharmacotherapy for long-term care. *Caring for the Ages, 5*(12), 1, 72, 75.

Hunter, T., Droege, M., Marsh, W., & Droege, W. (2005). Effectively managing pharmaceutical returns and waste. *Drug Topics, 149*(2), 36–45.

Joint Commission on Accreditation of Healthcare Organizations. (2006). *2006–2007 Comprehensive accreditation manual for home care.* Oakbrook Terrace, IL: Author.

Joint Commission on Accreditation of Healthcare Organizations. (2006). *2006–2007 Standards manual for pharmacy dispensing, clinical/consultant pharmacist, long-term care pharmacy, and freestanding ambulatory infusion services.* Oakbrook Terrace, IL: Author.

Kaiser Family Foundation. (2005). *The effect of formularies and other cost management tools on access to medications: An analysis of the MMA and proposed regulations.* [On-line] KFF. Available: www.kff.org.

Kaiser Family Foundation. (2005). *Issues for Medicare beneficiaries in long-term care settings: An analysis of the MMA and proposed regulations.* [On-line] KFF. Available: www.kff.org.

Lipowski, E. (2006). Medicare Part D for patients with special needs. *Drug Topics, 150*(15), 18.

McMahan, R. (2006). Demystifying medication therapy management. *Drug Topics, 150*(1), 39–48.

Palley, S. (2005). Pain research specific to long-term care. *Caring for the Ages, 6*(5), 16, 21–22.

Pettey, S. (2005). MMA to influence LTC prescribing practices. *Caring for the Ages, 6*(1), 12–14, 17–18.

Sipkoff, M. (2004). Idaho offers incentive to spur resale of returned drugs. *Drug Topics, 148*(22), 47.

Terrie, Y. (2004). Understanding and managing polypharmacy in the elderly. *Pharmacy Times, 7*(12), 84–85.

United States Department of Justice. Drug Enforcement Administration. (2005), *Code of Federal Regulations Title 21, Sections 1300, 1301, 1304, 1307—Preventing the accumulation of surplus controlled substances at long-term care facilities.* [On-line] U.S. Department of Justice. Available:www.dea.gov.

United States Department of Justice. Drug Enforcement Administration. (2005). *Code of Federal Regulations Title 21, Section 1306—Pharmacy.* [On-line] U.S. Department of Justice. Available: www.dea.gov.

United States Department of Labor. Occupational Safety and Health Administration. (2006). *Hazard Communication Standards.* [On-line] U.S. Department of Labor. Available: www.osha.gov.

United States Environmental Protection Agency. (2006). *Hazardous waste.* [On-line] EPA. Available: www.epa.gov.

United States Pharmacopeial Convention. (2006). *The United States pharmacopeia* (29th ed.) and *The national formulary* (24th ed.). Rockville, MD: Author.

Vivian, J. (2006). Federal anti-kickback laws. *U.S. Pharmacist, 31*(5), 72–76.

Wyeth, J., & Kozak, D. (2005). Laying the cornerstone for Medicare Part D. *Drug Topics, 149*(16), 37–46.

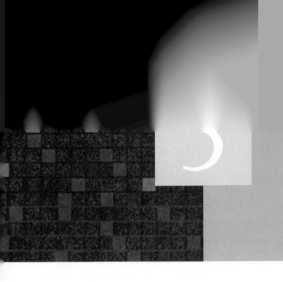

# Pharmacist and the Pharmacy Technician in Long-Term Care

## Learning Objectives

Upon completion of this chapter, the student should be able to:

- Explain consultant pharmacy practice.
- Understand the difference between consultant services and provider services.
- Define *consultant pharmacist*.
- Describe the different services of a consultant pharmacist.
- Understand the drug regimen review and its importance.
- Discuss the importance of the pharmaceutical care plan.
- Describe the purpose of a medication pass observation.
- Summarize consultant pharmacist activities in alternative long-term care settings.
- Discuss the pharmacy technician's role in long-term care pharmacy.

## Key Terms

care plan

consultant pharmacist

consultant pharmacy practice

drug regimen review

medication pass observation

pharmaceutical care plan

## Introduction

The long-term care pharmacist has a tremendous ability to affect resident outcomes in the long-term care facility. Pharmacists have been recognized as drug therapy experts through federally mandated, pharmacist-performed drug regimen review. Today, pharmacists oversee all aspects of medication use in the long-term care facility. An alternative area of pharmacy practice has evolved as a result. Consultant pharmacy practice involves the provision of pharmaceutical care services to long-term care facility residents by a consultant pharmacist. Consultant pharmacists provide many types of services to residents in nursing homes and in

many other different types of long-term care settings. Likewise, pharmacy technicians in long-term care perform many activities, both in the long-term care pharmacy and in the long-term care facility. This chapter focuses on the unique roles
of the consultant pharmacist and the pharmacy technician in long-term care. ■

## OVERVIEW OF CONSULTANT PHARMACY PRACTICE

The role of the consultant pharmacist in long-term care had its beginnings during the 1960s when the Medicare and Medicaid programs established standards
for pharmacy services. There were some pharmacists at that time who recognized
medication misuse in long-term care facilities and who tried to correct it. But it
was not until 1974 that federal regulations required that a pharmacist evaluate
the drug regimens of long-term care residents at least monthly and report any
irregularities to the director of nursing, attending physician, or both. Major nursing home legislation, in the form of OBRA 87 and its revisions, expanded the role
of the consultant pharmacist beyond drug regimen review. Today, the consultant
pharmacist is required to oversee all aspects of drug use in the long-term care facility. The role of the pharmacist in long-term care has developed into an alternative area of pharmacy known as consultant pharmacy. **Consultant pharmacy
practice** can be defined as the practice of pharmacy in which pharmacists provide pharmaceutical care services to achieve definite outcomes of drug therapy
and to improve the quality of life for the long-term care resident. In pharmacy, as
in any other health care area, there has been a shift from merely providing services to meeting the unique needs of the patient. Consultant pharmacy or consultant services are separate from, but complementary to, dispensing pharmacy, also
referred to as provider services. The two are not the same. Dispensing services are
performed in any pharmacy that serves long-term care residents. They focus on
the dispensing of medications and drug delivery systems. In addition to dispensing, they involve all other related pharmacy services, such as ordering, delivery,
storage, handling, and medication disposal. Dispensing services involve all pharmacy personnel. Consultant services, on the other hand, are usually performed
in the long-term care facility, not in the long-term care pharmacy. They focus on
pharmaceutical care and involve clinical activities. They are performed only by
the consultant pharmacist. Consultant services have been recognized as different
and separate from provider services, with separate contracts and fees.

Consultant services and provider services can be provided by the same long-
term care pharmacy or pharmacist, or they can be provided by a different long-term
care pharmacy or pharmacist. There is debate as to whether the two services
should be provided by the same or different pharmacy organizations. Services
provided by the same organization can lead to conflict of interest situations. For
example, the consultant pharmacist can make recommendations that generate
increased prescription revenues for the pharmacy. These combined services can
also lead to discounting or bundling of services. One advantage is that there can
be better communication between the dispensing and consulting pharmacists.
Services provided by different organizations eliminate conflict of interest situations and result in adequate fees for consulting services. However, communication problems can occur between two different organizations.

## THE CONSULTANT PHARMACIST

There is no doubt as to the separation of the consultant role from the provider role in long-term care pharmacy. The consultant pharmacist has emerged as a drug distribution and information expert, a problem solver, and a patient advocate. In the United States, there are over 10,000 consultant pharmacists, and the demand is expected to grow as the number of elderly persons needing long-term care increases.

A **consultant pharmacist** is defined as a pharmacist who is specially trained to provide pharmaceutical care services to long-term care facility residents. The training is obtained through post-graduate residencies, clinical rotations, and certificate and continuing education programs. The consultant pharmacist has knowledge concerning the long-term care environment, the aging population and their special medication needs, federal and state laws and regulations that pertain to long-term care, and specialized drug distribution systems. A consultant pharmacist may be board certified in geriatrics. The Commission for Certification in Geriatric Pharmacy (CCGP) has established a voluntary certification program for geriatric pharmacy practice, leading to a Certified Geriatric Pharmacist (CGP) designation.

Consultant pharmacists practice in a wide variety of long-term care settings, including nursing homes, subacute care units, psychiatric hospitals, correctional facilities, assisted living facilities, board and care homes, home infusion organizations, hospice organizations, senior centers, and others. The consultant pharmacist can be employed by a long-term care pharmacy organization or can be self-employed and practice as an independent consultant.

## CONSULTANT PHARMACIST SERVICES

Consultant pharmacists provide a wide range of services. These services help improve outcomes and improve the quality of life for long-term care facility residents. These services are collectively referred to as pharmaceutical care services. Pharmaceutical care services can be divided into several different areas: education, medication systems management, and clinical.

### EDUCATIONAL ACTIVITIES

Consultant pharmacists engage in a variety of educational activities in the long-term care facility. The educational role is a highly visible role and one that brings respect and credibility to the consultant pharmacist. There are several educational services offered by consultant pharmacists.

- Nursing education—in the form of in-service programs. In-services are presentations on pertinent topics to the nursing staff. These can include, for example, particular disease states, new medications, medication administration, federal regulations, adverse drug reactions, and policies and procedures. They are usually tailored to meet the particular needs of the staff.

- Interdisciplinary team education—in the form of important information given to team members, primarily at team meetings held within the facility, or on an individual basis when needed. An example would be the consultant pharmacist's making a recommendation to the dietician concerning a potential food-drug interaction.

- Physician education—in the form of recommendations made as a result of the drug regimen review or personal communication by phone or at meetings and conferences. This activity helps build relationships and increases the pharmacist's credibility with the physician. An example would be a consultant pharmacist's informing a physician about a new drug on the market that could benefit one of the patients.

- Resident education—in the form of direct resident counseling and the use of educational materials. The consultant pharmacist often extends this education to the resident's family and into the community. There are many areas of education. Examples include the patient's drug therapy, medication compliance, side effects, disease prevention, health promotion, admission interviews in the facility, and discharge counseling on discharge from the facility.

- Drug information—in the form of research and personal response to any drug information request.

- Written communication—in the form of newsletters to residents and staff; also monthly and quarterly reports.

- Miscellaneous educational activities—in the form of legislative involvement; educating the public about consulting pharmacy through television, radio, or publishing; and involvement in professional associations and colleges of pharmacy.

## MEDICATION SYSTEMS MANAGEMENT ACTIVITIES

The consultant pharmacist engages in several medication systems management activities that result in high-quality pharmacy services and help the facility comply with federal and state regulations. These activities include the following:

- *Drug distribution systems.* The consultant pharmacist assists the long-term care facility in developing and implementing a drug distribution system that meets its needs and helps educate the staff on all aspects of its use.

- *Medication storage.* The consultant pharmacist assists the facility in the appropriate and secure storage of medications in the facility through the provision of medication and treatment carts, medication room and nursing station inspections, and education of the staff.

- *Emergency medications.* The consultant pharmacist assists the facility in maintaining an appropriate supply of emergency medications in the facility and in developing policies and procedures for their use.

- *Drug product selection.* The consultant pharmacist helps select drug products for use in the facility on the basis of quality as well as cost-effectiveness.

- *Drug formulary.* The consultant pharmacist assists the facility in developing and maintaining a formulary specific to the needs of its residents.

- *Policies and procedures.* The consultant pharmacist assists the facility in developing and revising policies and procedures for medication use in the facility, such as policies and procedures for procuring medications, storing medications, prescribing and ordering medications, administering medications, documenting medication activity, and disposing of medications. Policies and procedures provide uniform standards for medication use in the facility and also serve as a teaching and evaluation tool.

- *Controlled substances.* The consultant pharmacist assists the facility in maintaining accountability for controlled substances, including their acquisition, storage, administration, and record keeping.

- *Medication administration.* The consultant pharmacist assists the facility in ensuring accurate and appropriate medication administration to residents through medication pass observation, review of the medication administration record during drug regimen review, and staff education.

- *Medication errors.* The consultant pharmacist assists the facility in ensuring that it is free of significant medication errors and in calculating its medication error rate by helping to develop a system for detecting, reporting, and reviewing medication errors in the facility and by the correct use of the facility's drug distribution system.

- *Information technology.* The consultant pharmacist assists the facility in implementing and using the latest information technology, such as personal digital assistants and laptop and desktop computers.

## CLINICAL ACTIVITIES

The consultant pharmacist offers a wide variety of clinical services, also referred to as cognitive services. The drug regimen review is the most important clinical service, but it is only one of many clinical services provided. These clinical activities include the following:

- *Pharmaceutical care plan.* The consultant pharmacist develops, implements, and monitors a pharmaceutical care plan that is part of the resident's overall care plan.

- *Participation on committees.* The consultant pharmacist, as an important member of the long-term care interdisciplinary team, participates on several committees in the long-term care facility. These committees include the pharmacy services or pharmacy and therapeutics committee, quality assurance committee, infection control committee, care planning committee, utilization review committee, and restraint committee.

- *Disease management.* The consultant pharmacist assists the facility in developing disease management programs and protocols to improve care in certain disease states.

- *Nutrition monitoring.* The consultant pharmacist assists the dietician in monitoring the resident's nutritional status in addition to providing information on food-drug interactions or medications that can affect appetite.

- *Pain management.* The consultant pharmacist assists the facility in assessing and treating pain in residents, especially residents nearing the end of life, through pain medication therapy recommendations and education of the staff and other health care professionals.

- *Pharmacokinetic dosing.* The consultant pharmacist uses pharmacokinetics to determine the appropriate dosages and frequency of certain medications such as aminoglycoside antibiotics.

- *Noncompliance.* The consultant pharmacist assists the facility in trying to eliminate medication noncompliance by its residents by determining the reasons for noncompliance and making recommendations.
- *Laboratory test monitoring.* The consultant pharmacist evaluates and, in some states, orders laboratory tests to monitor drug therapy and to make recommendations based on the results of these tests.
- *Monitoring outcomes.* The consultant pharmacist develops ways to monitor the outcomes of his recommendations for changes in the resident's medication regimen.
- *Drug therapy protocols.* The consultant pharmacist assists the facility in developing protocols for the safe and effective use of certain drug therapies that are highly toxic or can cause adverse drug reactions.
- *Participation in the survey process.* The consultant pharmacist assists the long-term care facility during its survey process by being present to answer surveyor questions regarding pharmacy services in the facility or to provide other information.
- *Psychotropic drug monitoring.* The consultant pharmacist assists the facility in monitoring behaviors and adverse drug reactions to psychotropic drugs in order to support the appropriate use of these drugs.
- *Research activities.* The consultant pharmacist assists the facility in improving its services by participating in research projects in areas that are related to falls, hip fractures, osteoporosis, Alzheimer's disease, and Parkinson's disease.

## DRUG REGIMEN REVIEW

The **drug regimen review** has been defined as the process of reviewing all of a resident's medications and corresponding medical information, formulating a clinical recommendation, and communicating that recommendation. It has been performed by consultant pharmacists for over 30 years now. It is the most important and time-consuming duty of a consultant pharmacist. Federal regulations require that a drug regimen review be performed for each resident at least monthly in a long-term care facility (and at least quarterly in an intermediate-care facility for the mentally retarded). In addition, the interpretive guidelines state that more frequent reviews may be necessary, depending on the needs of the resident, the medications the resident is taking, or the contract that exists between the consultant pharmacist and the facility. For example, more frequent reviews are required in subacute care units, transitional care units, and inpatient hospice facilities due to the short patient stays and more frequent patient turnaround.

The drug regimen review is a systematic process of review to assess a resident's medication therapy and make recommendations concerning that therapy. It is often referred to as a *chart review*. The drug regimen review has several characteristics. It is individual; that is, it is performed specifically for each individual resident. It is all-inclusive, taking into account all aspects of a resident's care, not just his drug therapy. It is continuous; that is, it is part of an ongoing process that takes place month after month. It is interdisciplinary, using information regarding the resident's care from other members of the long-term care interdisciplinary team. Finally, it is organized; that is, it proceeds in a systematic manner based on the personal method of the consultant pharmacist.

There are three types of drug regimen reviews. A *general review* is a drug regimen review that involves an overview of an individual resident's medication therapy to ensure appropriate medication use and to look for any medication use problems. A *focused review* is a drug regimen review that concentrates on a specific medication, medication class, medication problem, or medical problem within the entire long-term care facility. An example would be a drug regimen review focused on all residents with a diagnosis of diabetes or on all residents taking hyperglycemic medications. A *problem-centered review* is a drug regimen review that concentrates on a resident's particular medical problem and its medication therapy. It is a combination of a general review and a focused review. An example would be a drug regimen review focused on a resident's diagnosis of diabetes and a plan of therapy for that problem only. The type of drug regimen review performed is determined by the consultant pharmacist, taking into consideration the needs of the resident or the facility. Regardless of the type of review that is performed, all drug regimen reviews have the same goal: to improve the resident's health outcomes and quality of life through the best possible medication use.

The performance of the drug regimen review involves several steps. Information is collected from a variety of sources, such as the physician order form, the medication administration record, the treatment administration record, physician progress notes, nurse's progress notes, laboratory reports, and patient interviews. This information is then evaluated by the pharmacist. The consultant pharmacist uses the federal guidelines or indicators when performing the review. These indicators are meant to be minimum standards and serve as only the basis for a thorough drug regimen review. Finally, the consultant pharmacist documents and communicates his findings and makes recommendations for changes. There are several different types of forms that the consultant pharmacist may use in performing the drug regimen review and reporting his findings. Examples of these are found in Figures 5–1 and 5–2.

The goal of the drug regimen review is appropriate medication use. Table 5–1 gives examples of inappropriate medication use discovered during the performance of a drug regimen review.

There are also specific drugs that are frequently involved in drug regimen review irregularities and recommendations. These drugs have a narrow therapeutic range; they require frequent laboratory monitoring; or they have a high potential for drug interactions or adverse drug reactions. These drugs are listed in Box 5–1.

The drug regimen review has been shown to reduce medication errors; decrease drug-related problems, especially adverse drug reactions; decrease overall medication use; and decrease hospitalizations. It has been shown to have a positive effect on patient outcomes, and it has resulted in decreased health care costs. These are all reasons that the need for drug regimen review is being recognized in other long-term care settings, community and home-based, as well as other institutional-based long-term care settings.

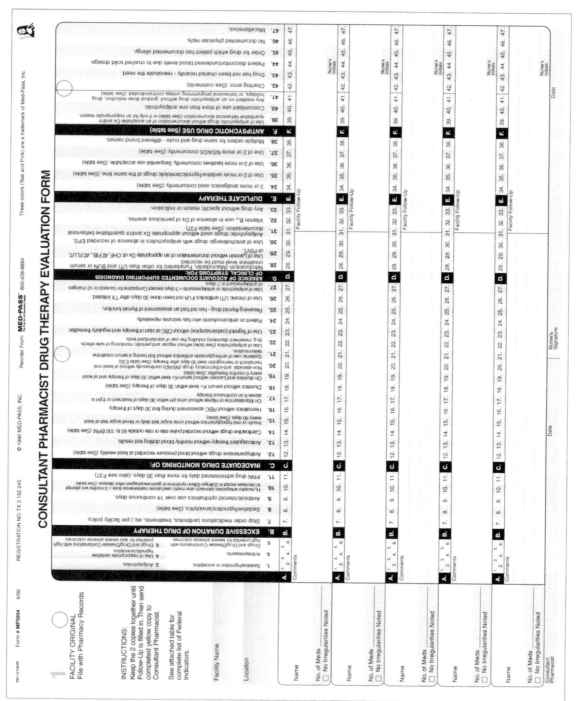

**FIGURE 5-1** Consultant Pharmacist Drug Therapy Evaluation Form. (Courtesy of MED-PASS, Inc.)

## DRUG REGIMEN REVIEW RECOMMENDATIONS TO PHYSICIANS

Resident Name _____

Facility Name _____

Month / Year _____

No. of Meds. _____

PHYSICIAN NAME: _____

FINDINGS: _____

_____

_____

_____

_____

_____

RECOMMENDATION: _____

_____

_____

_____

_____

_____

_____         _____

Consultant Pharmacist                              Date

PHYSICIAN RESPONSES: _____

_____

_____

_____

_____

_____

_____

_____

_____

_____         _____

Physician                                             Date

WHITE COPY: SEND TO PHYSICIAN          YELLOW COPY: CONSULTANT

**FIGURE 5–2**   Drug Regimen Review Recommendations to Physicians.

**TABLE 5–1**   Examples of Inappropriate Drug Use Discovered During a Drug Regimen Review

| REGIMEN REVIEW FINDING | CONSULTANT PHARMACIST DRUG RECOMMENDATION |
| --- | --- |
| Medication no longer necessary Example: Antibiotic continued after infection cleared | Discontinue medication |
| Duplicate medications Example: Two stimulant laxatives prescribed | Discontinue one medication |
| Drug allergy Example: NSAID administered to patient with aspirin allergy | Discontinue medication and switch to alternative medication |
| Use of drug without a reason Example: H2-receptor antagonist prescribed without supporting diagnosis | Ask physician to evaluate the need for the drug |
| Use of drug without adequate monitoring: Example: Anticoagulant medication prescribed without monthly blood clotting function test | Ask physician to order the appropriate laboratory tests |

**BOX 5–1    Drugs Frequently Involved in Drug Regimen Review Irregularities**

Coumadin (warfarin)
Synthroid (levothyroxine)
Digoxin
Dilantin (phenytoin)
Theophylline
Prednisone
Potassium
Lasix (furosemide)
Lithium
Steroid eye medications
NSAIDs

# PHARMACEUTICAL CARE PLAN

Care planning is defined as the process that uses information about a long-term care resident to form an individual plan of care for that resident. The purpose of care planning is to address each resident's medical, nursing, mental, and social needs and try to meet those needs. The **care plan** is defined as a plan that identifies a resident's problems being treated and the strategies for treatment. It sets goals or outcomes to work toward for each problem. The care plan is developed for each resident by the long-term care interdisciplinary team, including the consultant pharmacist, with input from the resident and his family. The care plan addresses the medications prescribed for each resident and their intended outcomes. In order to achieve the best possible outcomes from medication therapies, the consultant pharmacist develops a pharmaceutical care plan. The **pharmaceutical care plan**, also called a drug therapy plan of care, is a part of the overall care plan that sets goals for each medication prescribed for a resident. For example, if an antibiotic were prescribed for a urinary tract infection, the consultant pharmacist would set the goal for this medication as clearing of the infection. The pharmacist also monitors the plan to determine if goals are being met or if any drug-related problems occur. The consultant pharmacist is knowledgeable about medication therapy and is the most appropriate health care professional to make recommendations regarding this therapy and to develop the pharmaceutical care plan. An example of a form that assists the pharmacist in developing a drug therapy plan of care is shown in Figure 5–3.

## MEDICATION THERAPY MANAGEMENT

Medication therapy management (MTM) as mandated by the Medicare Modernization Act of 2003 in conjunction with the Medicare Part D Prescription Drug Benefit must be performed for long-term care residents who meet the criteria for this service. It is another set of clinical services in addition to the federally mandated drug regimen review and should be the responsibility of the consultant pharmacist, who is the drug therapy expert for the long-term care resident. Although standards for this service are not fully developed, medication therapy management in the facility may take several forms: a supplemental consultant review to reduce drug costs for these patients by looking at brand and generic drug use; a study of the incidence of falls in these residents; or a collaboration between the consultant pharmacist and the physician in establishing potential drug problem "alerts," for example, an alert concerning the length of therapy of certain drugs. The addition of MTM services to the drug regimen review will be shown to produce more positive outcomes for drug therapy in these residents and possibly a decrease in the number of medications and their costs.

## MEDICATION PASS OBSERVATION

According to CMS regulations, the long-term care facility must provide pharmaceutical services, including procedures that ensure the accurate administration of medications. Proper medication administration is critical for a medication to reach its maximum effectiveness. Part of the survey process for a long-term care facility is the observation by a surveyor of medication administration to residents by the nursing staff. The consultant pharmacist, in providing consultation on all aspects of pharmacy services in the facility, also observes the medication administration process in what is referred to as a **medication pass observation,** also called a med-pass observation. The goal of the med-pass observation is to ensure that medications are being administered in an

## DRUG THERAPY PLAN OF CARE

**CARE PLAN REVIEW focuses on:**

- Appropriate diagnosis/goal of therapy present
- Evaluation of use of non-drug approach where possible
- Drug, dose, frequency, & route appropriate to this resident
- Evaluation of presence of potential side effects or possibility of drug/drug or drug/food interactions
- Effectiveness of therapy
- Discontinuance of medications no longer in use

| Review Date | Initials | Signature of Reviewer | Review Date | Initials | Signature of Reviewer | Review Date | Initials | Signature of Reviewer |
|---|---|---|---|---|---|---|---|---|
| | | | | | | | | |

**ROUTE of ADMINISTRATION**
☐ No limitations
☐ Limitations due to: ______
☐ Crush pills, open caps ☐ Liquid meds
☐ IM
☐ ______
☐ See POC problem # ______
☐ ______

**SELF-ADMINISTRATION of MEDS:**
I.D.T. review date: ______
I.D.T. determined
☐ ABLE to self-administer meds responsibly
☐ UNABLE to self-administer meds responsibly due to:
☐ Cognitive status (POC problem # ______ )
☐ Physical factors (POC problem # ______ )
☐ Visual ability (POC problem # ______ )
Resident ☐ does ☐ does not wish to self-administer meds

**DRUG HOLIDAY**
☐ No
☐ Yes (Specify med & orders for Holiday)

**PSYCHOACTIVE PROTOCOL**
☐ Does not apply to this resident
☐ Protocol initiated, date: ______
See Psychoactive Drug Assessment and Behavior & Side Effects Monitoring Records for Specific Information
☐ Protocol discontinued, date: ______

| Date Ordered | Date D/C | Drug Order (Name, Dose, Frequency) | Reason Ordered or Goal of Therapy | Potential Side Effects | Monitoring Parameters | Initial |
|---|---|---|---|---|---|---|
| | | | | | | |

| Initial | Signature | Initial | Signature | Initial | Signature |
|---|---|---|---|---|---|
| | | | | | |
| | | | | | |
| | | | | | |

| Physician | Facility | | Allergy |
|---|---|---|---|
| Resident Name | Room No. | Resident ID # | Diagnosis |

LGM007537

LASER GRAPHICS MIDWEST INDIANAPOLIS, IN 007537 (8/18/98) MED-PASS C1–0 = BLUE FACE PMS 320 C2–0 = RED FACE PMS 233

**FIGURE 5–3** Drug Therapy Plan of Care. (Courtesy of MED-PASS, Inc.)

appropriate and accurate manner in the facility. In this way the pharmacist helps to prepare the facility for the survey by helping to correct medication administration problems. There are many dosage forms of medications that are prone to adminstration errors, such as eye and ear drops, metered-dose inhalers, transdermal patches, oral liquids, and injectables.

The med-pass observation process involves accompanying a nurse during medication administration. The consultant pharmacist tries not to call attention to himself or to disturb the nurse in performing his duties. The purpose is to observe and to evaluate the medication administration process. There are several areas that the consultant pharmacist may focus on, including:

- Medication administration errors—such as the wrong dose, the wrong drug, the wrong patient, the wrong time, or the wrong route of administration

- Sanitation—such as handwashing between patients or the touching of medication

- Security—such as locking the medication cart when it is not attended

- Inappropriate crushing of medications—such as crushing time-released forms of medications

- Documentation—such as properly charting the administration immediately afterward

The medication pass observation is a way for the consultant pharmacist to identify medication administration problems, to educate the nursing staff one-on-one, and to observe the patient. Most important, the consultant pharmacist assists the facility in complying with federal regulations and in providing quality care to its residents. Special forms are used to assist in performing the observation (Figure 5–4).

## CONSULTANT PHARMACIST SERVICES IN ALTERNATIVE LONG-TERM CARE SETTINGS

Routine medication review by a consultant pharmacist is lacking in most long-term care settings outside of the nursing facility because consultant pharmacist services are not federally mandated in these settings. Many long-term care settings can benefit from the services of a consultant pharmacist. There are high levels of medication use and consequently an increased potential for drug-related problems in these settings. All long-term care organizations wish to achieve the best possible outcomes of medications and manage their health care costs. The knowledge and expertise that the consultant pharmacist uses in the nursing home can also be applied to other settings. The consultant pharmacist can identify, prevent, and resolve drug-related problems. As in the nursing facility, the key is for the pharmacist to become an invaluable member of the team. Each type of long-term care setting presents different opportunities and challenges for the consultant pharmacist. The educational, medication systems management, and clinical services provided by consultant pharmacists can help to improve outcomes and decrease costs in all long-term care settings.

## MEDICATION PASS OBSERVATION REPORT

| | | | |
|---|---|---|---|
| Facility | Station/Wing | | Page of |
| Staff Observed | Time Started | Time Finished | Date |

* ERROR TYPE CODES
1. **Omissions** (Drugs ordered but not administered at least once)
2. **Unauthorized Drug** (Drugs administered without a physician's order)
3. **Wrong Dose**
4. **Wrong Route of Administration**
5. **Wrong Dosage Form**
6. **Wrong Drug**
7. **Wrong Time**
8. **Mfg. Specs. and/or Professional Standard (below)**

| RESIDENT | DRUG/DOSE AS PASSED | CURRENT DRUGS AS ORDERED | ERROR TYPE * 1 | 2 | 3 | 4 | 5 | 6 | 7 | 8 | S/NS |
|---|---|---|---|---|---|---|---|---|---|---|---|
| | | | | | | | | | | | |
| | | | | | | | | | | | |
| | | | | | | | | | | | |
| | | | | | | | | | | | |
| | | | | | | | | | | | |
| | TOTAL NO. OF MEDS PASSED | TOTAL NO. OF DRUGS ORDERED | ERROR GRAND TOTALS | | | | | | | | |
| See explanation on reverse for error types and examples of significant and non-significant errors (S/NS) | | PAGE ERROR TOTALS | | | | | | | | | |
| | | CUMULATIVE ERROR TOTALS (This plus previous pages) | | | | | | | | | |

**Type 8 = Medication Errors Due to Failure to Follow Manufacturers Specifications or Accepted Professional Standards (check each that was observed)**

- ☐ Failure to "shake well" products so labeled.
- ☐ Failure to properly mix insulin suspensions (e.g., "rolling") without creating air bubbles.
- ☐ Crushing tablets or capsules where manufacturer states "do not crush" [Exceptions - (a) if MD explains in the clinical record why crushing will not adversely affect patient, or; (b) if Facility can provide manufacturer or professional literature to justify why modification of dosage form will not compromise patient care]
- ☐ Failure to administer adequate (i.e., 8 oz) fluids with medications when manufacturer so specifies (e.g., with administration of bulk laxatives, NSAIDs or solid/liquid potassium supplements).
- ☐ Failure to administer medications with food or antacids when so specified by manufacturer (either before or with medication). This is especially important with NSAID medications.
- ☐ Administration of medications immediately before, during or immediately after administration of enteral nutritional formulas (ENFs) without, as a minimum,
  (1) checking placement of nasogastric or gastrostomy tube (cited under F281);
  (2) pre- and post-flushing of tube with at least 30 ml of preferably warm water (cited under F332/F333).
  NOTE - if Dilantin (phenytoin) is being given immediately before, during or immediately after ENF, check clinical record to assure patient is not experiencing loss of seizure control or side effects such as sedation.
- ☐ Failure to properly administer ophthalmic products wherein either (a) contact of the product with the eye occurs, or; (b) insufficient time (3-5 minutes) is allowed between administration of multiple ophthalmic products.
- ☐ Allowing resident to swallow sublingual tablets.
- ☐ Failure to properly administer medication via metered dose inhalers (MDIs). Proper administration includes: (a) shaking MDI well; (b) positioning MDI 2 finger widths in front of resident's mouth (or using spacer); (c) having resident exhale first then take a slow, deep breath as MDI is activated; (d) holding breath for a count of 10 after inhalation before slowly exhaling, and; (e) waiting a minute between puffs if multiple puffs are ordered.
  NOTE - if resident is unable to cooperate with the above procedures (e.g., due to dementia) this should not be considered an error.
- ☐ Other (please explain including potential for resident's discomfort or jeopardy to his or her health and safety). ______
- ☐ ______
- ☐ ______
- ☐ ______

Conclusion/Recommendation(s)

CALCULATED ERROR RATE = NUMBER OF ERRORS OBSERVED (Significant + Non Significant) ☐ / OPPORTUNITIES FOR ERRORS (Doses Given + Doses Ordered But Not Given) ☐ X 100 = ____ %

Consultant Pharmacist/Observer



**FIGURE 5–4** Medication Pass Observation Report. (Courtesy of MED-PASS, Inc.)

## SUBACUTE CARE

Consultant pharmacist services in the subacute setting focus on the drug regimen review. The drug regimen review is performed more frequently in this setting than in the nursing home, that is, more frequently than once a month, because patients move into and out of this area quickly. Subacute care patients are generally quite ill and are on many medications. Drug regimen review helps reduce medication therapy failures; decrease drug-related problems, especially adverse drug reactions and drug interactions; and improve the patient's overall medical condition.

In addition to this and other clinical services such as care planning and pain management, the consultant pharmacist in the subacute care setting also provides direction in all areas of medication systems management, such as the drug distribution system in use, medication storage and handling, and the use of emergency and controlled substance medications. The consultant pharmacist also serves as an educational resource to the interdisciplinary staff.

## PSYCHIATRIC HOSPITALS

The consultant pharmacist provides many services in a psychiatric hospital. The pharmacist performs drug regimen reviews, provides psychotropic drug monitoring, and provides individual and group medication consulting. The consultant pharmacist serves on several committees within the hospital, such as the infection control committee or the restraint committee, helps develop psychotropic medication use policies, and provides education and consultation to other health care professionals.

## CORRECTIONAL FACILITIES

There are many areas of involvement for the consultant pharmacist in a correctional facility. The pharmacist can counsel inmates concerning their medications, medication compliance, health promotion, and disease prevention and can provide drug information services to the staff. The pharmacist can play a role in medication management in the facility by helping to select an appropriate drug distribution system, monitoring the handling and record keeping of controlled substances, and developing and maintaining a formulary. The pharmacist also performs drug regimen reviews, sometimes including an interview with the inmate, monitors psychotropic drug use, and participates on committees, especially infection control and pharmacy services committees. The consultant pharmacist assists the correctional facility in complying with state and federal regulations concerning medications.

## ASSISTED LIVING

The assisted living market is one the fastest growing markets in health care and presents a growing opportunity for the consultant pharmacist as well. There are several challenges for consultant pharmacists in this setting. There are currently no specific federal regulations concerning pharmacy services in assisted living facilities. Only a few states require routine medication review by a consultant pharmacist for assisted living residents. Medication problems are very common in the assisted living setting. Assisted living residents usually have several chronic medical conditions and take multiple medications. On average, elderly residents of assisted living facilities use almost as many medications as nursing facility residents. Medically untrained caregivers often assist the residents with their medications. Some assisted living facilities may use a single pharmacy to obtain medications for their residents, while others may allow residents to obtain their medications from different pharmacies. This policy results in the use of several drug distribution systems in the facility, with the potential for medication errors. Although not mandated, consultant pharmacist services are urgently needed in this setting.

The consultant pharmacist can provide many educational services to the assisted living facility. The pharmacist can provide in-service training for the staff in areas such as proper medication administration, the appropriate crushing of medications, and adverse drug reactions to be aware of. He can provide counseling to residents on topics such as individual medication regimens, medication compliance, side effects, and wellness. The consultant pharmacist can assist the facility in the area of medication systems management by helping the facility choose and implement a single, easy-to-use drug distribution system, including one for controlled substances, and by providing forms for record keeping. There are numerous clinical services that the consultant pharmacist can provide in an assisted living facility. These include drug regimen review (current guidelines suggest once every 3 months), medication monitoring, and participation on committees to assist in all aspects of patient care. Finally, the consultant pharmacist can provide the facility with information concerning services that should be provided to assisted living residents and information concerning developing assisted living regulations that pertain to pharmacy services.

## BOARD AND CARE HOMES

The role of the consultant pharmacist in the board and care home is not legally required. The residents of board and care homes also have chronic medical conditions and take multiple medications. The personnel in these homes are not medically trained to help with medication administration. The residents usually obtain their medications from different community pharmacies, and medications are often not stored properly, not labeled properly, or outdated. These residents are at risk for drug-related problems due to incomplete pharmacy services. A consultant pharmacist can provide services such as drug regimen review, medication monitoring, staff education, and general oversight of medication use in this setting.

## OTHER COMMUNITY AND HOME-BASED LONG-TERM CARE SETTINGS

Other community-based long-term care settings, such as adult day care, respite care, continuous care retirement communities, and retirement housing, and home-based care can also benefit from the services of a consultant pharmacist. Although these patients or residents may live relatively independently or with their families, they have many unmet medication needs. They may need review of their drug regimens, assistance with confusing medication schedules, counseling concerning their medication regimens, advice on correct medication storage, and educational programs such as a "brown bag" program. This is a one-on-one discussion between the pharmacist and the patient, in which the pharmacist reviews all the medication that a patient brings to him in a brown bag. The pharmacist then counsels the patient on the use, storage, and expiration of these medications. A new term has emerged to describe the consultant pharmacist involved in the care of the elderly in these settings, the senior care pharmacist, a pharmacist who recognizes the unique medication needs of senior citizens in the community.

# THE ROLE OF THE PHARMACY TECHNICIAN IN LONG-TERM CARE

The role of the pharmacy technician in long-term care pharmacy is an important one. Pharmacy practice in long-term care has expanded the role of the pharmacist in providing pharmaceutical care. In order to provide this care, the pharmacist needs the assistance of the pharmacy technician. Many dispensing tasks previously performed by the pharmacist in long-term care are now being delegated to qualified pharmacy technicians. According to the definition of a pharmacy technician, the pharmacy technician in long-term care can assist the pharmacist in activities that do not require the professional judgment of the pharmacist. As in almost all other types of pharmacy practice, the long-term care pharmacist maintains control over all aspects of medication handling, including dispensing. However, there are many nonjudgmental tasks that the pharmacy technician can perform in long-term care. These can be divided into two areas: roles in the long-term care pharmacy and roles in the long-term care facility.

## THE PHARMACY TECHNICIAN IN THE LONG-TERM CARE PHARMACY

The pharmacy technician working in a long-term care pharmacy can perform many tasks related to dispensing medications. In order to perform these tasks, the pharmacy technician must possess traditional pharmacy knowledge and skills as well as special knowledge and skills specific to a long-term care pharmacy such as:

- Knowledge of the different methods of drug distribution systems used in long-term care
- Familiarity with the medications, different dosage forms, and over-the-counter products used in long-term care
- Medication repackaging skills
- Knowledge of medication labeling requirements, especially beyond-use dating
- Knowledge of the special forms and reports used in long-term care
- An understanding of the legislation and regulations pertaining to long-term care pharmacy practice

It is important for the pharmacy technician to remember that in assisting with the dispensing of medications, the long-term care pharmacist must perform the final check. Sample responsibilities for the pharmacy technician in the long-term care pharmacy include:

- Entering computer data on prescription drug and nondrug orders
- Repackaging and labeling medications

- Packaging and labeling prescriptions
- Ordering, receiving, and stocking medications and supplies
- Processing returned medications for reuse
- Maintaining repackaging and other equipment
- Maintaining a drug information library
- Maintaining computerized information such as patient profiles, committee reports, and drug information requests
- Preparing reports for the pharmacist and the facility
- Billing
- Providing forms to the facility
- Transporting medications to the facility or patient
- Maintaining delivery records
- Performing general pharmacy housekeeping

## THE PHARMACY TECHNICIAN IN THE LONG-TERM CARE FACILITY

The pharmacy technician may perform several tasks outside of the long-term care pharmacy in the long-term care facility. Here the pharmacy technician works very closely with the consultant pharmacist. Pharmacy technicians working inside the facility are usually highly trained and motivated. They possess special knowledge and skills very specific to the areas in which they are working. The importance of their functions is stressed. Pharmacy technicians in this setting report increased job satisfaction associated with the increased responsibility and importance of their work. It should again be mentioned that pharmacy technicians may not perform any task that involves clinical judgment. Pharmacy technician tasks in the long-term care facility can be divided into three areas: inspections, maintenance, and data collection.

### Inspections

Medications stored in the long-term care facility are inspected regularly as a part of the medication systems management services of a consultant pharmacist, for several reasons: to ensure efficient medication use, to reduce the chance of medication errors, and to help the facility prepare for surveys. The pharmacy technician can perform this service. Standardized forms are available to guide the technician and to ensure a thorough inspection of all areas where medications are stored, such as mobile medication and treatment carts, emergency boxes, refrigerators, drawers, and cabinets (Figure 5–5). Special attention is focused on storage conditions, medication security, and expired medications.

### Maintenance

All of the specialized equipment used in the long-term care facility, such as automated dispensing machines, medication and treatment carts, emergency boxes, and refrigerators, needs to be maintained. Maintenance is part of the medication systems management service provided to the facility. This service can be performed by the pharmacy technician as well. It involves the regular inspection of equipment, preventative maintenance, and resolving problems as they occur. The pharmacy technician must be thoroughly familiar with the specific equipment used in the facility.

DIRECTIONS: Enter appropriate review code in column provided below.
Use "Comment" section for additional narrative entries.

# MED ROOM INSPECTION
## NURSING STATION INSPECTION REPORT

| A | GENERAL APPEARANCE AND OBSERVATIONS | Review Codes |
|---|---|---|
| 1 | Metric-Apo conversion chart | |
| 2 | Drug reference available/current | |
| 3 | Poison antidote chart | |
| 4 | Policy/Procedures appropriate | |
| 5 | Previous deficiencies corrected | |
| 6 | Storage space organized | |
| 7 | Lighting/Ventilation adequate. | |
| 8 | Ordering procedures adequate. | |
| 9 | General appearance ☐ Good ☐ Poor | |
| 10 | Proper licenses posted | |
| 11 | Under sink-cleansers only | |
| 12 | Absence of drug samples | |
| 13 | D/C'd drugs listed & destroyed | |
| 14 | Internals/Externals separated | |
| 15 | No personal items stored. | |
| 16 | OTC - Stock drugs adequate/proper. | |
| 17 | Label on box & inside vials. | |
| 18 | Emergency O₂ equip. & cannula | |
| 19 | All Rx drugs labeled | |
| 20 | Med room locked when not in use. | |

| B | MED CARTS | Review Codes |
|---|---|---|
| 21 | Carts locked when not in use. | |
| 22 | Drawers neat, clean & orderly. | |
| 23 | D/C'd meds removed & stored. | |
| 24 | Multi-dose vials dated/signed. | |
| 25 | Re-packed meds within 6 mo. exp. | |
| 26 | Evidence of borrowing meds. | |
| 27 | MAR's entries proper & orderly. | |
| 28 | MAR's condition ☐ Good ☐ Fair | |
| 29 | Drawers labeled... Name/room #. | |
| 30 | Label over essential information | |

| C | CONTROLLED DRUGS | Review Codes |
|---|---|---|
| 31 | Drawers properly locked. | |
| 32 | Keys with Charge Nurse. | |
| 33 | Usage report. | |
| 34 | Inventory count each shift. | |
| 35 | Destroyed properly as necessary. | |
| 36 | Inventory records balance. | |

| D | EMERGENCY KIT | Review Codes |
|---|---|---|
| 37 | Current list posted properly. | |
| 38 | "Emergency Kit" sign on outside | |
| 39 | Meds within date of expiration | |
| 40 | Meds short | |
| 41 | Kit kept sealed | |
| 42 | Proper sign-out procedures | |
| 43 | Locks stored in DON's office | |

| E | REFRIGERATOR | Review Codes |
|---|---|---|
| 44 | Clean - no food | |
| 45 | Temperature (36° to 46° F) | |
| 46 | Daily temperature chart on door | |
| 47 | Expired medication | |
| 48 | Overstocked (Insulin, etc.) | |
| 49 | Opened vials - dated & initials | |
| 50 | Labels on box and inside vials | |

| F | MISCELLANEOUS | Review Codes |
|---|---|---|
| 51 | | |

Facility

Nursing Station

Pharmacist

Nurse

Date

Comments

Follow-up

Has the facility corrected problems from previous report? ☐ Yes ☐ No

Has the pharmacy corrected problems from previous report? ☐ Yes ☐ No

**REVIEW CODES:**
C - SEE COMMENTS      / - N/A (NOT APPLICABLE)      N - NURSING ATTENTION NEEDED
S - SATISFACTORY      R - RECOMMENDATION      P - PHARMACY ATTENTION NEEDED

WHITE - Pharmacist      CANARY - Facility

(Rev. 03/07)

Form # MP5502

Reorder From: **MED-PASS** 800-438-8884

These colors (Teal and Pink) are a trademark of Med-Pass, Inc.

© 1991 MED-PASS, Inc.

INH 100500

**FIGURE 5–5** Med Room Inspection Nursing Station Inspection Report. (Courtesy of MED-PASS, Inc.)

## Data Collection

The drug regimen review performed by the consultant pharmacist requires a lot of preparation. Some of this preparation involves the collection of data that the pharmacist uses in evaluating drug therapy. A highly trained and motivated pharmacy technician can assist the consultant pharmacist in this task. It requires that the pharmacy technician accompany the consultant pharmacist in performing the drug regimen review. The pharmacy technician assembles all of the forms needed by the pharmacist. The technician also collects data such as laboratory reports, records of pulse and blood pressure readings, physician and nurse's progress notes, reports from consulting physicians, the medication and treatment administration records, and dietician and other reports such as physical, occupational, and speech therapy. In many instances, because these pieces of information are found in many different places, data collection is difficult and time-consuming for the pharmacist. The pharmacist then uses these data in performing the drug regimen review.

There are other areas of data collection in which the pharmacy technician can be of help. These involve data required for meetings attended by the consultant pharmacist, data needed for pharmacy reports, data pertaining to drug information requests, and materials needed for pharmacist in-service education in the facility.

## KEY CONCEPTS

- Consultant pharmacy involves pharmaceutical care services performed by the pharmacist to achieve definite outcomes and improve the quality of life of a long-term care resident.
- Consultant services are separate from, but complementary to, dispensing services.
- The consultant pharmacist is a pharmacist who provides pharmaceutical care services in a wide variety of institutional, community, and home-based long-term care settings.
- The consultant pharmacist provides pharmaceutical care services in several areas, including education, medication systems management, and clinical services.
- The drug regimen review is a federal requirement for long-term care residents and the most important duty of a consultant pharmacist.
- The consultant pharmacist develops a pharmaceutical care plan as part of a long-term care resident's overall care plan.
- A medication pass observation by a consultant pharmacist is an important tool in ensuring accurate medication administration in the facility.
- The consultant pharmacist provides educational, medication systems management, and clinical services in various alternative long-term care settings.
- The pharmacy technician in long-term care performs many unique tasks both in the long-term care pharmacy and in the long-term care facility, including inspections, maintenance, and data collection.

## SELF-ASSESSMENT QUESTIONS

**MULTIPLE CHOICE**

1. Consultant services:
   a. are usually performed in the long-term care pharmacy
   b. are usually performed in the long-term care facility
   c. focus on drug distribution systems
   d. involve all pharmacy personnel

2. A consultant pharmacist can practice in which of the following settings?
   a. psychiatric hospitals
   b. subacute care units
   c. assisted living facilities
   d. all of the above

3. Which is not a medication systems management activity?
   a. drug information
   b. drug storage
   c. drug distribution systems
   d. drug formularies

4. All of the following are drugs that are frequently involved in drug regimen review irregularities except:
   a. penicllin
   b. warfarin
   c. phenytoin
   d. digoxin

5. Pharmaceutical care services consist of:
   a. medication systems management
   b. clinical services
   c. education
   d. all of the above

6. The consultant pharmacist serves on which of the following committees in the long-term care facility?
   a. care planning committee
   b. infection control committee
   c. restraint committee
   d. all of the above

7. Which is not a clinical service performed by the consultant pharmacist?
   a. pharmacokinetic dosing
   b. nutrition monitoring
   c. pain management
   d. emergency medication supply

8. All of the following are true statements concerning the drug regimen review except:
   a. it follows the organized system of the pharmacist
   b. it is performed individually for each resident

c. it takes the resident's total care into account

d. it is performed on an occasional basis

9. Drug regimen review has been shown to:

a. increase adverse drug reactions

b. increase medication errors

c. decrease hospitalizations

d. increase health care costs

10. An example of an activity performed by a pharmacy technician in the long-term care pharmacy is:

a. maintaining repackaging equipment

b. providing forms and reports to the facility

c. repackaging medications

d. all of the above

## TRUE/FALSE (CORRECT THE FALSE STATEMENTS)

1. _____ There are federal regulations for the provision of consultant pharmacist services in assisted living facilities.

2. _____ OBRA 87 expanded the role of the pharmacist beyond the drug regimen review.

3. _____ The goal of observing a medication pass is to ensure that medications are being administered in the proper manner.

4. _____ The drug regimen review is the most important and time-consuming duty of a consultant pharmacist.

5. _____ The consultant pharmacist develops a pharmaceutical care plan for each resident as a part of the overall plan of care.

6. _____ The role of the consultant pharmacist in board and care homes is legally required.

7. _____ The "brown bag" program is an example of a consultant pharmacist service.

8. _____ The pharmacy technician can perform many tasks in the long-term care facility as well as in the long-term care pharmacy.

9. _____ Consulting services are separate from provider services.

10. _____ Pharmacy technicians can perform tasks involving professional judgment regarding medication therapy.

## FILL-IN

1. _____ _____ is the process that results in the individual plan of care.

2. A pharmacist who is specially trained to provide pharmaceutical care services to long-term care residents is called a _____ _____.

3. A drug regimen review is referred to as a _____ _____.

4. The _____ role of the consultant pharmacist is a highly visible role.

5. Clinical services are also referred to as _____ services.

6. The type of drug regimen review that concentrates on a particular medical problem is a _____ review.

7. The goal of drug regimen review is _____ _____ _____.

8. Consultant pharmacist services in a subacute care unit focus mainly on the _____ _____ _____.
9. It is suggested that a drug regimen review be performed every _____ months in an assisted living facility.
10. The pharmacy technician can perform _____ of medication storage in the long-term care facility.

## CRITICAL THINKING

1. What is the difference between consultant and provider services in long-term care, and why is there a distinction made?
2. Give an example of each type of drug regimen review: general, focused, and problem-centered.
3. Why is a medication pass observation so important?
4. Compare and contrast the duties of a pharmacy technician in a long-term care pharmacy with those in a traditional community retail pharmacy.
5. What could be some negative findings during an inspection of medication storage in a long-term care facility?

## ■ BIBLIOGRAPHY

American Society of Consultant Pharmacists. (2004). *Consultant pharmacist handbook*. Arlington, VA: Author.

American Society of Consultant Pharmacists. (2004). *Fundamentals of consultant pharmacy practice*. Arlington, VA: Author.

American Society of Consultant Pharmacists. (2005). *ASCP guidelines on the role of pharmacy technicians in long-term care*. [On-line] ASCP. Available: www.ascp.com.

American Society of Consultant Pharmacists. (2005). *Medication management in assisted living: A report from the American Society of Consultant Pharmacists*. Arlington, VA: Author.

Brushwood, D. (2004). Drug therapy monitoring in assisted living facilities. *Pharmacy Today, 10*(3), 36.

Chandler, M., & Kirkwood, K. (2006). Pharmacist's role in long-term acute care hospitals. *Drug Topics, 150*(4), 56.

Erickson, A. (2005). Consultant pharmacist solves patients' medical mysteries in community setting. *Pharmacy Today, 11*(9), 18.

Frampton, K. (2004). Pain assessment and management in LTC requires a thorough, team-oriented care plan. *Caring for the Ages, 5*(5), 26, 29–30, 35.

Gebhart, F. (2004). New survey shows value of consultant pharmacists. *Drug Topics, 148*(23), 56.

Jerrard, J. (2005). Professional partners: There are many ways for consultant pharmacists and medical directors to collaborate. *Caring for the Ages, 6*(9), 34–39.

Pharmacy Technician Certification Board. (2005). *Your guidebook to PTCB certification 2005*. Washington, DC: Author.

Spooner, J. (2005). Medication therapy management services for long-term care patients: No road maps for those trying to find their way. *Journal of Managed Care Pharmacy, 11*(7), 586–587.

Trygstad, T., et al. (2005). Pharmacist response to alerts generated from Medicaid pharmacy claims in a long-term care setting: Results from the North Carolina Polypharmacy Institute. *Journal of Managed Care Pharmacy, 11*(7), 575–583.

# Home Health Care

## Learning Objectives

Upon completion of this chapter, the student should be able to:

- Define home health care.
- Give reasons for the growth in home health care.
- List some of the organizations that provide home health care services.
- Describe the interdisciplinary home health care team.
- Explain the funding for home health care.
- Describe the types of home health care services available.
- Describe the types of specialty home health care programs.
- Characterize the home health care patient.
- Understand the criteria for the selection of a home health care patient.
- Explain the home health care process.
- Explain the role of pharmacy in home health care.

## Key Terms

admission assessment
functional limitation
homebound

home care pharmacy
   practice
home health care

initial assessment
referral

## Introduction

Home health care is one of the fastest growing segments of the health care market. Today, more and more serious medical problems are treated outside of the hospital setting and in the home. Home health care is an important part of the continuum of care. It allows patients to be comfortable and independent while providing safe and effective therapies in the home. Home health care is also a less expensive way to provide care. Home health care includes a wide variety of services, including pharmaceutical services. Pharmacists and pharmacy technicians must be knowledgeable about the home health care environment in order to understand their roles in it. This chapter discusses home health care and provides the background for the discussion of home infusion pharmacy. ▪

## OVERVIEW OF HOME HEALTH CARE

**Home health care,** sometimes simply referred to as home care, is defined as health care services and health-related products provided to a patient at home. Home health care is a small segment of the health care system, but it is one of its fastest growing segments. This growth is due to several factors, including:

- *An increase in the number of the elderly.* This in turn increases the need for home care services.
- *Patient preference.* Patients prefer to be treated or cared for in their own homes. Home care allows the patient to stay in a familiar and supportive setting.
- *Personal attention.* Home care is more personal care. It helps the patient maintain her comfort, dignity, and independence.
- *Lower costs.* Home care is less expensive than hospital or nursing home care.
- *New and improved technology.* New and safer delivery systems make it possible to deliver complex treatments and traditional inpatient treatments in the home.
- *Managed care.* The diagnosis-related group (DRG) system of hospital reimbursement has led to early discharge of patients from hospitals to their homes.
- *Physician acceptance.* Physicians have become more comfortable with treating their patients at home.

The home care setting is often referred to as a "hospital without walls" because many treatments previously provided only in the hospital are now being provided at home. Patients with chronic illnesses who would otherwise be admitted to a hospital are now being taken care of at home. In some instances, treatments are started at home, completely eliminating hospitalization.

Home care has existed for over 100 years. Services back then consisted of midwife care for childbirth and nursing care for tuberculosis and influenza. Home infusion began in the 1970s, when total parenteral nutrition (TPN) started to be provided on an outpatient basis. In the 1980s, the home care industry expanded into other services as this cost-effective alternative to hospitalization was recognized. Today, home health care covers a wide range of services, from personal care and home equipment to high-technology medical care such as cardiac monitoring and intravenous infusion therapy. Home care has also expanded into alternative sites, that is, sites other than the patient's home, such as long-term care facilities, subacute care units, outpatient infusion centers (also called ambulatory infusion centers), physician office-based infusion centers, diagnostic centers, laboratories, outpatient clinics, outpatient surgery facilities, rehabilitation facilities, and emergency care facilities.

Home health care services are provided through a home health care organization. There are many types of home health care organizations that provide home health care services. Home health care services can be provided by home medical equipment companies, home infusion companies, independent home health care agencies, hospital-based home health care agencies, hospices, physician groups such as oncology groups, and community retail pharmacies, both independent and chain. It is interesting to note that many hospitals have set up their own home health care agencies to increase hospital revenues and to enable them to discharge patients earlier. Different types of home health care services are provided by different home health care organizations. It is important to note that not all home health care providers offer home health care pharmacy services, in particular, home infusion services, which is discussed in Chapter 7.

The home health care industry is interdisciplinary in nature; that is, it involves an interdisciplinary health care team. The home health care team consists of pharmacists, pharmacy technicians, physicians, nurses, allied health professionals such as physical therapists, occupational therapists, speech therapists, respiratory therapists, dieticians and social workers, and home health aides. Other home care personnel include case managers, intake coordinators, customer service representatives, delivery personnel, and billing personnel. Each team member has a specific and important role to perform. The pharmacist is an important member of this team and is involved with the physician, nurses, dietician, and, often, other therapists in planning, directing, providing, and monitoring certain home health care services.

Funding for home health care services comes from many sources. Private health insurance (managed care) is the number one source of payment. Health insurance companies often determine what home health care services are appropriate and covered. Medicare covers home health care services provided by Medicare-certified home health care agencies. In addition to Medicare, Medicaid covers some home health care services, but coverage varies from state to state. Finally, some home health care services are paid for by the patient, referred to as private pay. Regardless of the source of payment, it is important that home health care providers be reimbursed for their services because they are expensive, costing hundreds or thousands of dollars per day of treatment. Therefore, home health care providers usually verify that patients have appropriate coverage and that they will be reimbursed for services before providing them.

## TYPES OF HOME HEALTH CARE SERVICES

There are many types of home health care services that may be offered by home health care organizations. The types of services may be divided into several areas:

- Pharmaceutical services—drug products and pharmaceutical care services provided by pharmacists
- Nursing services—skilled and unskilled nursing care, including hospice care, provided by nurses
- Personal care services—nonmedical activities such as bathing, dressing, housekeeping services, cooking, and shopping provided by nonmedical personnel called home health aides

- Rehabilitation services—physical therapy, occupational therapy, speech therapy, respiratory therapy, and other health-related services performed by allied health professionals

- Home medical equipment services—maintenance or provision of reusable medical equipment, referred to as durable medical equipment (DME). Respiratory technicians are often included under this type of service and provide clinical respiratory services along with respiratory equipment.

## SPECIALTY HOME HEALTH CARE PROGRAMS

There are many home health care programs that provide specialized therapies to patients in the home. These programs focus on a specific condition or diagnosis. Specialty programs provide therapies for conditions and diagnoses such as heart disease, diabetes, cancer, stroke, and infection. Not all specialty programs, however, may be offered by every home health care organization. Specialty programs include:

- *HIV/AIDS programs.* HIV/AIDS programs provide therapy for the chronic and recurrent infections associated with these conditions, which often require prolonged courses of intravenous antibiotics, antifungals, or antivirals.

- *Oncology programs.* Oncology programs provide complete services for cancer patients in the home. They include, but are not limited to, chemotherapy, antiemetic therapy, parenteral nutrition therapy, pain management therapy, hydration therapy, education, support, and side effect monitoring. The patient, caregiver, and staff receive thorough education concerning the safe handling, administration, and disposal of chemotherapy.

- *Infertility programs.* Infertility programs provide injectable fertility medications, support, and education to couples in the more advanced stages of attempting to achieve a pregnancy.

- *Pain management programs.* Pain management programs provide appropriate assessment and management of pain for patients with chronic pain due to cancer, surgery, or a recurrent painful illness. They include medications, monitoring, and patient counseling under the guidance of a pharmacist.

- *Rehabilitation programs.* Rehabilitation programs provide many types of rehabilitation services in the home to avoid or shorten hospitalization. Physical therapy, occupational therapy, and speech therapy are provided under the guidance of physical therapists, occupational therapists, and speech therapists, respectively.

- *Noninvasive diagnostic studies.* There are many noninvasive diagnostic studies that can be performed in the home. These studies are performed through the use of diagnostic equipment such as electrocardiograph machines, Holter monitors, portable x-ray machines, and portable ultrasound machines. The results of these studies are then interpreted by a physician.

- *Maternal and infant care programs.* Maternal and infant care programs offer support and teaching through all stages of pregnancy and early parenting. They include the management of preterm labor, gestational hypertension, hyperemesis gravidarum (excessive nausea and vomiting during pregnancy) and gestational diabetes, rapid postpartum discharge, postcesarean section wound care, breast-feeding support, fetal monitoring, and infant sleep apnea monitoring. Special equipment, such as sleep apnea monitors, fetal monitors, and bilirubin lights, is supplied.

- *Cardiac programs.* Cardiac programs offer diagnosis and monitoring of heart conditions, including over-the-telephone arrhythmia and pacemaker monitoring. Special equipment includes electrocardiograph machines and Holter monitors. The results are interpreted by a cardiologist or other physician. Intravenous therapy with dobutamine, an intravenous drug that improves heart function, is also provided for end-stage congestive heart failure patients.

- *Durable medical equipment.* Durable medical equipment, or DME, is reusable medical equipment provided to patients in the home. The provision of DME involves the selection, delivery, setup, and maintenance of the equipment and patient education. The equipment can be rented or purchased. Equipment includes hospital beds, commodes, wheelchairs, crutches, canes, and walkers, as well as high-technology equipment such as oxygen tanks, intravenous infusion pumps, respiratory equipment, glucose monitoring devices, cardiac monitors, fetal monitors, bilirubin lights, sleep apnea monitors, and others.

- *Ostomy and incontinence programs.* Ostomy and incontinence programs provide support, education, and ostomy and incontinence supplies to help patients manage these conditions.

- *Wound care programs.* Wound care programs provide support, education, supplies, and nursing services to patients with wounds, surgical incisions, or decubitus ulcers.

- *Preoperative management programs.* Preoperative management programs attempt to reduce the risks associated with surgery by identifying and correcting problems preoperatively. These programs include taking complete patient medical histories, performing physical assessments of the patient, performing preadmission laboratory testing, and teaching or explaining the anticipated surgical procedures.

- *Breast cancer recovery programs.* Breast cancer recovery programs provide support, education, information, and referral services after a diagnosis of breast cancer has been made. These programs attempt to decrease fear, identify a patient's treatment options, and promote early intervention.

- *Psychiatric home care programs.* Psychiatric home care programs offer comprehensive mental health services, including psychotherapy, case management, and coordination of treatment. They are usually under the guidance of a psychiatric nurse who has an advanced degree.

- *Respiratory programs.* Respiratory programs provide respiratory therapy and equipment for patients with chronic lung conditions, such as chronic obstructive lung disease (COLD), emphysema, cystic fibrosis, and asthma. They include oxygen administration, nebulizer treatments, cystic fibrosis treatments, training in the use of metered-dose inhalers, and asthma management. These programs are under the guidance of a respiratory therapist.

- *Diabetic monitoring programs.* Diabetic monitoring programs provide support, education, and supplies for diabetics. They offer diabetic care plans and blood glucose monitoring. Equipment includes blood glucose monitors and test strips and insulin pumps.

- *Posttransplant programs.* Posttransplant programs involve specialized postoperative therapies, support, and education for kidney, heart, bone marrow, and other transplant patients.

- *Anticoagulation programs.* Anticoagulation programs provide education and monitoring for patients taking oral (warfarin) or injectable (heparin) blood thinners. These programs result in improved therapeutic control and a reduction in the adverse drug reactions associated with these medications.

- *Hemotherapy programs.* Hemotherapy is the treatment of a medical condition through the administration of blood products. It involves the infusion of blood products such as packed red blood cells, platelets, and clotting factors to patients with diseases such as hemophilia and cancer.

- *Iontophoresis.* Iontophoresis involves the delivery of small doses of drugs through the skin without an injection. A special device transports the drug by means of a mild electric current. It is used to deliver anti-inflammatory drugs, local anesthetics, and chemotherapy for a wide range and variety of conditions.

- *Nursing care programs.* Nurses have been caring for patients in the home for years through home visits. Nursing care programs provide many types of nursing services for home care patients that include patient teaching, patient assessment and monitoring, treatments, and medication administration. Specific examples include starting intravenous lines; caring for the intravenous site; taking vital signs such as blood pressure, pulse, and temperature; and drawing blood.

- *Dialysis programs.* Dialysis programs provide support, education, supplies, and nursing care to patients undergoing dialysis procedures in the home.

- *Hospice programs.* Hospice programs provide management of symptoms such as pain, nausea, and bowel problems for terminally ill patients, rather than treatment of the disease. The focus is on patient comfort. The pharmacist is especially involved in the area of pain management.

- *Personal care and homemaker programs.* Personal care and homemaker programs provide assistance with activities of daily living such as bathing, dressing, walking, eating, and toileting and instrumental activities of daily living such as cooking, shopping, banking, and housekeeping. These services are provided by home health aides.

- *Nutrition programs.* Nutrition programs provide enteral and parenteral nutrition, including the equipment, such as infusion devices, and the supplies, such as bags and tubing, needed to infuse these types of nutrition. These programs involve a dietician and home infusion pharmacist.

- *Intravenous therapy programs.* Intravenous therapy programs involve the safe and effective preparation and administration of intravenous medications and solutions to patients in the home. They involve nurses who are specially trained to administer intravenous medications and the home infusion pharmacist. Examples of intravenous therapies include antibiotics, chemotherapy, hydration, and pain management.

## BOX 6–1    Functional Limitations

Amputation
Mental confusion
Poor vision or hearing
Obesity
Paralysis
Bowel or bladder incontinence
Surgical incision
Poor circulation
Plaster cast on arm or leg
Fatigue
Severe pain
Mental retardation
Swelling in the extremities
Limited range of motion
Difficulty breathing
Urinary catheter
Open or draining wound
Numbness or weakness in the legs
Poor balance
Dizziness

## THE HOME HEALTH CARE PATIENT

The home health care patient, or home care patient, can be an infant, a child, or an adult. Most often the home care patient is elderly, has multiple chronic medical conditions, and is under the care of more than one physician. The home care patient may have some type of functional limitation. A **functional limitation** is defined as a condition that limits a person's ability to function in a normal manner. It limits the person's ability to perform activities of daily living and instrumental activities of daily living. A functional limitation can be physical or mental. Examples of functional limitations are given in Box 6–1.

The home care patient may also be homebound. **Homebound** is defined as the inability to leave the home under normal conditions. A patient can be homebound for several reasons. She may have one or more functional limitations, may be unable to walk, may have limited endurance, may have restrictions on her activity such as no climbing of stairs or no lifting over a certain weight, or may need physical assistance to leave the home.

## CRITERIA FOR SELECTION FOR HOME HEALTH CARE

A patient does not choose home health care as a health care option for herself. A patient is typically *referred* to a home health care organization for services. A **referral** is defined as a request for care made on behalf of a patient. A referral can be made by a physician, nurse, social worker, hospital discharge planner, friend, or family. Once a referral is made, an employee of the home health care organization, called the intake coordinator, gathers data concerning the patient. These data are used by the interdisciplinary home health care team to perform an initial assessment. The **initial assessment** determines if the patient is an appropriate candidate for home care and if home health care is the correct choice. Generally, a patient will be eligible for home care if she is homebound, is under the care of a physician who prescribes a treatment, or needs some type of rehabilitation or nursing care. However, not all patients are appropriate candidates for home care. Before the patient is accepted by the home health care organization for home care services, several other factors must be considered, such as:

- The type of therapy to be provided
- The patient's health insurance and reimbursement
- The patient's ability to move about
- The patient's social, work, and economic histories
- The patient's medical condition
- The patient's mental and emotional condition
- The patient's medication regimen
- The patient's support system
- The patient's home environment

Certain criteria must be met for a patient to be accepted for home health care. These criteria include:

- The therapy must be appropriate for home care.
- The home care services will be reimbursed.
- The patient's medical condition must be stable.
- The patient must be able to assist in her care.
- The patient must be willing to take responsibility for her care.
- The patient must have a caregiver, such as a friend or family member, to assist in her care.
- The patient must have the proper home environment, which has clean space and storage conditions for medications, supplies, and equipment and a telephone, refrigerator, and running water.

Once the patient's insurance and coverage have been verified and the required criteria have been met, she is admitted to the home health care organization to receive services. This admission is referred to as intake. Intake is the beginning of the home health care process.

## THE HOME HEALTH CARE PROCESS

The home health care process is a series of steps in the provision of home health care services. It is an extensive process that starts on admission or intake and continues until the patient is discharged from the program or service. An **admission assessment**, which is different from the initial assessment, is the first step in the process. It is more extensive than the initial assessment and contains detailed information about the patient and her medical history. The elements of the admission assessment are found in Box 6–2.

The care plan, or plan of care, is the next step in the process. It is defined as all of the identified problems being treated and the strategies for treatment. The care plan is developed by the interdisciplinary home health care team along with input from the patient and family. It includes the therapy selected, the type and frequency of monitoring, and the desired therapeutic outcome or goal. It is developed and used to guide therapy and to reduce the problems associated with therapy. Furthermore, any home health care organization that seeks accreditation must develop and use a plan of care. The care plan is updated regularly as the patient's health status changes. The specific elements of a care plan are found in Box 6–3.

Services are provided after the plan of care is developed. A schedule is set up for the delivery of services, equipment, and supplies. It is hoped that this schedule meets the needs of the patient as well as of the home health care organization.

Monitoring is the next step in the home health care process. The patient's progress is continuously monitored, documented, and reported to the interdisciplinary team throughout the patient's therapy. Monitoring is accomplished by

---

### BOX 6–2  Elements of an Admission Assessment

Name, address, phone number
Sex, date of birth
Responsible party
Height and weight
Allergies
Diagnosis
Prognosis
Therapy
Referring physician
Medical and surgical histories
Medication history
Nutritional assessment
Mental status
Physical assessment

---

### BOX 6–3  Elements of a Care Plan

Diagnosis
Current medication regimen
Therapy
Goals of therapy
Monitoring required
Nutrition
Permitted patient activities

assessing the patient's response to therapy, compliance with therapy, and any problems with therapy. Nurses, allied health professionals, or home health aides visit the patient at home at regular intervals throughout the therapy. These home visits allow treatments to be provided; medications, equipment, and supplies to be delivered; and laboratory or diagnostic work to be performed. Most important, they provide an opportunity to assess and reassess the patient and to provide additional reinforcement or training if needed.

The final step in the process is the discharge assessment. It is the final assessment performed at the completion of therapy. The patient is evaluated to determine if the outcome or goal of therapy was achieved. A report, referred to as a discharge summary, is provided to the referring physician. It is a summary of the home health care services provided to the patient and the status of the patient's problem over the course of the therapy. The patient is then discharged from the home health care organization. The entire home health care process is shown in Figure 6–1.

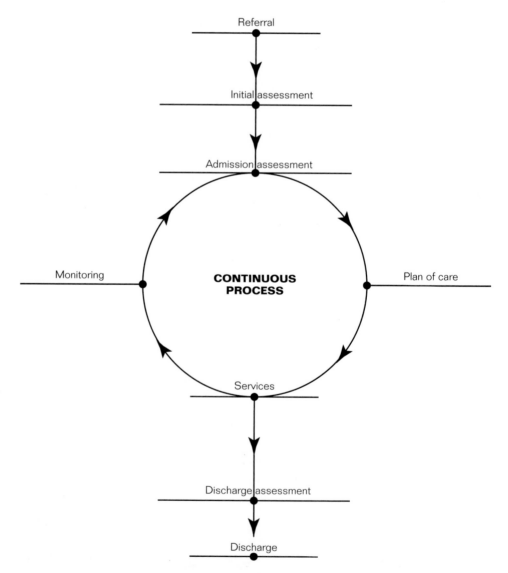

**FIGURE 6–1**    The Home Health Care Process.

## THE ROLE OF PHARMACY IN HOME HEALTH CARE

Pharmacists in retail pharmacy practice have provided home health care for decades by providing canes, crutches, walkers, and other supplies along with prescription and over-the-counter medications to patients at home. Along with the growth in the home health care industry, some pharmacists have expanded the home health care services they provide. Some pharmacists provide a full range of durable medical equipment. Some provide nutritional care and are recognized by the Board of Pharmaceutical Specialties as nutritional support pharmacists. Other pharmacists provide home infusion therapies. However, all pharmacists who provide home health care services share the same goal: to ensure the safe, appropriate, and effective use of medications and home health care products and services in the home.

**Home care pharmacy practice** has emerged and is defined as the practice of pharmacy that provides medications, home health care products and services, and pharmaceutical care to patients in the home. These products and services range from traditional durable medical equipment, such as canes, crutches, and walkers, to oxygen, nutritional products, and intravenous therapies. Home care pharmacists provide pharmaceutical care in addition to the products and services. Pharmaceutical care is in the form of patient monitoring to ensure the best possible outcomes of these products and services.

There are many home health care products and services provided by pharmacies today, usually in the retail setting. These include:

durable medical equipment

oxygen therapy

wound care and decubitus ulcer products

ostomy and incontinence products

prosthetic devices—artificial limbs, mastectomy supplies

orthopedic supplies—braces, supports, trusses

first aid supplies

medical instruments—stethoscopes, blood pressure kits

home diagnostic products

prescription medications not for self-administration—respiratory drugs

nutritional therapy

intravenous therapy

Nutritional therapy and intravenous therapy are collectively referred to as infusion therapy. Home infusion therapy has evolved into a separate and unique practice area of pharmacy known as home infusion pharmacy. Home infusion pharmacy is discussed in Chapter 7.

## KEY CONCEPTS

- Home health care is the provision of health care services and health-related products to a patient at home.

- Home health care is one of the fastest growing areas of health care because of several factors, including an increase in the number of the elderly, patient preference for home care, and lower costs.
- Many different types of home health care organizations provide home health care services.
- Home health care involves an interdisciplinary health care team.
- Funding for home health care comes from several sources but primarily private insurance.
- The types of home health care services that are available are pharmaceutical, nursing, and personal care; rehabilitation; and home medical equipment services.
- Many home health care organizations provide specialty programs that focus on specific conditions or diagnoses.
- The home health care patient usually has a functional limitation or is homebound.
- There are several criteria that must be met before a patient can receive home health care services.
- Home health care services are provided in a series of steps in conjunction with a plan of care.
- Pharmacists provide many home health care services and products.

## ■ SELF-ASSESSMENT QUESTIONS

### MULTIPLE CHOICE

1. A home health aide provides:
   a. skilled nursing care
   b. personal care services
   c. rehabilitation services
   d. pharmaceutical services

2. Which is a false statement about home health care?
   a. it is more expensive than inpatient care
   b. it uses advanced technology
   c. it is a fast-growing segment of health care
   d. it is preferred by the patient

3. A source of funding for home health care is:
   a. Medicare
   b. private health insurance
   c. Medicaid
   d. all of the above

4. Which is not a functional limitation?
   a. paralysis
   b. obesity
   c. diabetes
   d. poor vision

5. Most home care patients are:

   a. children
   b. elderly
   c. women
   d. none of the above

6. A patient meets the criteria for home health care if:

   a. the therapy is appropriate for home care
   b. she has the proper home environment
   c. her medical condition is stable
   d. all of the above

7. Which is not a home health care site?

   a. the patient's home
   b. ambulatory infusion centers
   c. hospitals
   d. a physician's office

8. All of the following are home health care organizations except:

   a. home infusion companies
   b. home health care agencies
   c. long-term care facilities
   d. home medical equipment companies

9. An example of a specialty home health care program is:

   a. maternal and infant care program
   b. breast cancer recovery program
   c. intravenous therapy program
   d. all of the above

10. Which is not a home care pharmacy service?

    a. intravenous therapy
    b. durable medical equipment
    c. nutritional therapy
    d. dental products

## TRUE/FALSE (CORRECT THE FALSE STATEMENTS)

1. _____ Increases in the number of the elderly will increase the need for home health care services.
2. _____ Psychiatric care can be delivered in the home.
3. _____ Personal care services include ADLs and IADLs.
4. _____ Functional limitations are physical in nature.
5. _____ An admission assessment is the same as an initial assessment.
6. _____ Patient monitoring is not a part of the home health care process.
7. _____ Insurance verification is an important part of the home health care process.
8. _____ The admission assessment includes a nutritional assessment.
9. _____ Any home health care organization that seeks accreditation must develop and use a plan of care.
10. _____ Not all specialty home health care programs are offered by every home health care organization.

## FILL-IN

1. A patient who cannot leave home under normal conditions is called _____.
2. Reusable medical equipment is called _____ _____ _____.
3. A _____ _____ is defined as all of the identified problems being treated through home health care.
4. A condition that limits a person's ability to function normally is called a _____ _____.
5. A _____ _____ is the final report of care and services provided to the physician at the end of the patient's therapy.
6. The type of home health care service performed by allied health professionals such as physical therapists, occupational therapists, speech therapists, and respiratory therapists is called _____ _____.
7. The delivery of small amounts of drug through the skin without an injection is _____.
8. The admission process into a home health care organization is referred to as _____.
9. The primary source of payment for home health care services is _____ _____ _____.
10. Respiratory programs are under the supervision of a _____ _____.

## CRITICAL THINKING

1. What are the results of the shift from hospital care to home health care?
2. Compare and contrast the interdisciplinary health care team in home health care with that in long-term care.
3. Select an example of a specialty home health care program and create a patient scenario.
4. How does a home health care patient differ from a long-term care patient?
5. Compare and contrast an initial assessment and an admission assessment within the home health care process.

## ■ BIBLIOGRAPHY

McCarthy, R., & Schafermeyer, K. (2004). *Introduction to health care delivery: A primer for pharmacists.* Gaithersburg, MD: Aspen Publishers, Inc.
Pal, S. (2005). Home health care services. *U.S. Pharmacist, 30*(6), 12–14.
Wertheimer, A., et al. (2005). Increasing profits with home health care products. *Pharmacy Times, 71*(10), 42–44.
Zagaria, M.A. (2006). Family caregiving. *U.S. Pharmacist, 31*(12), 23–29.

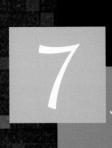

# 7 Home Infusion Pharmacy

## Learning Objectives

Upon completion of this chapter, the student should be able to:

- Define home infusion pharmacy.
- List the types of home infusion therapies.
- Describe the elements of a home infusion pharmacy.
- Describe the home infusion therapy process.
- Explain the pharmaceutical care plan.
- Describe the prescription-filling process in a home infusion pharmacy.
- Understand vascular access and the types of vascular access devices.
- Describe infusion devices and other delivery systems used in home infusion.
- List the special supplies used with home infusion therapies.
- Describe enteral nutrition therapy.
- Describe parenteral nutrition therapy and the special challenges in home care.
- Understand the legislation and regulations that pertain to home infusion pharmacy.
- Describe the roles of the pharmacist and the pharmacy technician in home infusion.

## Key Terms

compounding record

enteral nutrition

home infusion pharmacy

infusion device

parenteral nutrition

vascular access

vascular access device

## Introduction

Home infusion pharmacy is a unique practice area for pharmacists and pharmacy technicians. It resembles hospital pharmacy in its preparation of sterile products, but it differs in several ways. Home infusion pharmacy is complex

147

because of the services it offers, the wide range of patient ages and medical conditions that it treats, and the coordination with other health care professionals that is required. Home infusion pharmacy also offers an expanded pharmaceutical care role for the pharmacist. In order to work in this area of pharmacy, pharmacists and pharmacy technicians must possess unique knowledge and sterile compounding skills. They must also be familiar with the specific legislation and regulations that pertain to home infusion pharmacy practice. This chapter focuses on the home infusion pharmacy and the unique roles of the pharmacist and pharmacy technician in this area. ▪

## OVERVIEW OF HOME INFUSION PHARMACY

A **home infusion pharmacy** is defined as a pharmacy that prepares and dispenses infusion therapies to patients in the home and alternative sites. These infusion therapies include intravenous (IV) solutions, other injectable drugs, and enteral nutrition therapy. Home infusion pharmacy began in the 1970s with the preparation of home total parenteral nutrition (TPN), when it was discovered that patients did not have to be hospitalized in order to receive long-term intravenous therapy. The same factors responsible for the overall growth in the home health care industry are also responsible for the growth in home infusion pharmacy. In particular, there have been rapid advances in technology, such as automated compounding devices, new types of vascular access devices, and safer, smaller, and more lightweight infusion devices. Equally as important, there is now updated knowledge concerning the compounding and stability of IV therapies. Today, home infusion pharmacies compound a wide variety of complex IV therapies that were previously prepared and administered only in hospitals.

Home infusion pharmacy has emerged as a separate and distinct pharmacy practice. Home infusion pharmacy involves the safe compounding of an IV therapy and its delivery to the patient. It also involves the provision of the equipment and supplies needed to infuse the therapy. Most important, it involves the provision of pharmaceutical care services by the home infusion pharmacist in the form of clinical care planning and monitoring.

Home infusion pharmacy is essentially a sterile compounding practice. It resembles a hospital pharmacy practice, but it differs in several ways. It does not involve the preparation or dispensing of oral dosage forms of medications, as part of a hospital pharmacy practice does. Home infusion pharmacy has a highly recognized clinical component. It follows a strict process that parallels the home health care process. Home infusion pharmacy involves different sterile compounding and safety issues. It adheres to very strict standards, especially concerning labeling, expiration dating, and record keeping. Home infusion pharmacy may use different equipment and supplies than hospital pharmacy practice, such as specialized IV containers or systems.

Home infusion pharmacies can be found in a variety of settings, ranging from community pharmacies, long-term care pharmacies, and hospital pharmacies to regional or national home infusion companies. Home infusion therapy can be the only type of pharmacy business for a particular pharmacy, or it can be just a part of its business. Regardless of the setting, home infusion therapy is provided only by a licensed pharmacy, with one exception. The exception is a physician practice that provides infusion therapy in the office. In this setting, a nurse, not a pharmacist, compounds the IV medication. This exception is most commonly seen in oncology and infectious disease practices.

# TYPES OF HOME INFUSION THERAPIES

There are many types of infusion therapies prescribed by physicians that are suitable for home infusion. As mentioned previously, infusion therapies include IV therapies, other injectable drug therapies, and enteral nutrition therapy. Diagnoses associated with these therapies include infection, malnutrition, chronic pain, cancer, dehydration, and congestive heart failure. Many of these therapies were once thought to require hospitalization or repeated physician office visits. However, with appropriate home infusion pharmacy services and nursing services to support them, it is possible to safely and effectively provide standard as well as complex infusion therapies in the home.

## ANTI-INFECTIVE THERAPY

Anti-infectives are the most common type of home infusion therapy. They include antibiotics, antifungals, and antivirals. Home infusion therapy with antibiotics is used to treat infections that require long-term IV therapy, such as cellulitis (an infection of soft tissue), osteomyelitis (an infection of the bone), pneumonia, urinary tract infections, and AIDS-related infections. Examples of antibiotics commonly used in the home include cephalosporins, penicillins, and vancomycin.

Antifungal therapy is used to treat persistent or serious fungal infections that are not responsive to oral therapy. Examples are amphotericin B, fluconazole, and caspofungin. Antiviral therapy is used to treat viral infections such as hepatitis and AIDS and includes ganciclovir, foscarnet, and cidofovir.

## PAIN MANAGEMENT THERAPY

Pain management therapy involves the continuous intravenous, subcutaneous, or epidural infusion of controlled substance analgesics to provide relief from chronic pain, in particular, chronic terminal cancer pain. Examples of analgesics used include morphine and hydromorphone.

## CHEMOTHERAPY

Home chemotherapy involves antineoplastic drugs that need to be infused over several hours or days. An example of this type of chemotherapy is 5-fluorouracil. Chemotherapy can be performed in the home as a result of safer practices and better patient, caregiver, and staff education.

## NUTRITION THERAPY

There are two types of nutrition therapy that are infused into the patient at home: enteral nutritional therapy and parenteral nutrition therapy. They are two of the most common home infusion therapies. Enteral nutrition therapy is infused into the gastrointestinal (GI) tract by means of a tube. Enteral formulas are not compounded in the home infusion pharmacy but are commercially available. Parenteral nutrition therapy is infused into the patient through a vein. Parenteral formulas are compounded in the home infusion pharmacy. Enteral and parenteral nutrition therapies are discussed later in this chapter.

## HYDRATION THERAPY

Hydration therapy involves the intravenous replacement of fluids, electrolytes, and vitamins lost as a result of dehydration. Dehydration can be due to medical conditions such as the vomiting of early pregnancy, the diarrhea associated with irritable bowel syndrome, or cancer states. Hydration therapy is usually a short-term therapy.

## BIOTECHNOLOGY THERAPY

Biotechnology therapy involves the administration of biotechnology drug products, also called biotech drugs, for various conditions, such as multiple sclerosis, rheumatoid arthritis, and growth disorders. These drugs are produced through genetic engineering. They are usually given for long periods of time and therefore are ideally suited for administration in the home setting. These drugs are usually administered through subcutaneous and conventional IV injection rather than by infusion. Examples of these drugs include growth hormone, erythropoietin, filgrastim, and interferon.

## MISCELLANEOUS THERAPIES

Several other infusion therapies are provided in the home. Not all of these are administered by intravenous infusion; some are administered by subcutaneous or conventional IV injection. Examples of these therapies include heparin, diuretics, steroids, H2-receptor antagonists, proton pump inhibitors, terbutaline (for premature labor), and dobutamine.

## ANCILLARY DRUGS

There are several injectable drugs that are provided to home infusion patients to assist in their therapy. Line maintenance drugs, such as low-dose heparin and sterile normal saline, are used to maintain intravenous lines. They flush IV catheters to prevent occlusion, or blockage. Anaphylaxis drugs, such as antihistamines, steroids, and epinephrine, usually in a kit form, are provided in the event of a severe allergic reaction, called anaphylaxis, to a home-administered drug. Patient-additive drugs are drugs that must be added to an intravenous infusion, usually a TPN, by the patient just before infusing. These are drugs that have limited stability or that can affect the overall stability of the IV infusion product if added too far in advance of administration. These drugs include vitamins, trace elements, insulin, heparin, and H2-receptor antagonists.

## ELEMENTS OF A HOME INFUSION PHARMACY

There are many elements that make up a home infusion pharmacy. Some of these elements are the same elements that are found in a traditional hospital pharmacy. However, some of these elements are unique.

### PERSONNEL

A wide variety of personnel are needed in the home infusion pharmacy to ensure its efficient operation. Pharmacists, pharmacy technicians, drivers, and other support personnel are found in a home infusion pharmacy.

A pharmacist who practices in a home infusion pharmacy is referred to as a home infusion pharmacist or, simply, an infusion pharmacist. The home infusion pharmacist has specialized knowledge of the home health care industry in general; home infusion pharmacy practice and management; and sterile drug product selection, compounding, and reimbursement. The pharmacy technician is an important member of the home infusion pharmacy team. The technician assists the pharmacist in compounding sterile drug products as well as in purchasing, assembling equipment and supplies, performing clerical duties, and ensuring quality control.

A driver is needed to deliver the infusion therapies, equipment, and supplies to patients in their homes or alternative sites in a safe, timely, and courteous manner. There are also several types of support personnel who contribute to a home infusion pharmacy operation. These include an intake coordinator, customer service representatives, billing personnel, and administrative personnel. The appropriate number of pharmacists, pharmacy technicians, and other personnel in the home infusion pharmacy depends on the size of the pharmacy, the number of patients it serves, and the types of infusion therapies that are offered.

### INVENTORY

The drug inventory in a home infusion pharmacy is limited and specialized. It differs from the inventory found in a traditional hospital pharmacy in that it does not include oral dosage forms of medications. The inventory consists of injectable drugs, intravenous fluids needed to compound sterile IV products, and ancillary drugs. The inventory in the home infusion pharmacy is customized for the types of infusion therapies offered by the pharmacy.

### PHARMACY DESIGN

In general, the design of a home infusion pharmacy resembles the design of the sterile products preparation area of a traditional hospital pharmacy. It is divided into different areas. The home infusion pharmacy has an IV compounding area or clean room for the preparation of sterile products, an anteroom, and an adjacent secure area for the storage of drugs, especially controlled drugs, and IV compounding supplies. The home infusion pharmacy has a separate area for the storage of equipment and supplies. This can be an open storage area, but in many home infusion pharmacies, there is a separate room or warehouse for this purpose. The home infusion pharmacy must also have a separate area for contaminated equipment and supplies. It is a type of holding area for receiving equipment, unused supplies, and waste that is returned from patients. The home infusion equipment is cleaned, repaired, and maintained in this area before being placed back into general storage. Overall, the home infusion pharmacy must be clean and secure and must provide patient confidentiality.

## EQUIPMENT AND SUPPLIES

A variety of equipment is found in the home infusion pharmacy. Most of this equipment can also be found in a traditional hospital pharmacy and includes horizontal and vertical laminar flow hoods, glove boxes, automated compounding devices, a large industrial refrigerator with a locked compartment for the storage of refrigerated Schedule II controlled substances, computer hardware and printers, facsimile machines, copiers, phone systems, and paging devices for drivers. A home infusion pharmacy uses specialized computer software that is capable of prescription processing, inventory management, clinical record keeping, and billing. Other specialized equipment consists of infusion devices and IV poles that are sent to the patient's home for administration of the infusion therapies.

Traditional hospital pharmacy supplies found in the home infusion pharmacy consist of syringes; needles; dispensing pins; IV containers; filters; transfer sets; IV tubing; alcohol prep pads; gowns; gloves; masks; beard and shoe covers (if using a clean room); prescription labels; and bags, boxes, or other packaging for transporting the finished sterile products. There are a few specialized IV containers or systems used predominately in home infusion, such as elastomeric balloons. There are also some specialized forms and reports and individual patient charts that are used in the home infusion pharmacy for clinical purposes.

## DELIVERY SERVICE

The safe and timely delivery of IV products, equipment, and supplies to the patient at home or at an alternative site is critical to a home infusion pharmacy operation. Timely delivery is necessary to avoid interruption of therapy and to guarantee the integrity of the sterile products. Changes in temperature can affect the stability of sterile products. Refrigerated products should be shipped in coolers. Chemotherapy should be shipped in protective containers in case of leakage. The delivery service also includes the pickup of equipment, unused supplies, and waste from the patient's home at the completion of therapy. A home infusion pharmacy should have protocols for the safe transport of all products, equipment, supplies, and waste.

# THE HOME INFUSION THERAPY PROCESS

The home infusion therapy process is a clinical process that parallels the home health care process in general. The various steps in the process are the same, but require the additional and separate input of the home infusion pharmacist.

## PHARMACY PATIENT ASSESSMENT

The pharmacy patient assessment is completed by the home infusion pharmacist on the patient's admission to the home infusion service. It is the basis for clinical decisions by the pharmacist. It includes patient demographic information, the primary diagnosis, medical history, functional limitations, initial laboratory work, and a review of body systems. A nutritional assessment and a drug regimen review are also part of this assessment. The nutritional assessment is an evaluation of the patient's nutritional status. It is performed to identify the patient's risk for malnutrition and is a Joint Commission standard. The drug regimen review is performed to determine if the prescribed infusion therapy is appropriate and to identify any drug-related problem, such as duplicate drug therapy, drug interactions, and actual or potential adverse drug reactions. It is also a Joint Commission standard. Any problems that are identified are included on the pharmaceutical care plan. The pharmacy patient assessment is part of the patient's medical record.

## PHARMACEUTICAL CARE PLAN

A pharmaceutical care plan, also referred to as a drug-related problems plan of care, is developed by the pharmacist at the start of therapy as part of the overall care plan for the home health care patient. The purposes of the pharmaceutical care plan are to achieve the goals of drug therapy and to minimize drug-related problems. Information from the pharmacy patient assessment is used to develop the pharmaceutical care plan.

There are five elements of a pharmaceutical care plan.

1. *Problems.* These include the problems being treated with medications as well as actual or potential drug-related problems that may occur.
2. *Goals.* These are the desired therapeutic outcomes associated with each problem.
3. *Interventions.* These are pharmacy-related activities that can achieve the desired goals.
4. *Monitoring.* This is information that can indicate if the interventions are producing the desired goals.
5. Resolution. This is documentation that the problems have been resolved.

Examples of the elements of a pharmaceutical care plan are given in Table 7–1.

**TABLE 7–1** Elements of a Pharmaceutical Care Plan

| PROBLEMS | GOALS | INTERVENTIONS | MONITORING | RESOLUTION |
|---|---|---|---|---|
| Cellulitis | Infection resolved | Vancomycin 1 gram IV every 12 hours for 4 weeks | Patient assessment | Infection cleared |
| Nephrotoxicity due to vancomycin | Nephrotoxicity avoided | Pharmacokinetic dose calculations and adjustments | Laboratory: vancomycin peak and trough levels | Negative nephrotoxicity |

The pharmaceutical care plan is reviewed and updated continuously throughout the patient's therapy. The pharmaceutical care plan is also part of the patient's medical record.

## MONITORING

The pharmacist monitors the patient's IV drug therapy according to the pharmaceutical care plan to ensure that the drug produces the desired effect and to avoid any problems. Monitoring is a continuous process. It involves several areas. The patient is monitored by a nurse during home visits to assess the response to the drug and any signs of drug-related problems, especially adverse reactions, and the nurse's findings are communicated to the pharmacist. Laboratory work is also monitored, such as serum drug levels, vancomycin peak and trough levels, and blood chemistries such as potassium or albumin levels. On the basis of monitoring, the pharmacist may make recommendations to adjust, change, continue, or discontinue IV drug therapy.

The results of monitoring are communicated by the pharmacist to the other health care professionals involved in the patient's care. In fact, a key element of home infusion pharmacy is the communication and sharing of information between the home infusion pharmacist and nurse. One type of communication is the patient care conference, which is a periodic meeting to discuss the patient and his care. Other forms of communication are written progress notes and telephone updates.

## DISCHARGE ASSESSMENT

The discharge assessment is performed by the home infusion pharmacist at the end of IV drug therapy. It is hoped that the drug therapy has resulted in the desired outcome. A discharge summary is completed to document that the goals of the IV drug therapy have been reached, and the patient is then discharged from the home infusion service.

## DOCUMENTATION

Home infusion pharmacy requires the complete documentation of pharmacy services. In addition to the normal prescription and dispensing records, a clinical record called the medication record or a chart must be developed for each patient. This requirement is unique to home infusion pharmacy. The chart contains documentation of all pharmacy activities and includes the pharmacy patient assessment, such as the nutritional assessment and the drug regimen review, IV prescription orders, pharmaceutical care plan, laboratory monitoring data, patient's medication profile, pharmacy compounding records, progress notes, patient care conference notes, supply list, and discharge summary. Maintaining the patient's chart is the responsibility of the home infusion pharmacist. The chart should be current and complete, and it should be easy to follow.

## THE PRESCRIPTION-FILLING PROCESS IN A HOME INFUSION PHARMACY

The process of filling and dispensing a prescription order in a home infusion pharmacy differs in several ways from the process used to dispense a prescription in any other type of pharmacy practice.

A prescription order for an infusion therapy originates with a physician. It is usually received in the home infusion pharmacy by facsimile machine, but it may also be received by phone or electronically. The prescription order must contain all of the necessary information. It is screened by the home infusion pharmacist, who then begins the home infusion therapy process. The prescription information is entered into the computer, using highly specialized computer software, by the pharmacist or pharmacy technician. This step leads to the generation of the prescription label and possibly packing lists and mixing reports. The prescription label for a home infusion therapy is different from the prescription label required for an infusion therapy used in the hospital setting. A home infusion prescription is considered to be an outpatient prescription, so it must be labeled according to state and federal requirements for outpatient prescriptions. It must contain a prescription number, date, patient's name, physician's name, drug name, concentration of the drug, diluent, rate and frequency of administration, pharmacist's initials, and expiration date. The total amount of drug or nutrient in each container and any pump settings should be included on the label (if the medication is to be administered by an infusion device). The patient and the caregiver should be able to understand the prescription label.

The prescription order is then compounded by a home infusion pharmacist or a pharmacy technician. Sterile compounding of a home infusion therapy involves greater risk than sterile compounding of a hospital infusion therapy. Home infusion therapies are usually prepared in batches, with several days' worth of product being prepared at one time. There is a longer period of time between when the drug is compounded and when it is administered to the patient. Therefore, there is a greater chance of contamination through the growth of bacteria in the product. Excellent aseptic technique is required to safeguard the sterility of the infusion mixture.

Complete documentation of the compounding process is required. A **compounding record,** also referred to as a mixing report, is a form used in the home infusion pharmacy to document compounding activities and is part of the patient's chart. It records the lot number and expiration date of the components in a sterile infusion product and any specific compounding instructions, as well the stability of the final product. Examples are shown in Figures 7–1 and 7–2. The entire compounding process is under the supervision of the pharmacist.

The labeling and expiration dating of the finished product constitute the final step in the prescription-filling process. An expiration date, or beyond-use date, is assigned to the infusion product by the pharmacist. Assigning an expiration date to a home infusion product is also different from assigning an expiration date to an infusion product for use in the hospital setting. The expiration dates for home infusion products are based on stability and sterility data. Physical and chemical changes can take place in the infusion product. The stability of a sterile product can be affected by temperature, light, material of the product container, combination of drugs within a mixture, order of mixing, method of infusion, and storage conditions in the home. The sterility of the product can be affected by the aseptic technique used in the preparation of the product and by the amount of time between the preparation and administration of the sterile product. The home infusion pharmacist must take all of these factors into consideration in assigning an expiration date. The expiration date that the pharmacist assigns should be the maximum date that falls within the appropriate

## MIXING REPORT

| Stability: | Patient Name: |
|---|---|
| Reference:  *Handbook of Inj. Drugs* | Origin Rx Number: |
| Other: | |
| Calculations: | Place copy of Rx label here: |
| Checked By | |

| Refill Date | Ingredients (one per line) | Volume used | Units used | Prepared date–time | MFG lot no. | Exp. date | Prep. by: |
|---|---|---|---|---|---|---|---|
| | | | | | | | |
| | | | | | | | |
| | | | | | | | |
| | | | | | | | |
| | | | | | | | |
| | | | | | | | |
| | | | | | | | |
| | | | | | | | |
| | | | | | | | |
| | | | | | | | |
| | | | | | | | |
| | | | | | | | |

**FIGURE 7–1**   Mixing Report.

stability limits for the individual components of the mixture based on USP guidelines. The final check of the prescription is made by the home infusion pharmacist. The infusion therapy is then packaged into bags or insulated boxes for delivery.

# TPN MIXING REPORT

| Patient Name: | | | RX No: | | | | | |
|---|---|---|---|---|---|---|---|---|
| **Pooled Electrolytes** | | Dose/Liter | (Vol. of Dose × | L) × 1.1 = Tot. Vol. | | Qty. | Lot No. | Exp. Date |
| Calcium Gluconate 10% | 0.48 mEq/ml | mEq | ( | ml × | L) × 1.1 = | | | |
| Magnesium Sulfate | 4 mEq/ml | mEq | ( | ml × | L) × 1.1 = | | | |
| Potassium Chloride | 2 mEq/ml | mEq | ( | ml × | L) × 1.1 = | | | |
| Potassium Acetate | 2 mEq/ml | mEq | ( | ml × | L) × 1.1 = | | | |
| Sodium Acetate | 2 mEq/ml | mEq | ( | ml × | L) × 1.1 = | | | |
| Sodium Chloride 23.4% | 4 mEq/ml | mEq | ( | ml × | L) × 1.1 = | | | |
| Copper | 0.4 mg/ml | mg | ( | ml × | L) × 1.1 = | | | |
| Manganese | 0.1 mg/ml | mg | ( | ml × | L) × 1.1 = | | | |
| Chromium | 4.0 mcg/ml | mcg | ( | ml × | L) × 1.1 = | | | |
| Selenium | 40.0 mcg/ml | mcg | ( | ml × | L) × 1.1 = | | | |
| Multiple Trace Elements Mix: | | ml | ( | ml × | L) × 1.1 = | | | |
| | | | ( | ml × | L) × 1.1 = | | | |
| | | | ( | ml × | L) × 1.1 = | | | |

| Number of IV Bags to be Prepared | | | Total Pooled Volume | ml | Volume per IV Bag: | | ml | |
|---|---|---|---|---|---|---|---|---|
| **Non Pooled Electrolytes** | | Dose/Liter | (Vol. of Dose × | L) × 1.1 = Tot. Vol. | | Qty. | Lot No. | Exp. Date |
| Potassium Phosphate | 4.4 mEq/m | ml | ( | ml × | L) × 1.1 = | | | |
| Sodium Phosphate | 4 mEq/ml | ml | ( | ml × | L) × 1.1 = | | | |
| | | | ( | ml × | L) × 1.1 = | | | |
| | | | ( | ml × | L) × 1.1 = | | | |

| IV Solution | Strength | Vol/Liter × Liters Prep = Total Volume | | | Final Conc. | Qty. | Lot No. | Exp. Date |
|---|---|---|---|---|---|---|---|---|
| Amino Acids | % | ml × | L = | ml | % | | | |
| Dextrose | % | ml × | L = | ml | % | | | |
| Sterile Water for Inj. | ml | ml × | L = | ml | | | | |
| Fat Emulsion | % | ml × | L = | ml | % | | | |
| **IV Bags** | Calculations by: | | | Prepared by: | | | | |
| 1 Liter | Date: | | | Date: | | | | |
| 2 Liter | Checked by: | | | | | | | |
| 3 Liter | Date: | | | | | | | |

**ATTACH COPY OF LABEL ON BACK OF THIS FORM**

**FIGURE 7–2**  TPN Mixing Report.

## THE PROVISION OF EQUIPMENT AND SUPPLIES FOR HOME INFUSION

Home infusion therapy requires special equipment and a variety of disposable supplies. The home infusion pharmacy provides the appropriate equipment and supplies necessary to infuse the prescribed home infusion therapy. One of the main duties of the pharmacy technician in the home infusion pharmacy is the processing of equipment and supply orders. The choice of supplies depends on several factors: the type of medication being infused, the container that holds the drug, the vascular access device in place in the patient, and the infusion device being used. The amount of supplies sent also depends on the duration, or the day's supply, of the therapy being sent and the frequency of deliveries, for example, weekly delivery. In order to perform this activity, the pharmacy technician must be familiar with several topics relevant to intravenous infusion in order to correctly choose and assemble the appropriate equipment and supplies. The pharmacy technician must be familiar with vascular access and vascular access devices, infusion devices, and other IV delivery systems.

### VASCULAR ACCESS DEVICES

**Vascular access**, also referred to as venous access, is defined as access to the bloodstream. Vascular access must be established in order to infuse intravenous medications. The type of vascular access depends on several factors, such as the age and mobility of the patient, condition of the patient's veins, type and volume of the IV infusion therapy to be infused, and length of IV therapy. There are two types of vascular access: peripheral vascular access and central vascular access. Peripheral vascular access is access to the bloodstream through a peripheral vein, such as the veins in the arm. Peripheral access is used for short-term IV therapy. Central vascular access is access to the bloodstream through a large vein in the chest that empties into the superior vena cava, the large blood vessel that leads into the heart. Central access is used for long-term IV therapy or for IV drugs that are irritating to the vein. Vascular access is achieved through a vascular access device.

A **vascular access device** is defined as a catheter inserted directly into a vein through which intravenous medication is infused. It provides vascular access, that is, access to a vein. The vascular access device is inserted and maintained for the duration of IV therapy, which can be from several days to several months or possibly several years. Maintenance consists of proper cleaning of the IV access site to prevent infection and flushing of the access device to prevent blockage. The amount and frequency of flushing and the choice of line maintenance drug (heparin, sterile normal saline) for flushing depend on the type of vascular access device in place and the protocol of the home infusion organization or pharmacy. The following sections discuss several types of vascular access devices.

### Peripheral Catheters

A peripheral catheter, also referred to as a peripheral line, is a short, flexible intravenous catheter that is inserted into a peripheral vein in the arm. It is up to an inch in length and is used for short-term IV therapy, generally for less than 10 days.

## Midline Catheters

A midline catheter is a long, flexible intravenous catheter that is inserted into a peripheral vein in the arm and threaded approximately 6 inches up the arm. It can be left in place for up to 4 weeks. A midline catheter is used for IV medication that is irritating to the vein or for therapy of a few weeks' duration.

## Central Venous Catheters

A central venous catheter is a rigid intravenous catheter that is surgically inserted into a large vein in the chest, with the tip positioned in the superior vena cava (Figure 7–3). A central venous catheter can remain in place for months to years. It is used for an IV therapy that requires a large volume of fluid, such as TPN, or for a very irritating IV therapy, such as chemotherapy. There are several well-known examples of central venous catheters: Leonard, Hickman, Broviac, and Groshong catheters. These central venous catheters are actually referred to as tunneled catheters. A tunneled catheter is a catheter that is tunneled, or burrowed, under the skin for a short distance before being inserted into a large vein in the chest. It provides stability and acts as a barrier to infection. Hickman and Broviac catheters require daily flushing with heparin. A Groshong catheter has a valve on the end and does not require heparin flushes but can be flushed with sterile normal saline.

## Peripherally Inserted Central Venous Catheters

A peripherally inserted central venous catheter, or PICC line, is a flexible intravenous catheter that is inserted peripherally into a vein in the arm and threaded into a large vein in the chest (Figure 7–4). It does not need to be inserted surgically but can be inserted by a specially trained nurse. An x-ray is required to verify the placement of the catheter. A PICC line can remain in place for months, possibly up to a year. It can be used for any type of IV therapy, including TPN and chemotherapy. A PICC line requires daily dressing changes and flushing with heparin.

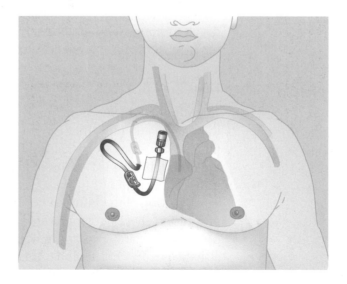

**FIGURE 7–3**   Central Venous Catheter.

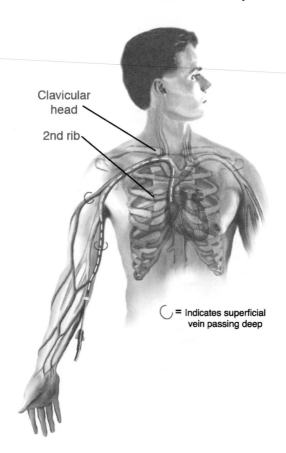

Clavicular head

2nd rib

ↄ = Indicates superficial vein passing deep

**FIGURE 7–4**    PICC Line.

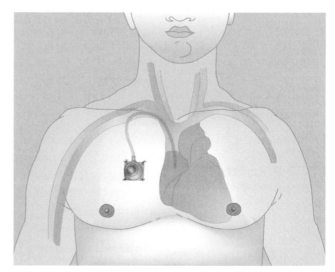

**FIGURE 7–5**    Subcutaneous Port.

### Subcutaneous Ports

A subcutaneous port is a vascular access device that is surgically implanted into a large vein in the chest, with all parts of the device under the skin (Figure 7–5). It consists of a reservoir covered by a rubber diaphragm and an attached catheter that is positioned in the vein. A port is accessed by inserting a special needle, called a Huber needle, into the port through the skin. This type of needle is a *non-coring* needle; that is, it does not produce a core or rubber plug with each insertion through the diaphragm. A Huber needle must be used with this type of device. A port is used for long-term, periodic IV therapy. It requires weekly flushing with sterile normal saline, if used, or monthly flushes, if not used.

### INFUSION DEVICES

An **infusion device** is defined as a device that regulates the infusion of an intravenous therapy, that is, that regulates the flow of the medication into the patient. Infusion devices, also referred to as infusion pumps or, simply, pumps, are especially needed in the home care setting to ensure the safe and accurate infusion of therapies in the absence of around-the-clock medical supervision. The selection of the infusion device depends on several factors, such as the type of infusion therapy being infused, patient's condition and lifestyle, ease of use of the pump, and cost and reimbursement. The choice of infusion device will also dictate the choice of the IV container (IV bag, syringe, elastomeric balloon) and the corresponding infusion supplies. There are two types of infusion devices: stationary infusion pumps and ambulatory infusion pumps.

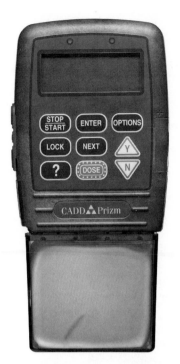

**FIGURE 7–6** Ambulatory Infusion Device. (Courtesy of Smiths Medical MD, Inc.)

A stationary infusion pump is an infusion device that attaches to an IV pole. Stationary pumps were developed for hospital use but are also used in home care. They are used for patients who are bedridden or for patients who receive infusion therapy during the night. Over the years, new technology has made these pumps lighter and smaller. They can be programmed automatically and use standard IV administration sets.

An ambulatory infusion pump is an infusion device that is small, lightweight, and portable and can be worn by the patient. It is used for patients who are ambulatory. There are two types of ambulatory pumps: therapy-specific pumps and multiple-therapy pumps. A therapy-specific pump is an ambulatory infusion pump designed to infuse a specific type of infusion therapy, such as TPN or antibiotics. As an example, there are several therapy-specific pumps in the CADD infusion pump line by Smiths Medical MD, Inc. The CADD-Legacy pump is for infusing antibiotics; the CADD-TPN pump is for infusing TPN; and the CADD-Legacy PCA pump is for patient-controlled analgesia, or PCA. A multiple-therapy pump is designed to infuse a variety of infusion therapies. An example is the CADD-Prizm VIP pump by Smiths Medical MD, Inc. (Figure 7–6).

New infusion pump technology has emerged that combines the latest in drug delivery technology with software that focuses on patient safety and medication error reduction. These new pumps have been referred to as "smart" pumps by the Institute for Safe Medical Practices. A "smart" pump is an infusion device that incorporates computer software to perform a variety of functions in addition to drug delivery. One of the most important features of these pumps is pre-set dosage levels. Computer software checks the dose of the drug being programmed into the pump against pre-set limits specific for the drug. Therefore, if the infusion pump is programmed incorrectly, the programmer is alerted that the dose is outside of the recommended range. It has been found that "smart" pumps reduce the occurrence of potentially fatal IV dosing errors. Additional features are the pump's ability to monitor a patient's vital signs, such as temperature and heart rate, while infusing; the ability to be programmed from a remote site; bar code scanners; and the ability to interface with other home infusion software. Advances in infusion pump technology will continue well into the future.

There are several other delivery systems used in home care to administer infusion therapies, such as the following:

- *Gravity infusion system.* The medication is contained in a minibag and is infused by gravity. It is regulated by controlling the number of drops. It is used for patient self-administration and is a stationary system.
- *Syringe infusion system.* The intravenous medication is contained in a syringe and is infused by means of a special syringe pump. This system is used to infuse small volumes and is also a stationary system.
- *Elastomeric balloon system.* The drug is contained inside a pressurized balloon reservoir and is infused by deflating the device. The rate of infusion is controlled by the use of special tubing. This device is small, lightweight, disposable, and simple to use. It is an ambulatory system. An example of an elastomeric device is shown in Figure 7–7.
- *IV push system.* The drug is contained in a syringe and is infused by manually depressing the plunger of the syringe. Drugs administered by IV push are infused very rapidly.

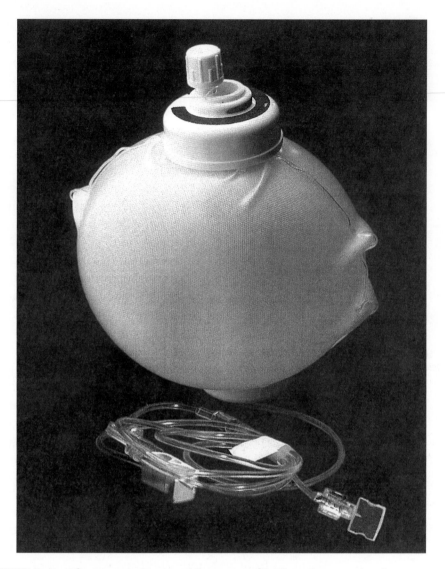

**FIGURE 7–7**    Elastomeric Device. (Courtesy of I-Flow Corporation.)

## HOME INFUSION SUPPLIES

There are many different types of disposable supplies used in home infusion and delivered to the patient along with the infusion therapy. These supplies include:

- IV start kits—self-contained packets of supplies used to insert a peripheral catheter or to change the dressing at the site
- CVC dressing kit—central venous catheter dressing change kit; also self-contained packets of supplies for changing the dressing at the site
- IV tubing—also called IV sets
- Extension tubing—also called extension sets
- IV clave—a universal connector using a needle-less system. A CLC connector is a special connector for Groshong products.
- IV filters—used for central lines
- Injection caps—used to close the end of a catheter

- Needle-less syringe systems—used to flush catheters
- IV poles—for stationary infusion pumps
- Sterile dressings—include sterile gauze dressings and occlusive dressings
- Antibacterial cleaning solutions—for cleaning IV sites; include alcohol pads, povidone iodine swab sticks, or chlorhexedrine
- Sharps containers—for used syringes and needles
- Infectious waste bags or receptacles—for infectious waste, which is considered to be biohazardous waste
- Tape—used to secure dressings
- Masks—used during changing dressings
- Gloves—include nonsterile gloves for drawing blood or handling chemotherapy and sterile gloves for changing dressings
- Batteries—for infusion devices that are battery-operated
- Chemotherapy spill kits—used in case of a chemotherapy spill in the home
- Ancillary drugs

## NUTRITION THERAPY

There are two types of nutritional therapy provided by a home infusion pharmacy: enteral nutrition therapy and parenteral nutrition therapy. Enteral therapy is not an intravenous therapy; however, it is infused into the patient, so it is included here. It is also the most common home infusion nutritional therapy. Pharmacists and pharmacy technicians must be familiar with this type of infusion therapy and with the various enteral nutrition products, access devices, and equipment and supplies associated with enteral nutrition therapy.

### ENTERAL NUTRITION THERAPY

**Enteral nutrition** is defined as nutrition delivered into the GI tract through a tube. Often referred to as *tube feeding,* enteral nutrition is the most common home infusion nutritional therapy. It is the next approach when oral nutrition is not appropriate or possible. Enteral nutrition can be used to supplement oral or parenteral nutrition, or it can be used to meet the patient's entire nutritional needs. Home enteral nutrition is prescribed for patients with swallowing problems due to dementia, stroke, or trauma or for patients with AIDS, cancer, or other debilitating diseases. Enteral nutrition formulas are not compounded in the home infusion pharmacy but are commercially available.

#### Access to the Gastrointestinal Tract

Infusing enteral nutrition requires some type of access into the GI tract. A hollow tube, called a feeding tube, provides access. It is placed into the stomach or the upper part of the small intestine (the duodenum or the jejunum) through the nose or through the skin. The feeding site (stomach or small intestine) and the method of placement are determined by the duration of the enteral therapy, type and volume of the enteral formula to be infused, amount of the patient's GI function, feeding schedule, ease of placement, and cost.

**TABLE 7–2**   Types of Enteral Feeding Tubes

| FEEDING TUBE | ABBREVIATION | PLACEMENT | SITE |
|---|---|---|---|
| Nasogastric tube | NG tube | Nose | Stomach |
| Nasoduodenal tube | ND tube | Nose | Duodenum |
| Nasojejunal tube | NJ tube | Nose | Jejunum |
| Percutaneous endoscopic gastrostomy tube | PEG tube | Skin (guided into place by endoscopy) | Stomach |
| Percutaneous endoscopic jejunostomy tube | PEJ tube | Skin (guided into place by endoscopy) | Jejunum |

For example, feeding tubes placed into the stomach through the nose are used for short-term enteral therapy of up to 3 or 4 weeks. They are low in cost and easy to place. However, they cause irritation, are easily blocked or occluded, and are easily displaced. Feeding tubes placed into the stomach or small intestine through the skin are used for long-term enteral therapy because they are not as irritating and are not easily displaced. The types of feeding tubes correspond to the site and method of placement. These are listed in Table 7–2 and pictured in Figure 7–8. It is important for the pharmacy technician to know the type, including the brand, and size of the feeding tube that has been placed in the patient in order to select the appropriate enteral infusion device and supplies.

**Enteral Formulas**

There are a number of commercially available enteral formulas. Different types of formulas meet different patient needs. Enteral formulas do not require a prescription and are considered an over-the-counter item. When they are infused into the patient through an infusion device, however, they are considered a home infusion therapy. The pharmacy technician must be familiar with the different types of enteral formulas.

Standard formulas—for the majority of patients

Lactose-free formulas—for patients who are lactose-intolerant

High-calorie formulas—for patients who have an increased need for calories, such as burn or trauma patients, or for patients who are on fluid restriction

High-protein formulas—for patients who have an increased need for protein, such as patients with wounds or decubitus ulcers

Fiber-containing formulas—for patients who need increased fiber to help maintain bowel functioning

Hydrolyzed protein formulas—formulas containing protein that has been broken down into amino acids; for patients who are unable to digest and absorb proteins owing to some type of GI dysfunction

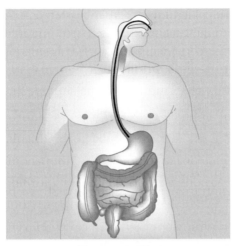

Nasogastric Tube

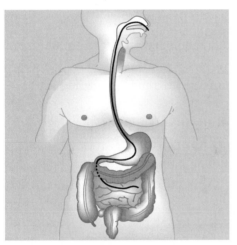

Nasojejunal Tube

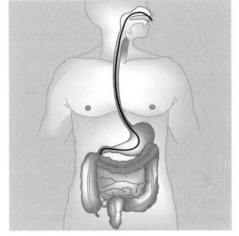

Nasoduodenal Tube

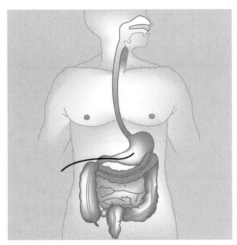

Percutaneous Endoscopic
Gastrostomy Tube

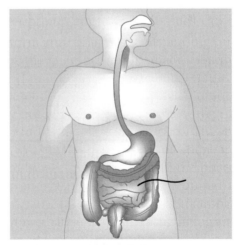

Percutaneous Endoscopic
Jejunostomy Tube

**FIGURE 7–8** Enteral Feeding Tubes.

Specialized formulas—referred to as *disease-specific* formulas; for patients who have a specific disease or condition, for example, hepatic formulas, renal formulas, pulmonary formulas, diabetic formulas, and trauma or high-stress formulas

Modular formulas—single supplements of carbohydrate, protein, or fat to be added to another enteral formula or to enhance a regular food diet

The selection of the appropriate enteral formula for the patient depends on several factors, such as:

- The patient's ability to digest and absorb a formula
- The patient's nutritional status
- The patient's current medical conditions
- The patient's ability to tolerate fluid
- The patient's electrolyte status
- The route of delivery
- The patient's current drug regimen (there is the possibility of a nutrient-drug interaction)
- The ease of use (no mixing or added ingredients required; the formula is easy to find)
- The cost of and reimbursement for the formula

The home infusion pharmacist also monitors enteral nutrition. The pharmacist continuously assesses the patient and examines laboratory data to ensure that the enteral formula selected for use is the most appropriate choice. Oftentimes a change in the enteral formula is necessary. The American Society for Enteral and Parenteral Nutrition has established Standards for Home Nutition Support and Standards for Nutrition Support Pharmacists. A nutrition support pharmacist is a pharmacist with specialized training in providing nutritional care.

### Enteral Infusion Equipment and Supplies

Enteral infusion therapy requires special equipment and supplies. An infusion device is necessary to infuse enteral nutrition. The infusion device regulates the flow of the enteral formula into the GI tract. Enteral infusion devices, also referred to as enteral nutrition pumps or enteral feeding pumps, are used only to deliver enteral formulas. They are different from and not interchangeable with intravenous infusion pumps. Enteral pumps are usually marketed by enteral formula companies, which also supply enteral bags and tubing. An example of an enteral infusion pump is shown in Figure 7–9.

Special supplies are also needed to administer enteral nutrition therapy. Special bags, called enteral bags, which resemble intravenous bags, hold the volume of enteral nutrition to be infused. Special tubing, called enteral tubing, which also resembles intravenous tubing, conducts the formula into the patient. These enteral supplies are not interchangeable with intravenous supplies.

## PARENTERAL NUTRITION THERAPY

**Parenteral nutrition** is nutrition delivered directly into the bloodstream through a vein. TPN was the first type of home infusion therapy and is the

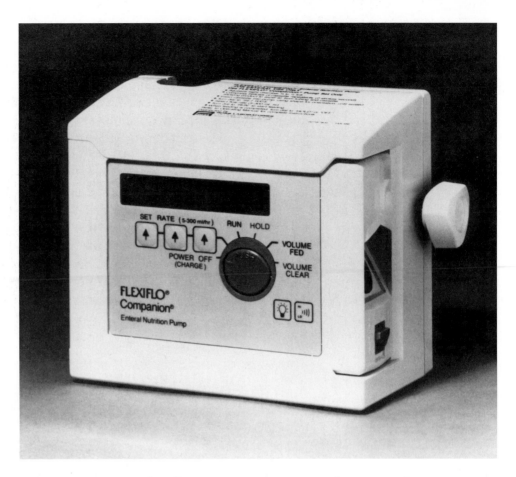

**FIGURE 7–9** Enteral Infusion Pump. (Courtesy of Ross Products Division, Abbott Laboratories.)

second most common home infusion therapy today. There are a few noteworthy differences between parenteral nutrition compounded for use in the home care setting and parenteral nutrition compounded for use in the hospital setting.

Parenteral nutrition, or TPN, for home infusion is usually compounded as a 3-in-1 solution; that is, the amino acid, dextrose, and lipid sources are all contained in the same bag. This type of solution is more convenient for the patient and caregiver, and it requires less manipulation and fewer supplies. There are, however, compounding and stability concerns associated with the use of 3-in-1 solutions.

TPN formulations are highly complex, and proper mixing, either manually or by means of an automated compounding device, is important. An improper order of mixing ingredients can cause drug precipitates to form or the emulsion to break. A safe and effective order of mixing ingredients should be followed. Each completed TPN should be visibly inspected. In addition, the nurse, patient, and caregiver should be instructed to perform a visual inspection of the product before infusing and to recognize a "broken" formulation.

TPN formulations for home infusion are usually prepared several days before they are administered. During that time, changes can take place in the solution. Many variables can affect the stability of the TPN, such as temperature, the delivery process, storage conditions in the home, and the mixture in general. There are some ingredients in a TPN that have limited stability. They can degrade or lose their potency. Loss of potency occurs with vitamins, trace elements, heparin, and insulin. The H2-receptor antagonist drug ranitidine loses its potency by binding to the plastic IV bag. These drugs should be added by the patient or caregiver on a daily basis just before infusing. These drugs are indicated as "patient additives" on the prescription label. There are other ingredients that can affect the overall stability of the TPN over the course of time. They can cause a reaction that destabilizes or breaks the formulation. Again, everyone involved in the handling and administration of the TPN should be instructed to perform a visual inspection of the product before infusing. Last, the use of in-line filters should be encouraged to prevent administration of particles, microorganisms, and air to the patient. The American Society for Parenteral and Enteral Nutrition (ASPEN) has published safety guidelines for TPN formulations that deal with the prescribing, compounding, labeling, and administration of TPN solutions. Home infusion pharmacists and pharmacy technicians should be aware of the problems associated with TPN formulations for home infusion and should consult these guidelines to improve the safety of home TPN.

## LEGISLATION AND REGULATIONS FOR HOME INFUSION PHARMACY

Home infusion pharmacies are licensed and regulated by their respective state boards of pharmacy. In a number of states, home infusion pharmacies are licensed as "retail" pharmacies because these states do not have a separate license category for home infusion pharmacies. However, the majority of states now have a separate license category for home infusion pharmacies with specific requirements unique to this type of pharmacy practice. These requirements relate to personnel, equipment, staffing, the physical environment of the pharmacy, and the compounding of sterile products. Some states require a home infusion pharmacy to have an additional license to dispense sterile products to patients who reside in other states.

Home infusion pharmacies must comply with all state and federal laws and regulations, especially those concerning the compounding of sterile products, in particular, documentation. Model Rules for Sterile Pharmaceuticals, developed by the National Association of Boards of Pharmacy, serve as a guide. These model rules require that the manufacturer's lot number and the expiration date of the individual components used in compounding a sterile drug product be recorded. Recording is performed through the use of the compounding or mixing report. Even though some states may not legally require this documentation, it is required by the USP.

Currently, there is no federal requirement for a home health care agency to obtain consultant pharmacist services, such as drug regimen review, as in the long-term care facility. However, because most home health care accrediting organizations require a pharmacist's involvement, most home health care agencies employ or contract with a pharmacist to provide pharmaceutical care services. Following are several specific federal regulations that govern home infusion pharmacy.

## MEDICARE PRESCRIPTION DRUG BENEFIT

The Medicare Prescription Drug Benefit, or Medicare Part D, presents a challenge to the Medicare beneficiary who requires home infusion therapy and to the home infusion pharmacy. Medicare Part D covers home infusion drugs not already covered under the Medicare Part B Durable Medical Equipment (DME) benefit, as long as they are on the plan's formulary. As in long-term care pharmacy, the cost of home delivery is incorporated into a higher dispensing fee for the home infusion pharmacy. However, Medicare Part D does not cover pharmacy or nursing services, supplies, or the equipment necessary to administer these drugs. This drug-only coverage is inconsistent with the practice and accreditation standards followed by home infusion pharmacies. These standards are followed to ensure the safe administration of home infusion therapies. It is hoped that in the future, the CMS will reconsider complete coverage for home infusion therapies, perhaps under Medicare Part B, where limited coverage for some therapies already exists.

## OMNIBUS BUDGET RECONCILIATION ACT OF 1990

OBRA 90 mandates patient counseling. This counseling requirement applies to home infusion pharmacy practice. A home infusion pharmacist is required to counsel the home infusion patient about the safe and effective use of the infusion drug therapy. This counseling may be provided by means of consultation over the phone, by home visits, or through written or printed information in the form of a computer-generated printout.

## DRUG ENFORCEMENT AGENCY REGULATIONS

There is an exception to the DEA requirement for a written prescription for an injectable Schedule II controlled substance for a home infusion patient. The exception applies if the prescription is for a Schedule II controlled substance that is compounded for administration to a patient by IV, SQ, epidural, or intraspinal infusion. A copy of the prescription may be faxed to the home infusion pharmacy, and the facsimile copy is considered a written prescription. It is not necessary for the original written prescription to be delivered to the home infusion pharmacy, either before or after the delivery of the drug to the patient's home. The facsimile copy must contain all the information required for a normal written Schedule II prescription, including the physician's signature. The home infusion pharmacy is required to retain the facsimile copy in the same manner as a normal written Schedule II prescription. This exception is intended to make it easier for a home infusion pharmacy to obtain prescriptions for patients requiring frequently changed injectable Schedule II controlled substances. This exception does not apply to the dispensing of oral dosage forms of Schedule II controlled substances.

## UNITED STATES PHARMACOPEIA (USP) CHAPTER <797>

USP Chapter <797>, "Pharmaceutical Compounding—Sterile Preparations," was published in 2003 and went into effect in 2004, with proposed revisions to be published in 2007. This chapter sets standards for the compounding, preparing, and labeling of sterile drug preparations and applies to all practice settings that compound sterile preparations, including the home infusion pharmacy. Prior to Chapter <797>, most home infusion pharmacies were voluntarily following safe compounding practice standards. However, new standards are now required and enforced by the FDA and state boards of pharmacy, and compliance is expected by accrediting organizations. The purpose of these new sterile compounding regulations is to ensure the accuracy and sterility of compounded sterile drugs in order to protect the patient from inaccurately prepared or contaminated drugs.

There are several areas of concern that have been addressed in Chapter <797>. The most important issues that apply to a home infusion pharmacy are beyond-use dating and maintaining the quality of the sterile drug preparation once it leaves the pharmacy. These are important, because many sterile products compounded in the home infusion pharmacy are prepared several days before administration and are stored.

The beyond-use date, according to USP, is calculated from the time a sterile drug product is compounded until the product is administered to the patient. This expiration date is based on the three risk levels for contamination of sterile products published by the USP: low, medium, and high risk. For example, a TPN is considered a medium-risk sterile product, and the maximum beyond-use date under refrigeration for a medium-risk product is considered to be 7 days. This could pose a problem when more than a 7-day supply of a TPN is compounded, delivered, and stored. Table 7–3 lists the USP beyond-use dating guidelines for sterile compounded products.

Maintaining the quality and integrity of the sterile product once it leaves the home infusion pharmacy is important. Suitable packaging for transport is required, especially for refrigerated products and chemotherapy. Compounded sterile products should not be shaken or exposed to excessive heat or light, during both delivery and storage. The patient or caregiver must be trained as to the proper storage of the sterile drug product in the home.

Ensuring the accuracy and sterility of compounded sterile drugs is the purpose of USP Chapter <797>. The home infusion pharmacist, pharmacy technician, and driver play an important role in maintaining the quality of these drugs.

### FDA ALUMINUM MANDATE

In 2004, the Food and Drug Administration mandated new requirements for TPN formulations in regard to the aluminum content. Aluminum is an

**TABLE 7–3** USP Beyond-Use Dating Guidelines for Compounded Sterile Products

| RISK LEVEL | ROOM TEMPERATURE | REFRIGERATION | FREEZER |
| --- | --- | --- | --- |
| Low | 48 hours | 14 days | 45 days |
| Medium | 30 hours | 7 days | 45 days |
| High | 24 hours | 3 days | 45 days |

Adapted from *The United States Pharmacopeia* (29th ed.) and *The National Formulary* (24th ed.), Rockville, MD: Author.

element that may be toxic to patients with impaired kidney function. Variable amounts of aluminum are present in the raw materials used to make TPNs or are produced during the compounding process. In order to assure the safety of TPN formulations and to reduce the adverse reactions associated with them, FDA regulations require that the aluminum content of the products used to compound TPN solutions be labeled by the manufacturer and that the aluminum level of the finished TPN be calculated. Home infusion pharmacists are responsible for choosing the lowest-aluminum-containing raw materials, calculating the aluminum load for each component of a TPN and for the final solution, calculating the amount of aluminum that a patient is receiving based on the patient's body weight, and comparing that amount to published data to determine whether the aluminum level is safe, unsafe, or toxic for the patient.

## NATIONAL INSTITUTE FOR OCCUPATIONAL SAFETY AND HEALTH HAZARDOUS DRUG ALERT

The National Institute for Occupational Safety and Health (NIOSH), part of the U.S. Department of Health and Human Services, issued an alert in 2004 that sets guidelines for the preparation of chemotherapy and other cytotoxic agents. These drugs can be hazardous to health care workers who prepare them, especially pharmacists and pharmacy technicians, as well as to those who handle them, such as drivers who deliver these drugs to patients' homes. The guidelines were developed to protect health care workers. They call for the use of appropriate equipment, such as biological safety cabinets and closed-system drug transfer devices; proper gowning, including double gloves, when compounding as well as when unpacking shipments of hazardous drugs; standardized compounding procedures; and quality control procedures, such as the decontamination of work surfaces and the transportation of hazardous drugs in a closed container, to minimize or eliminate the potential danger associated with these drugs. The NIOSH alert has been incorporated into USP and ASHP practice standards.

## FDA SAFE MEDICAL DEVICES ACT

The FDA Safe Medical Devices Act of 1990 requires that all medical devices be tracked. Infusion pumps, IV and enteral, are medical devices. Under this law, the home infusion pharmacy must know the location of all of its infusion pumps at all times. A tracking system must be in place. Tracking can be accomplished by keeping a file or log on each device, including the serial number of the device, patient name and address, and dates of service. Tracking records must be maintained for the useful life of the device.

Joint Commission standards, although not legally required, also require that infusion devices be tracked in case of a recall or to perform preventative maintenance. The Joint Commission requires preventative maintenance once or twice a year or according to the manufacturer's recommendation, and requires that the devices be cleaned and checked after each patient use. The reliability of infusion pumps is critical to the safe and accurate administration of IV products. A sample of an infusion pump tracking record is shown in Figure 7–10.

## PUMP CERTIFICATION/TRACKING RECORD

| Pump Type | | Serial Number | | | | |
|---|---|---|---|---|---|---|
| Date Out | Patient/Facility/Address | Date In | Date Cleaned | Date Checked | Initial | |
| | | | | | | |
| | | | | | | |
| | | | | | | |
| | | | | | | |
| | | | | | | |
| | | | | | | |
| | | | | | | |
| | | | | | | |
| | | | | | | |
| | | | | | | |
| | | | | | | |
| | | | | | | |

Upon return all pumps will be cleaned and must pass all functional tests before being placed in inventory.

| Activity | Comments                        Date |
|---|---|
| 1. External Inspection<br>  • All controls are in good working order<br>  • Electrical cord and plug are in good order<br>  • Internal and external doors are in good working order | |
| 2. Equipment Cleaning (do not submerge pump)<br>  • Clean with mild soap solution<br>  • Disinfect with alcohol or hydrogen peroxide<br>  • Dry thoroughly with a soft cloth | |
| 3. Battery and Power Up Check<br>  • Plug pump in and turn on<br>  • Remove plug, and test battery operation | |
| 4. Motor Operation Check<br>  • Insert an administration set<br>  • Set volume to be delivered to 50 ml<br>  • Set rate to 50 ml/hr<br>  • Press run, hear pump run and display proper settings | |
| 5. Alarm Check<br>  • Press run and open outer door<br>  • Alarm sounds and proper error message is displayed | |

**FIGURE 7–10**    Infusion Pump Tracking Record.

## FREEDOM OF CHOICE LAW

The Freedom of Choice law allows a patient to select the pharmacy of his choice for services, including home infusion services. A patient who is referred to a home health care organization and ultimately to a home infusion pharmacy has the right to refuse that referral and to select the home health care organization and home infusion pharmacy of his choice.

## JOINT COMMISSION STANDARDS FOR HOME INFUSION PHARMACY

The Joint Commission is the primary accrediting organization for home infusion therapy. The Joint Commission has been accrediting home infusion pharmacies since 1988. Joint Commission accreditation for home infusion pharmacies is voluntary and not legally required. Accreditation is sought by the home infusion pharmacy itself and by its referral sources, payers, and patients. Accreditation implies quality and value. More important, the standards on which accreditation is based are a model for how a home infusion pharmacy should operate. These standards promote patient safety and optimum outcomes.

As with long-term care pharmacy accreditation, home infusion pharmacy accreditation is not intended for individual home infusion pharmacists but for the organization as a whole. The survey process is detailed and addresses all areas of home infusion pharmacy. The surveyor has experience specific to home health care and home infusion. The Joint Commission surveys the home infusion pharmacy for compliance with USP Chapter <797> regulations for sterile compounding. These standards relate to personnel training and evaluation, beyond-use dating and labeling, the use of automated compounding devices, aseptic compounding technique, and the checking and testing of finished products. In addition, to meet Joint Commission home infusion pharmacy standards, there are specific activities that the home infusion pharmacist must perform or be involved in. These include the nutritional assessment, the pharmaceutical care plan, the patient's medication profile as part of the chart, the determination of aluminum content, progress notes, written communications to physicians and nurses, the tracking and maintenance of infusion devices, and prescription labeling, including the labeling of line maintenance drugs, anaphylaxis drugs, and patient additive drugs. Pain management standards have been added, and home infusion pharmacists must seek to improve pain management for their home infusion patients through their pharmaceutical care services.

The Joint Commission has combined home infusion pharmacy, home care pharmacy, and long-term care pharmacy under home care accreditation. It was found that a significant number of long-term care pharmacies also provide home care or home infusion services. There are common standards as well as unique standards that apply to each type of pharmacy.

## OTHER ACCREDITATIONS FOR HOME INFUSION PHARMACY

There are two other organizations that accredit the home infusion pharmacy: the Community Health Accreditation Program (CHAP) and the Accreditation Commission for Health Care (ACHC). In addition, several national pharmacy organizations, including the National Home Infusion Association, have established the Pharmacy Compounding Accreditation Board (PCAB), a voluntary pharmacy accreditation program for all types of compounding, including sterile compounding. The purpose of this accreditation is to improve the quality and raise the awareness of compounding in all pharmacy settings. PCAB standards relate to all aspects of compounding: the pharmacist and pharmacy technician, the physical setup of the pharmacy, the compounding equipment, and the process. PCAB accreditation demonstrates to the FDA and state boards of pharmacy adherence to the highest standards of pharmacy compounding.

## THE ROLE OF THE PHARMACIST IN HOME INFUSION

Home infusion pharmacy practice offers a variety of roles for the pharmacist. These can be divided into clinical, dispensing, and administrative roles. In general, in order to practice successfully in the home infusion setting, the pharmacist should possess traditional pharmacy knowledge and skills; an overall knowledge of the home health care industry; and knowledge of home infusion, vascular access, and the selection, use, and maintenance of the drugs, equipment, and supplies used in home infusion.

### CLINICAL ROLE

The clinical role of the home infusion pharmacist is the most visible and important role. It involves the provision of pharmaceutical care services. Specific activities include identifying problems; assessing patients; developing care plans; performing interventions; monitoring therapy for appropriate response; collaborating with other home health care team members; providing nutrition support; detecting adverse drug reactions and drug interactions; participating in patient care conferences; documenting clinical activities; providing drug information to the home health care team members, especially physicians and nurses; and counseling patients and caregivers concerning their infusion therapies.

### DISPENSING ROLE

The dispensing role of the home infusion pharmacist is related to the compounding of home infusion therapies and the provision of related equipment and supplies. Specific activities include screening prescription orders; performing compounding calculations; compounding or supervising compounding; selecting ancillary drugs; determining the appropriate infusion device; selecting necessary supplies; and performing the final check on all medications, equipment, and supplies before dispensing them from the pharmacy.

### ADMINISTRATIVE ROLE

The administrative role of the home infusion pharmacist is related to the management of the home infusion pharmacy. Typical administrative activities include hiring, training, and testing pharmacists and pharmacy technicians; supervising all personnel; developing policies and procedures that pertain to home infusion pharmacy services; ensuring compliance with state and federal legislation and regulations and Joint Commission or other accreditation standards; purchasing drugs, equipment, and supplies; and maintaining records.

## THE ROLE OF THE PHARMACY TECHNICIAN IN HOME INFUSION

The role of the pharmacy technician in the home infusion pharmacy is an important one. The pharmacy technician performs many activities pertaining to the compounding of sterile products and the handling of home infusion equipment and supplies. Having the pharmacy technician perform these activities allows the home infusion pharmacist time to perform critical clinical activities.

In order to work in a home infusion pharmacy, the pharmacy technician must possess traditional pharmacy knowledge and skills as well as knowledge and skills specific to home infusion pharmacy, such as:

- Knowledge of home infusion therapies and nutritional products
- Knowledge of the home infusion process
- In-depth knowledge of sterile compounding
- Excellent aseptic technique
- Knowledge of pharmaceutical calculations
- Knowledge of vascular access devices
- Knowledge of home infusion equipment and supplies
- Knowledge of the documenting and record-keeping requirements in home infusion pharmacy
- General knowledge of reimbursement
- Excellent computer skills
- An understanding of the legislation and regulations pertaining to home infusion pharmacy

The pharmacy technician in a home infusion pharmacy works under the direct supervision of the home infusion pharmacist. The technician will not be involved in any activity that requires professional judgment. There are many varied activities that the pharmacy technician may perform in the home infusion pharmacy. These can be divided into three areas: compounding, equipment and supplies, and computer functions.

## STERILE COMPOUNDING

The traditional role of the pharmacy technician in a home infusion pharmacy is the compounding of sterile products. Other activities in this area include labeling sterile products; completing compounding records; performing quality control activities in the compounding area; cleaning and disinfecting the compounding area; completing cleaning logs; ordering, receiving, and stocking IV medications and compounding supplies; and cleaning and performing quality control checks on compounding equipment.

## EQUIPMENT AND SUPPLIES

The most important activity for the pharmacy technician in this area is the processing of home infusion equipment and supply orders. This involves the picking, assembling, and packaging of the appropriate equipment and supplies and arranging for their delivery. Other activities that the pharmacy technician may be responsible for are programming infusion devices; cleaning, tracking, and maintaining infusion devices and completing the proper documentation; maintaining inventory and warehouse areas; disposing of hazardous waste generated in the pharmacy and returned from patients; and ordering, receiving, and stocking home infusion equipment and supplies.

## COMPUTER FUNCTIONS

The pharmacy technician can perform several computer functions in the home infusion pharmacy. The pharmacy technician can enter new patient referrals, prescription orders, and orders for home infusion equipment, supplies, and ancillary drugs; can generate medication labels, packing lists, and compounding records; and can print educational materials for patients. The pharmacy technician also supports the pharmacist in clinical activities by collecting patient data and laboratory results, maintaining patient charts, and printing out progress notes and communications with other home health care team members.

## KEY CONCEPTS

- Home infusion pharmacy practice is a sterile compounding practice that also involves the provision of infusion equipment and supplies and pharmaceutical care.
- The types of home infusion therapies provided by a home infusion pharmacy include intravenous therapies, injectable drug therapies, and nutrition therapies.
- The home infusion pharmacy has traditional and unique elements.
- The home infusion therapy process is a clinical process that parallels the home health care process.
- A pharmaceutical care plan is developed by the home infusion pharmacist to help achieve the goals of drug therapy and to minimize drug therapy problems.
- The prescription-filling process in a home infusion pharmacy is different from this process in other types of pharmacies.
- Access to the bloodstream for intravenous therapy is accomplished peripherally or centrally through different types of vascular access devices.
- There are different types of devices and systems that regulate and deliver infusion therapy.
- There are a variety of disposable supplies needed for home infusion therapy.
- Enteral nutrition therapy is a type of infusion therapy that is administered into the GI tract rather than into the bloodstream.
- There are compounding and stability issues concerning home infusion parenteral nutrition therapy.
- There are legislation and regulations that pertain specifically to home infusion pharmacy.
- The home infusion pharmacy offers a strong clinical role for the pharmacist and several tasks for the pharmacy technician, the most important being the compounding of sterile products and the processing of home infusion equipment and supply orders.

## SELF-ASSESSMENT QUESTIONS

### MULTIPLE CHOICE

1. The term *3-in-1 solution* refers to a parenteral nutrition solution with:
   a. carbohydrate and lipids in a 3-to-1 ratio
   b. multivitamins, trace elements, and electrolytes in the same bag
   c. carbohydrate, protein, and lipids in the same bag
   d. none of the above

2. A care plan for a home infusion patient:
   a. is not necessary for TPN
   b. includes a pharmaceutical care plan
   c. is necessary only for chemotherapy
   d. cannot be revised

3. Which pharmaceutical care service is not provided by a home infusion pharmacist?
   a. monitoring therapy
   b. the pharmaceutical care plan
   c. cleaning and tracking infusion devices
   d. nutrition support

4. An example of a home infusion therapy is:
   a. blood products
   b. TPN
   c. analgesics
   d. all of the above

5. Home infusion pharmacy services involve the provision of infusion therapies along with:
   a. occupational therapy services
   b. infusion equipment and supplies
   c. pharmaceutical care services
   d. b and c only

6. The most complex home infusion therapy to compound is:
   a. antibiotic therapy
   b. parenteral nutrition therapy
   c. enteral nutrition therapy
   d. pain management therapy

7. A PICC vascular access device:
   a. must be inserted surgically
   b. does not require flushing with heparin
   c. can remain in place for weeks to months
   d. can be used only for TPN infusion

8. All of the following pertain to infusion devices except:
   a. tracking
   b. proper record keeping
   c. sterilizing
   d. cleaning and checking between uses

9. The shortest-dwelling vascular access device is a:
   a. PICC
   b. peripheral catheter
   c. midline catheter
   d. subcutaneous port

10. The selection of supplies for home infusion therapy depends on:
    a. the infusion device
    b. the IV container
    c. the type of vascular access device
    d. all of the above

## TRUE/FALSE (CORRECT THE FALSE STATEMENTS)

1. _____ Although a nasogastric tube is the least expensive type of access to the GI tract, it is not favored for home use because it can be displaced.
2. _____ Intravenous infusion pumps can also be used to deliver enteral therapy.
3. _____ The first home infusion therapy was TPN.
4. _____ A subcutaneous port must be surgically implanted.
5. _____ The drug inventory in a home infusion pharmacy includes oral and IV dosage forms of medications.
6. _____ Enteral nutrition is more involved than parenteral nutrition.
7. _____ The Joint Commission does not recognize the home infusion pharmacist as an important member of the home health care team.
8. _____ The home infusion therapy process is similar to the home health care process.
9. _____ An infusion device regulates the flow of infusion therapy into the patient.
10. _____ The DEA allows a faxed copy of an injectable Schedule II controlled substance to serve as the written copy.

## FILL-IN

1. The most common home infusion therapy is _____.
2. The most common home infusion nutritional therapy is _____ _____ _____.
3. In addition to normal prescription and dispensing records, a home infusion pharmacy must keep a _____ _____ on each patient to document pharmacy activities.
4. _____ _____ is access to the bloodstream.
5. A _____ _____ is used to document the preparation of sterile products.
6. Vascular access devices must be _____ to prevent blockage.
7. A _____ ambulatory infusion pump can be used only to deliver a particular type of IV therapy.
8. Intravenous medications prepared in syringes are infused by means of an infusion device called a _____ _____.
9. The system in which a drug contained in a pressurized balloon reservoir is infused by deflating is called an _____ _____ _____.
10. Drugs added by a patient or caregiver before infusion are referred to as _____ _____.

## CRITICAL THINKING

1. Compare and contrast pharmacy operations in a home infusion pharmacy with those in a traditional hospital pharmacy.
2. Apply *structure*, *process*, and *outcomes* to a home infusion pharmacy.
3. Compare and contrast a patient chart used in home infusion with a patient profile.

4. Compare and contrast the DEA final rule for the transmission of a Schedule II controlled substance prescription by facsimile in a home infusion pharmacy with that in a traditional community retail pharmacy.
5. Compare and contrast the duties of a pharmacy technician in a home infusion pharmacy with those in a traditional hospital pharmacy.

## ■ BIBLIOGRAPHY

American Society of Health-System Pharmacists. (2005). *ASHP guidelines on the safe use of automated compounding devices for the preparation of parental nutrition admixtures.* [On-line] ASHP. Available: www.ashp.org.

American Society of Health-System Pharmacists. (2005). *Best practices for hospital and health-system pharmacy: Position and guidance documents of ASHP, 2005–2006.* Bethesda, MD: Author.

Baker, K. (2006). Compounding Accreditation Board. *Infusion, 12*(3), 35.

Blank, C. (2005). Preventing harm from risky meds: Role of smart pumps. *Drug Topics, 149*(3), 56.

Caputo, R., Huffman, A., & Reich, R. (2005). USP Chapter <797>: Practical solutions for microbiology, sterility and pyrogen testing. *International Journal of Pharmaceutical Compounding, 9*(1), 11–14.

Coster, J. (2005). The Medicare Modernization Act Part 1: Introduction to the new prescription drug benefit. *U.S. Pharmacist, 30*(7), 39–46.

Counce, J. (2005). Home infusion and specialty pharmacy: A marriage whose time has come. *Infusion, 11*(1), 16–20.

Counce, J. (2005). Top ten things commercial payers should understand about home infusion. *Infusion, 11*(5), 12–18.

Counce, J. (2006). Digging deep. Infusion pharmacies bear the cost of USP <797> compliance. *Infusion, 12*(1), 15–19.

Counce, J. (2006). Infusion pump market gets busy. *Infusion, 12*(4), 10–18.

Douglass, K. (2005). Establishing sound practices for cleaning your cleanroom: Cleaning products and procedures for <797> compliance. *Pharmacy Purchasing and Products, 2*(5), 16–19.

Douglass, K. (2006). Training and competency considerations for pharmacies providing compounded sterile preparations. *International Journal of Pharmaceutical Compounding, 10*(4), 253–261.

Joint Commission on Accreditation of Healthcare Organizations. (2006). *2006–2007 Comprehensive accreditation manual for home care.* Oakbrook Terrace, IL: Author.

Joint Commission on Accreditation of Healthcare Organizations. (2006). *2006–2007 Standards manual for pharmacy dispensing, clinical/consultant pharmacist, long-term care pharmacy, and freestanding ambulatory infusion services.* Oakbrook Terrace, IL: Author.

Kaplan, L. (2006). Patient safety under the new medicare prescription drug benefit. *Infusion, 12*(1), 27–31.

Kastango, E. (2005). Using ACDs in the practice of pharmacy. *International Journal of Pharmaceutical Compounding, 9*(1), 15–21.

Kastango, E. (2006). USP Chapter <797>: The next phase. *Infusion, 12*(4), 25–29.

Kelley, L. (2005). Increasing pharmacy's role in the purchase of ambulatory infusion pumps. *Pharmacy Purchasing and Products, 2*(2), 26–27.

Leone, M. (2004). Compounding considerations: New alert on exposure to hazardous drugs in the workplace. *Infusion, 10*(5), 33–36.

Levy, S. (2005). Infusion providers brace for Medicare Part D benefits. *Drug Topics, 149*(9), 48.

McElhiney, L. (2005). USP Chapter <797> and preparing for a JCAHO survey. *International Journal of Pharmaceutical Compounding, 9*(1), 22–28.

Moyer, P. (2005). New "smart pumps" reducing IV medication errors. *Drug Topics, 149*(16), 10s.

Nakazawa, N. (2005). Pharmacological management of vascular access devices. *Infusion, 11*(1), 2–7.

Newton, D., & Trissel, L. (2004). A primer on USP Chapter <797> "Pharmaceutical Compounding—Sterile Preparations" and USP process for drug and practice standards. *Infusion, 10*(4), 38–41.

Ockerman, A. (2004). Compounded sterile preparations. An overview of the new standards in USP <797>. *U.S. Pharmacist, 29*(4), 46, 56–62.

Pharmacy Compounding Accreditation Board. (2004). *Standards for accreditation.* [On-line] PCAB. Available: www.pcab.org.

Reid, B. (2006). Smart pump features bar-coding for safer IVs. *Drug Topics, 150*(4), 42.

Richard, C. (2006). Proposed revisions to sterile compounding Chapter <797> released. *Pharmacy Today, 12*(6), 28.

Saladow, J. (2004). Trends in ambulatory infusion pumps. *Infusion, 10*(4), 16–19.

Tanguay, P. (2005). IT and beyond: Evolving technology and home infusion therapy. *Infusion, 11*(4), 31–41.

Thomas, D. (2005). Increasing your compounding speed and accuracy: Automated compounding devices and related software. *Pharmacy Purchasing and Products, 2*(5), 6–8.

Trissel, L. (2005). *Handbook on injectable drugs* (13th ed.). Bethesda, MD: American Society of Health-System Pharmacy.

Ukens, C. (2005). Compounding board gears up for accreditation. *Drug Topics, 149*(20), 29.

Ukens, C. (2006). Board for compounding accreditation debuts. *Drug Topics, 150*(12), 16.

United States Department of Health and Human Services. Food and Drug Administration. (2004). *Aluminum in large and small volume parenterals used in total parental nutrition.* [On-line] FDA. Available: www.fda.gov.

United States Department of Health and Human Services. National Institute for Occupational Safety and Health. (2004). *Preventing occupational exposure to antineoplastic and other hazardous drugs in healthcare settings.* [On-line] NIOSH. Available: www.cdc.gov/niosh.

United States Department of Justice. Drug Enforcement Administration. (2005). *Code of Federal Regulations Title 21, Section 1306—Pharmacy.* [On-line] U.S. Department of Justice. Available: www.dea.gov.

United States Pharmacopeial Convention. (2006). *The United States pharmacopeia* (29th ed.) and *The national formulary* (24th ed). Rockville, MD: Author.

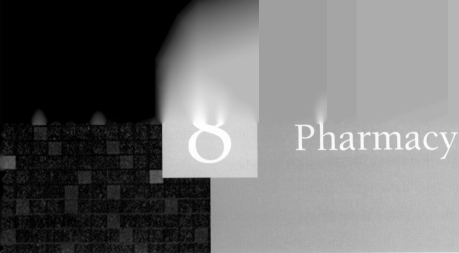

# 8 Pharmacy

Upon completion of this chapter, the student should be able to:

- Describe the prescription drug benefit.
- Describe the types of pharmacy provider networks.
- Discuss pharmacy reimbursement.
- Explain the decisions regarding covered and excluded drugs.
- Define the formulary system and explain the need for formulary exception processes.
- Explain the need for patient co-payments and describe the different types.
- List the different types of plan limitations.
- Discuss reasons for the rise in the cost of the prescription drug benefit.
- List several cost containment strategies.
- Discuss pharmacy benefit management.
- Describe managed care pharmacy practice and the pharmacist's role in it.
- Understand the legislation and regulations pertaining to managed care pharmacy practice.
- Describe the role of the pharmacy technician in managed care pharmacy practice.

## Key Terms

covered drug

disease management

drug utilization review

excluded drug

formulary

formulary exception process

managed care pharmacy practice

member co-payment

outcomes research

pharmacy benefit management company

pharmacy network

prescription drug benefit

reimbursement formula

therapeutic equivalent drug

therapeutic interchange

## Introduction

Managed care has had an impact on how prescription drugs are delivered in our health care system. The prescription drug benefit has become an important part of managed care health plans. It is designed to deliver high-quality, cost-effective drug therapy to members. However, the pharmacy benefit must be managed to ensure the best possible outcomes of drug therapy and to keep the cost of the drug benefit under control. Pharmacy benefit management involves managing the quality and cost of the prescription drug benefit through various activities. An area of pharmacy referred to as managed care pharmacy practice has emerged in which the pharmacist performs clinical and administrative activities in managing the drug benefit. Managed care pharmacy is unique in that it does not involve dispensing activities. Pharmacy technicians are also involved in managed care pharmacy practice. Both pharmacists and pharmacy technicians need to have a broad knowledge of managed care issues, especially the prescription drug benefit, in order to work in a managed care pharmacy setting. They also must be familiar with the legislation and regulations that pertain to the drug benefit. This chapter focuses on the prescription drug benefit and the unique roles of the pharmacist and pharmacy technician in managed care pharmacy. ■

## THE PRESCRIPTION DRUG BENEFIT

A **prescription drug benefit** is defined as prescription drug coverage provided as an employee benefit. The prescription drug benefit offered by employers to employees has grown over the past 40 years. Before 1960, very few health plans had a separate prescription drug benefit, also called a pharmacy benefit. Those that did required employees to pay the pharmacy for their prescriptions and then to submit the receipts for reimbursement. There were often large deductibles that had to be satisfied before any reimbursement was made. In the 1960s, prescription drug plans, also called card plans, emerged, in which an insurance company would contract with pharmacies to provide prescription drugs to its members. This benefit allowed the member to pay only a small charge to the pharmacy when a prescription was dispensed. The balance of the cost of the prescription was paid to the pharmacy by the insurance company, now referred to in this arrangement as the *third party*. Since then, the prescription drug benefit has become a major and important employee benefit.

A benefit is defined as a form of compensation other than wages paid to an employee. Benefits provide security to employees and their families. Some benefits are legally required, such as Social Security. However, most benefits are not. Health care benefits, including the prescription drug benefit, are not legally required but are highly sought because, while other countries have federally financed national health insurance, most employed Americans receive their health insurance from their employers. The prescription drug benefit is not a required part of a patient's health care coverage, but it is generally added on as a rider. Most employers today offer prescription drug coverage to their employees. It is a very visible health care benefit and one of the most frequently used.

The prescription drug benefit is available to the employee according to a contract. This contract is between the employer or the payer of the benefit and the insurance company or the managed care organization that administers the benefit. The employee is referred to as a member or enrollee, a participant in the prescription drug benefit plan.

The prescription drug benefit defines the prescription drug coverage provided to the member. This benefit varies dramatically among employers and health care plans. It is designed to meet the needs of the member, the employer, *and* the pharmacist and pharmacy. It is also designed to meet the goals of managed care: lowest *cost,* reasonable *access,* and high *quality.* The prescription drug benefit is designed so that members have access to the most appropriate and cost-effective drugs for their medical conditions. Several components of the prescription drug benefit are discussed in the following sections.

## PHARMACY PROVIDER NETWORKS

The pharmacy provider network is a critical component of the pharmacy benefit. A network has been defined as a group of health care providers that are linked through a contract to provide services. A **pharmacy network** is a group of pharmacies that sign a contract to provide pharmacy benefits to members in exchange for a specified reimbursement. The network is designed so that all members have access to a participating pharmacy within a reasonable distance from their homes. There are several types of provider networks.

### Community Pharmacy Network

A community pharmacy network is composed of chain and independent community retail pharmacies. It can be an open or a closed network. An open network is one in which all community pharmacies may participate in providing pharmacy services. This type of community pharmacy network provides the best access for members. A closed network is one in which only select community pharmacies may participate. It is also known as an exclusive network. The majority of managed care prescriptions are filled through community pharmacy networks.

### In-House Pharmacy Network

An in-house pharmacy network is composed of pharmacies owned and operated by a health maintenance organization (HMO). These pharmacies are usually located in HMO medical facilities and provide pharmacy services only for their own enrolled members.

### Mail-Order Pharmacy Network

A mail-order pharmacy network is composed of mail-order pharmacies owned and operated by a managed care organization. These pharmacies may be located far from a member's home, but the member receives prescriptions through the mail. A mail-order pharmacy network provides the member with an *option* to the community pharmacy network.

### Physician Dispensing Network

A physician dispensing network is composed of physicians who dispense medications in their office. This type of pharmacy network is relatively uncommon and is usually found only in rural areas where there is a lack of community pharmacies.

Managed care organizations often do not use one network exclusively to provide the pharmacy benefit for their members. Some contract with community pharmacies, as well as with a mail-order pharmacy. Other managed care organizations contract with community pharmacies in addition to having their own pharmacy within a medical center.

## REIMBURSEMENT

Another component of the drug benefit is the reimbursement to the participating pharmacy for providing pharmacy services to members. Pharmacies are reimbursed through a formula, referred to as the **reimbursement formula.** This formula is represented as:

$$\text{Ingredient Cost} + \text{Dispensing Fee}$$

The ingredient cost is the raw cost of the drug. It is based on a standard reference, such as the average wholesale price, or AWP. The AWP is the average cost of a drug. It is the *list* price of a drug and is higher than the price that most pharmacies pay for the drug. Therefore, the AWP is discounted by a percentage to lower the ingredient cost to what is believed to be the actual cost of the drug to the pharmacy. The formula then becomes:

$$[\text{AWP} - \% \text{ Discount}] + \text{Dispensing Fee}$$

The ingredient cost also can be based on another reference, the actual acquisition cost, or AAC. It is the *actual* cost of the drug to the pharmacy. It is not discounted in the reimbursement formula.

$$\text{AAC} + \text{Dispensing Fee}$$

When the prescribed drug has a generic equivalent, reimbursement can be based on the maximum allowable cost, or MAC. This is the maximum cost a plan will pay for a generic drug that is available from many sources or companies. It also is not discounted further in the reimbursement formula.

$$\text{MAC} + \text{Dispensing Fee}$$

The dispensing fee is a fixed dollar amount added to the ingredient cost. It reflects the costs associated with dispensing a prescription, a fair or competitive profit for the pharmacy, and a professional fee for the pharmacist. However, with pharmaceutical care activities by the pharmacist increasing, new methods of reimbursement are being discussed to adequately compensate pharmacists for their pharmaceutical care services. For example, the formula may be:

$$[AWP - \% \text{ Discount}] + \text{Dispensing Fee} + \text{Pharmaceutical Care Fee}$$

## COVERED AND EXCLUDED DRUGS

Covered and excluded drugs are another component of the prescription drug benefit. Each prescription drug plan defines which drugs are covered and which drugs are not. Covered and excluded drugs can vary widely among plans.

A **covered drug** is a drug that will be reimbursed or paid for under the prescription drug plan. An **excluded drug** is a drug that will not be reimbursed under the plan. The prescription drug plan is designed to include a wide range of covered drugs. Covered drugs usually include:

- Federal legend drugs (included on the plan formulary)
- State-restricted drugs
- Compounded medications containing a federal legend or state-restricted drug
- Insulin and, sometimes, needles and syringes

Most plans exclude or do not cover certain drugs, or certain drug classes, regardless of the fact that the physician writes a prescription for these drugs. These drugs are excluded for many reasons. The outcomes of some drugs are uncertain, such as investigational drugs. Some drugs are not considered to be medically necessary, such as cosmetic drugs. Some drugs are sometimes covered under the members' medical benefit, such as vaccines. Finally, some drugs are considered to be discretionary; that is, they involve personal choice, such as impotence drugs. Examples of drugs commonly excluded from pharmacy benefit plans are found in Box 8–1.

Over-the-counter drugs (except insulin), nutritional supplements, and some therapeutic devices, such as glucometers, have been traditionally excluded from

---

### BOX 8–1    Drugs Commonly Excluded from Pharmacy Benefit Plans

Investigational drugs
Vaccines
Oral contraceptives and diaphragms
Over-the-counter drugs (except insulin)
Fertility drugs
Smoking cessation drugs
Impotence drugs
Cosmetic drugs
Injectable drugs (except insulin)
Vitamins and nutritional supplements
Therapeutic devices
Hair growth drugs
Weight loss drugs

coverage because they are considered to be unpredictable, not medically necessary, and discretionary. However, they are now being considered for coverage by some prescription drug benefit plans because they are often less expensive than prescription drugs. The most commonly covered over-the-counter products are smoking cessation drugs and antihistamines.

## THE FORMULARY

A formulary is one of the most important components of the prescription drug benefit. A **formulary,** as it pertains to managed care and the prescription drug benefit, is defined as a list of medications approved for use or reimbursement under a prescription drug plan. It is designed to meet most reasonable patient needs while keeping drug costs in line. Each managed care organization develops its own formulary and promotes compliance with the formulary through controls such as variable co-payments and the prior authorization process. Almost all managed care organizations have some type of formulary. The use of a formulary is the most important way for a managed care organization to control the cost of the drug benefit. There are three different types of formularies used in managed care prescription drug plans.

### Open Formulary

An open formulary is a formulary in which a broad range of drugs is covered. It provides access to most medications. An open formulary contains several choices of drugs in each therapeutic category. Often, brand-name drugs are arranged in levels corresponding to different levels or tiers of cost sharing, and the drugs are usually referred to as *preferred* or *nonpreferred*. Preferred drugs have a lower co-payment than nonpreferred drugs as an incentive to use these drugs, which, along with generics, are usually lower in cost.

### Closed Formulary

A closed formulary is a formulary in which a very limited list of drugs is covered. Drugs that do not appear on the formulary are not covered. A closed formulary contains a limited choice of drugs in each therapeutic category. However, entire classes of drugs may be excluded. It is the most restrictive type of formulary. An exception process must exist so that a member can obtain a necessary nonformulary drug. Closed formularies offer the greatest cost savings for the managed care organization but are not well accepted by physicians and members. As a result, many states have passed legislation that addresses closed formularies.

### Restricted Formulary

A restricted formulary, also referred to as a selective, limited, partially closed, or managed formulary, is a formulary in which some nonformulary drugs are covered. It also is a limited list of drugs, but is not as restrictive as a closed formulary. Select nonformulary drugs can be covered through a formulary exception process.

## FORMULARY EXCEPTION PROCESSES

A **formulary exception process** is a component of any good prescription drug benefit. It is defined as a process that provides access to nonformulary drugs and certain formulary drugs when necessary. One type of formulary exception process is formulary override. Formulary override is a process that involves obtaining authorization to use a nonformulary drug. It is a way for a physician to prescribe a nonformulary drug in a prescription drug plan that has a closed formulary. Formulary override requires the physician to request approval for the use of the nonformulary drug and to document the reason for the use of the drug. Once the request is approved, the drug is available to the patient as a covered item. Formulary exception requests can be made, for example, when a patient has tried a formulary drug but it has failed or when a patient is intolerant or allergic to a formulary drug.

Another formulary exception process is called prior authorization or prior approval. Prior authorization is a process that involves obtaining authorization to use certain formulary drugs. It is a way to control or limit the use of certain drugs that are on the formulary but that are very expensive, overused, too toxic, have a high potential for abuse, or are beneficial to a limited number of people. Prior authorization also requires that the physician request approval and document the reason for the use of the drug. The plan allows coverage of the drug if certain predetermined conditions for its use are met. For example:

- An expensive new drug comes onto the market—the patient must have tried older, less expensive drugs first. If the patient's condition does not respond to the older drugs, the more expensive new drug will be covered. This is referred to as step therapy, that is, the use of various drugs in steps.
- Nail fungus is considered a cosmetic condition in healthy individuals—a drug for nail fungus is considered medically necessary only if a medical problem such as diabetes makes it necessary.
- Oral contraceptives are usually excluded drugs—they may be covered if they are not used for contraception but are used to correct a hormonal problem.

Some other examples of drugs that may require prior authorization are growth hormones, weight loss drugs, and erythropoietin. Prior authorization ensures that patients who really need a particular drug have access to it.

To be successful, formulary exception processes require physician and member education concerning the processes. They also require phone, facsimile, and computer processes and a trained staff within the managed care organization to handle and process the formulary exception requests.

## MEMBER CO-PAYMENT

The **member co-payment** is an important component of the prescription drug benefit. It is defined as the portion of the total cost of a prescription that the member must pay. It reflects the member's responsibility for the drug benefit. Most managed care organizations require that members pay a portion of the cost of their prescriptions. The co-payment is paid to the pharmacy at the time a prescription is dispensed. This amount is subtracted from the reimbursement formula, the balance then being paid by the managed care organization. Co-payments, also called co-pays, help lower the cost of prescriptions for the prescription drug plan. They also help discourage unnecessary use of the prescription drug benefit. The co-payment is designed so that it is not too high or so unaffordable that it prevents members from obtaining needed medications. Three different types of co-payments are discussed next.

### Fixed Co-payment

A fixed co-payment is a fixed or set dollar amount. It is the same dollar amount for any prescription, regardless of the drug. An example is a $10 co-payment for any prescription.

### Percentage Co-payment

A percentage co-payment is a fixed percentage of the total cost of the prescription. An example is a 20 percent co-pay per prescription. For a prescription that costs $50, the co-payment would be 20 percent, or $10. Percentage co-payments encourage patients to ask for less expensive drugs to be prescribed and dispensed.

### Variable Co-payment

A variable co-payment is a variable or different dollar amount based on the type of drug that is dispensed; for example, a generic drug vs. a brand-name drug, or a *preferred* brand-name drug vs. a *nonpreferred* brand-name drug. It is also called a multilevel co-pay or tiered co-pay. The most common type of variable co-pay is the *three-tiered co-pay*. It sets the lowest co-pay for a generic drug, the next highest co-pay for a preferred brand-name drug, and the highest co-pay for a nonpreferred brand-name drug. For example:

$5 co-pay    Generic drug

$10 co-pay  Preferred brand-name drug

$25 co-pay  Nonpreferred brand-name drug

A lifestyle drug, also referred to as a quality of life drug, is a drug that enhances the quality of a member's life but is not considered medically necessary. Examples are impotence drugs (Viagra), hair growth drugs (Rogaine), antiwrinkle creams (Renova), weight loss drugs, oral contraceptives, and smoking cessation drugs. Sometimes lifestyle drugs are excluded from a formulary altogether. However, a fourth co-payment tier for lifestyle drugs is being added by some managed care organizations. The co-pay for drugs in this tier will be the highest. An addition to the above example would be a $40 co-pay for a lifestyle drug.

Variable co-payments encourage the use of generic and formulary drugs. They allow better access to drugs. In effect, variable co-payments offer members and physicians an open type of formulary but one that makes them responsible for their drug choices through higher co-pays. Variable co-payments lower the cost of the prescription drug benefit to the employer or plan by shifting more of the cost of expensive drugs to the members, referred to as *cost shifting*.

## PLAN LIMITATIONS

The plan limitations are the final component of the prescription drug benefit. They are an important part of any prescription drug plan. Plan limitations are intended to control prescription drug use and reduce prescription drug costs. Limits are used because they are easy to incorporate into the plan and the savings can be easily measured. There are two types of plan limitations: limitations on individual prescriptions and limitations on the drug benefit.

### Limitations on Individual Prescriptions

There are limits on the amount of prescription drug that can be dispensed at one time. A quantity limit is the maximum quantity of a drug that can be dispensed at one time, for example, 30 units of a medication, or 30 tablets. A day supply limit is the amount of a drug that can be dispensed according to a certain day supply, for example, a 30-day or 90-day supply. Both quantity and day supply limitations lower the cost per prescription and are referred to as *prescription maximums*.

### Limitations on the Drug Benefit

There are limits on the dollar amount of prescription drugs that can be dispensed. A dollar limit is the maximum dollar amount of a prescription that can be dispensed at one time, for example, a dollar limit of $500 per prescription. The dollar limit can also be the maximum dollar amount of prescriptions that can be dispensed for a member over a particular period of time, such as monthly, quarterly, or annually; for example, a $1,000 limit per year. It is also referred to as a *spending* or *prescription cap*.

There also are limits on the number of prescriptions that can be covered during a certain period of time. A number limit is the maximum number of prescriptions that can be dispensed for a member over a particular period of time, usually per month, for example, six prescriptions per month.

Finally, there are limits on the amount of time that a prescription can be covered. A time limit is the maximum amount of time in which a prescription can be filled for a member; for example, prescriptions can be refilled for 6 months or 1 year. Dollar, number, and time limitations all lower the number of claims, thereby lowering the cost of the drug benefit. They are referred to as *drug benefit maximums*.

Plan limitations must be incorporated carefully into the prescription drug benefit. Limits can have a negative effect on total health care costs when patients who have exceeded their benefits stop obtaining and taking their medications.

## ◼ COST OF THE PRESCRIPTION DRUG BENEFIT

The prescription drug benefit is receiving much attention because of its high cost. It is the fastest-growing type of health care expenditure. Each year, managed care organizations spend a larger portion of their budget on the prescription drug benefit, and the cost of the prescription drug benefit is expected to continue to rise. There are many reasons for the rise in the cost of this benefit. These include:

- An increase in the number of people covered by a prescription drug plan
- An increase in the elderly population, who use more medications than the young
- General inflation
- An increase in the use of drugs
- Expensive new drugs and technology, such as biotechnology
- Drug manufacturer price increases
- The switch from prescribing older drugs to newer drugs
- Larger prescriptions sizes, for example, 90-day supplies vs. 30-day supplies
- Direct advertising of drugs to consumers

BOX 8–2   **Drug Classes That Contribute to Increased Drug Spending**

Nonsedating antihistamines
Selective seritonin reuptake inhibitors
"Statin" cholesterol-lowering drugs
Oral hypoglycemics
Oral inhalers
Proton pump inhibitors
"Triptan" migraine drugs
Nasal steroid inhalers

The increase in the utilization of drugs is the most important reason for the rise in the cost of the prescription drug benefit. More people are taking medications and for longer periods of time. More and more health care is being provided by drugs as they are being used as the first line of treatment for many medical conditions. New breakthroughs in drug development have resulted in medications that did not exist in the past, such as biotechnology drugs. Newer, more expensive medications are being used over older, less expensive medications because they may be more effective or have fewer side effects than older drugs. As a rule, new drugs cost more than old drugs and, because of patent protection, are not available in less expensive generic form. The high price of new drugs is the second most important reason for increased drug spending.

There are certain drugs and drug classes that are contributing to increased drug spending. The biggest increase actually comes from just a few therapeutic classes, which are being heavily advertised to consumers. These are oral antihistamines, antidepressants, cholesterol-lowering drugs, and antiulcer drugs. Box 8–2 lists the drug classes that are responsible for increased spending for the pharmacy drug benefit.

## COST CONTAINMENT STRATEGIES

Managed care organizations are under increasing pressure as a result of the increase in the cost of the prescription drug benefit. They must lower costs while ensuring the best possible outcomes of drug therapy and maintaining member and employer satisfaction with the drug benefit. Most managed care organizations use several strategies to lower the cost of the prescription drug benefit without sacrificing quality. Some are cost controls; that is, they control the costs associated with the drug benefit. Others are utilization controls; that is, they control the use of the drug benefit. Used together, cost and utilization controls reduce spending for the prescription drug benefit by lowering costs, decreasing unnecessary drug use, encouraging appropriate drug use, and improving the quality of care. Cost containment strategies include:

- *Restrictive pharmacy networks.* These reduce administrative costs and result in discount fee arrangements with the participating pharmacies.

- *Mail-order and Internet pharmacy.* This provides a less expensive way to fill prescriptions for maintenance drugs through decreased administrative costs, bulk purchasing of drugs, and automation. Mail-order pharmacy, including Internet pharmacy, is discussed in Chapter 9.

- *Electronic claims submission.* This is the most efficient way to process prescription claims. It lowers administrative costs and minimizes slow or lost claims as well as provides data for statistics and clinical uses.
- *Higher member co-payments.* These reduce the utilization of drugs and shift more of the cost of the drug benefit to the member. Studies show that higher co-pays are associated with lower drug use.
- *Tiered co-payments.* These encourage the use of less expensive generic and preferred brand-name drugs and discourage the use of nonpreferred brand-name drugs. These make members more responsible financially for their drug choices.
- *Aggressive formulary management.* This reduces inappropriate drug use by limiting drug choices. Price competition between pharmaceutical manufacturers for drugs in the same therapeutic class also helps lower drug costs.
- *Prior authorization.* This reduces unnecessary and inappropriate drug use by making sure that a member really needs a particular drug.
- *Competitive drug buying.* Pharmaceutical manufacturer discounts on drugs purchased for in-house or mail-order pharmacy networks decrease drug costs.
- *Benefit limitations.* These reduce total claim costs without negatively affecting the quality of care. Smaller quantities and shorter day supplies reduce waste from unused or discontinued drugs.
- *Mandatory generic substitution.* This strategy reimburses participating pharmacies only at generic prices, forcing the pharmacy to dispense the generic equivalent or the patient to pay the cost of the brand-name drug. It lowers drug costs and is one of the most effective way to control the cost of the prescription drug benefit.

## FUTURE INFLUENCES ON THE PRESCRIPTION DRUG BENEFIT

The prescription drug benefit is perceived to be a valuable employee benefit, and its use will continue to grow in the future. We can expect some influences in the future on the way this benefit is managed and expanded. Probably the two most important influences on the prescription drug benefit are the Internet and Medicare.

### The Internet

The Internet is changing the way pharmacy benefits are managed, especially in the areas of claim processing and consumer information. Members are choosing to access their prescription drug benefit on-line. They may enter their insurance information, order prescription refills, and pay the co-pay—all on-line. Prescriptions can then be delivered by a mail-order pharmacy or picked up at a participating community pharmacy. Likewise, members can obtain information concerning their prescription drug benefit and update their personal information on-line. The Internet also helps members take a more active role in their health by providing information on their medical problems and available treatments. This information can help them use their health benefit, especially their prescription drug benefit, more efficiently.

Physicians are also being connected on-line to managed care organizations and pharmacies. Through a physician-payer link, physicians can check the formulary status of a drug, drug cost information, practice guidelines, disease state management protocols, and the patient's drug use history. This link results in more rational prescribing and can help prevent problems such as duplicate or inappropriate drug therapy. A physician-pharmacy link allows electronic prescribing. This can improve prescribing, dispensing, and prescription claims processing and improve compliance with the formulary.

### Medicare Prescription Drug Benefit

The federally mandated prescription drug benefit for Medicare patients was enacted in 2006. Older Americans have more health conditions requiring drug treatment, consume more drugs and other health care services, and are at a higher risk for drug-related problems, especially adverse drug reactions, than younger Americans. The availability of a prescription drug plan for Medicare patients, some of whom were previously unable to afford necessary medications, has improved the quality of life for these patients, as well as decreased total health care costs.

Like any other prescription drug benefit, the Medicare drug benefit needs to be managed to promote appropriate drug use and to control its cost. Pharmacy benefit management companies, or PBMs, are using several cost containment strategies, such as formularies, co-payments, contracts with pharmacy networks, mail order, prior authorization, quantity limits, and manufacturer discounts or rebates. The complexity of the Medicare Prescription Drug Benefit and the large volume of claims will continue to challenge PBMs in their management of this program.

## PHARMACY BENEFIT MANAGEMENT

Pharmacy benefit management involves managing the cost as well as the quality of the pharmacy benefit. Like other health care expenditures, such as hospital and physician costs, the prescription drug benefit also can be managed. Managing the pharmacy benefit can help keep the cost of the benefit down without compromising the overall benefit in terms of quality and member satisfaction. The pharmacy benefit is managed through many types of services, programs, and management techniques. Managing costs is accomplished through cost containment strategies. Managing quality involves the use of clinical programs that help make the most of drug therapy.

The pharmacy benefit is very complex, and it can be difficult to manage. Some health plans manage their pharmacy benefit internally, or themselves. However, most managed care organizations separate or "carve out" the prescription drug benefit and contract with a company that specializes in managing the pharmacy benefit. PBM companies have the expertise and experience to effectively manage the pharmacy benefit using the managed care principles of cost, access, and quality.

### PHARMACY BENEFIT MANAGEMENT COMPANY

A **pharmacy benefit management company**, or PBM company, is a managed care organization that designs, administers, and manages only the prescription drug benefit. Pharmacy benefit management companies have existed since the early 1980s. Initially, their only services were claims processing and mail-order pharmacy service. Later, they found ways to control drug costs through negotiated discounts with pharmacy provider networks, the use of formularies, generic substitution, and rebates on brand-name drugs from pharmaceutical manufacturers. Today, the role of the PBM company has expanded into drug benefit design, disease management, outcomes reporting, and patient education programs. PBM companies have evolved over the last 20 years and have been shown to lower drug costs, increase member satisfaction, and improve drug outcomes within a prescription drug benefit program.

A PBM company provides services to a variety of customers, that is, anyone who sponsors a prescription drug plan or is a payer of a prescription drug plan. Its customers include self-insured employers, health insurance companies, government programs (Medicare and Medicaid), third-party benefit administrators, unions, large companies such as *Fortune* 500 companies, and managed care organizations such as HMOs and preferred provider organizations that do not have their own pharmacy benefit management programs. In fact, most HMOs choose to contract with a PBM company for some form of pharmacy benefit management. Most employers today use a PBM company because of their many services.

A PBM company may be owned by a number of different organizations, such as an independent company, pharmaceutical manufacturer, retail pharmacy chain, or HMO. Examples include Medco Health Solutions, Inc., Caremark Rx, Inc., and Express Scripts, Inc., the three largest PBMs, as well as smaller PBMs, such as Aetna Pharmacy Management, Walgreens Health Initiatives, and Medimpact Healthcare Systems, Inc.

A PBM company maintains a relationship with the member, the employer, or the plan sponsor; the participating pharmacy; and the pharmaceutical manufacturers, as shown in Figure 8–1. It administers and manages the prescription

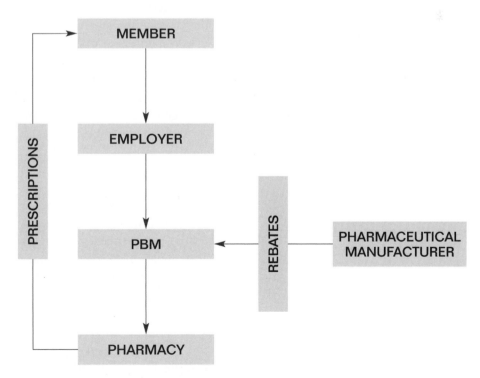

**FIGURE 8–1** The Pharmacy Benefit Management Network.

drug benefit that is designed according to the employer or plan sponsor. The actual prescription drug benefit is provided to members through participating pharmacies. Pharmaceutical manufacturers extend rebates to the PBM company on drugs dispensed through community pharmacy networks as rewards for increased market share or increased use of their drugs.

Pharmacy benefit management companies manage the pharmacy benefit through a wide range of services. These services can be divided into cost containment services, member services, and clinical services. Cost containment services are services that help reduce the cost of the prescription drug benefit. These services include processing and reimbursing claims, developing pharmacy networks, providing and promoting the mail-order pharmacy option, managing a formulary, requiring generic substitution, performing drug utilization reviews, negotiating pharmaceutical manufacturer discounts, obtaining rebates from pharmaceutical manufacturers, processing formulary override and prior authorization requests, and auditing participating pharmacies. Member satisfaction services are services that involve communicating with members, providing answers to questions regarding their drug benefit and helping them use it efficiently. These services include providing toll-free telephone help lines, performing mail surveys, and providing member education through written materials or a Web site. Clinical services are services that help ensure the best possible outcomes of drug therapy. These services include establishing disease management programs, performing drug utilization review, performing outcomes research, and providing wellness programs to members.

## OVERVIEW OF MANAGED CARE PHARMACY

The growth of managed care, the high cost of the prescription drug benefit, and the concept of pharmaceutical care as the basis for pharmacy practice have all combined to create a practice opportunity for pharmacists in managed care organizations. An area of pharmacy practice has evolved that is known as managed care pharmacy practice. **Managed care pharmacy practice** is defined as the practice of pharmacy that involves clinical and administrative activities performed in a managed care organization by a pharmacist. It is referred to as "pharmacy without walls" because it does not involve dispensing activities as in a traditional pharmacy. Instead, the pharmacist works in an office environment. In managed care pharmacy practice, the pharmacist helps manage the prescription drug benefit.

A managed care pharmacist is a pharmacist who specializes in managed care pharmacy practice. The managed care pharmacist practices outside of a traditional pharmacy. This pharmacist is directly employed by and is found in a managed care organization, such as a staff or group model HMO, where she may be referred to as a pharmacy director, supervisor, or administrator; an independent practice association; a pharmacy benefit management company, where she is known as a pharmacy benefit manager; an insurance company that provides a prescription drug benefit; or a multispecialty physician group. A managed care pharmacist must possess traditional pharmacy knowledge skills as well as clinical skills. In addition, the managed care pharmacist must have general business and management skills and excellent communication skills in order to perform administrative activities. The managed care pharmacist must also be familiar with the extensive legislation and regulations that pertain to the prescription drug benefit of managed care organizations. Because the role of the managed care pharmacist is essentially managed care pharmacy practice, it is discussed here.

# THE ROLE OF THE PHARMACIST IN MANAGED CARE

The pharmacist in a managed care organization primarily assists in managing the drug benefit. The managed care pharmacist performs many activities to ensure the rational and cost-effective use of drugs within a prescription drug plan. Combined clinical and administrative activities lead to improved patient outcomes and cost savings. The clinical role involves drug *therapy* management through clinical activities. The administrative role involves drug *benefit* management through various administrative activities.

## CLINICAL ROLE

The clinical role of the pharmacist in managed care pharmacy practice involves managing drug therapy for enrolled members. The managed care pharmacist works to improve outcomes of drug therapy through the appropriate use of drugs and the appropriate use of the drug benefit. The emphasis in this role is on pharmaceutical care.

Pharmaceutical care activities include developing and managing the formulary, developing disease management programs, performing outcomes research, performing drug utilization reviews, developing drug use guidelines, providing drug information services, and educating health care professionals and members. The most important of these clinical roles are discussed next.

### Formulary Development and Management

Formulary development refers to the selection of drugs for inclusion in a prescription drug plan formulary. Developing the formulary requires an understanding of drug therapy, drug costs, patient behavior regarding taking drugs, and physician prescribing habits. The formulary for a prescription drug plan is developed by a pharmacy and therapeutics committee or its equivalent or a separate formulary development committee within the managed care organization, of which the managed care pharmacist is an important member. It is developed on the basis of careful and thorough review of the most current drug literature, which includes the package insert, studies used for FDA approval, articles in journals, and postmarketing data. Drugs are selected on the basis of safety, effectiveness, and cost. Cost is not the first consideration but is considered when drugs are determined to be equal in terms of safety and effectiveness. Other guidelines used in formulary development include:

- The formulary should consider the needs or the unique characteristics of the enrolled members, for example, many elderly or AIDS patients.
- The formulary should include a broad range of dosage *forms,* such as tablets and capsules, suppositories, liquids, and injectables.

- The formulary should have a process to accommodate patients who cannot tolerate certain drugs or dosages.
- The formulary should complement disease management programs and drug use guidelines, that is, those drugs that are recommended for use in these programs, and guidelines should be included in the formulary.

Formulary management involves the continuous review and revision of the formulary as new information and drugs become available. The managed care pharmacist also educates other health care professionals concerning changes in the plan formulary.

Therapeutic interchange is a type of formulary management tool. **Therapeutic interchange** is the authorized substitution of a prescribed drug with a therapeutic equivalent drug. A **therapeutic equivalent drug** is a drug that has a different chemical structure but is in the same therapeutic class or drug class. An example is famotidine and ranitidine, two drugs that can be expected to have the same outcome when used in therapeutically equivalent doses. For example, famotidine 20 mg is equivalent to ranitidine 150 mg. Therapeutic interchange is performed by a dispensing pharmacist with the approval of the physician. The pharmacy and therapeutics committee or its equivalent oversees this program. It evaluates and selects drugs for therapeutic interchange that are the most appropriate for the members being served from the same perspectives of safety, efficiency, and cost. Therapeutic interchange is a way to control costs by controlling the number of drugs on the formulary in the same therapeutic class, especially when there is a wide variation in the costs of these drugs. However, the well-being of the patient must be the primary consideration. Therapeutic interchange should not alter the effectiveness of the patient's drug therapy in any way. Therapeutic interchange is most often permitted for antiulcer drugs, anti-inflammatory drugs, cholesterol-lowering drugs, antibiotics, and oral contraceptives (when covered).

The role of the pharmacist in formulary development and management is important. Pharmacists have the knowledge and skills to guide the pharmacy and therapeutics committee and the expertise to make formulary recommendations. As drug experts and educators, managed care pharmacists are essential in the entire formulary process.

## Disease Management Programs

**Disease management** is defined as a coordinated approach to treating a specific disease that involves the entire health care team. More simply stated, disease management is control of a chronic disease. Disease management uses a step-by-step treatment plan with care provided by many different health care providers to manage and improve the health of a patient with a particular disease. The goal is to select and deliver the most appropriate and cost-effective treatment. Disease management programs focus on diseases that are chronic, involve a large number of patients, consume a large amount of health care resources, are costly to treat, and usually have less than optimum outcomes when not managed well. Examples of diseases that are treated through disease management programs include asthma, diabetes, depression, osteoporosis, high cholesterol, hypertension, and congestive heart failure.

Disease management uses a combination of health care strategies. Drugs are one of these strategies. The managed care pharmacist is an important contributor to disease management programs within managed care organizations. As a medication expert, the pharmacist is involved in developing the medication component of disease management programs. The managed care pharmacist helps in drug management by:

- Evaluating drug therapies and making recommendations for drug use
- Providing advice on a disease and its management
- Evaluating drug costs
- Demonstrating the value of particular drug choices
- Monitoring the effects of drug choices
- Identifying drug-related problems
- Educating other health care professionals about drug treatment guidelines
- Educating patients concerning their drugs and the importance of compliance
- Ensuring that drug choices are included on the plan formulary

Disease management programs have been shown to decrease the complications of disease, prevent unnecessary hospitalization and emergency room visits, and improve the quality of life. The managed care pharmacist again helps to develop programs that result in improved outcomes for members.

## Drug Utilization Review

**Drug utilization review** (DUR), sometimes referred to as drug use review, is a process that examines whether prescription drugs are being used efficiently and appropriately within the prescription drug benefit. It is a retrospective study performed *after* drugs are dispensed to patients. DUR involves the analysis of prescription drug claims data that are available as a result of electronic claims processing. The managed care pharmacist is involved in analyzing these data and in identifying and correcting inappropriate drug use. The pharmacist examines physician prescribing, pharmacist dispensing, and patient utilization of prescription drugs. Several issues can be identified by this activity. These include:

- Underutilization of drugs
- Overutilization of drugs
- Incorrect drug dosages
- Duplicate drug therapy
- Inappropriate drug selection
- Inappropriate duration of drug therapy
- Drug interactions

For example, DUR may show that similar drugs are being prescribed for the same patient for the same condition; incompatible or duplicate drugs are being prescribed for the same patient by different physicians; a potentially inappropriate drug is being prescribed for an elderly patient; or an expensive new drug is being prescribed for a patient when there is a less expensive drug that is just as effective and has not been tried. The managed care pharmacist uses her expertise in identifying and advising physicians concerning inappropriate drug use and its related problems. This is another activity that improves the outcomes of drug therapy and reduces drug costs.

### Outcomes Research

**Outcomes research** is defined as the process of collecting information to determine the effectiveness of a therapy. As it applies to drugs, outcomes research studies the effects of drug therapy on a patient's quality of life. It evaluates drug therapy to determine if the desired outcome is produced. It is used to help managed care organizations make better decisions about drug therapy and improve the quality of the prescription drug benefit. Outcomes research involves pharmacoeconomics, which is the evaluation of the cost as well as the outcomes of drugs therapy. Pharmacoeconomics is more than just looking at the cost of the drug. It studies how a drug produces an outcome that can lower health care costs.

The pharmacist is involved in outcomes research within the managed care organization. The managed care pharmacist evaluates data from electronic claims submission, patient surveys, and the literature to identify trends. These findings are used within the prescription drug benefit to help develop practice guidelines and to make formulary decisions, among other programs. Pharmacists can be effective in evaluating drug outcomes and in helping to design other programs to improve patient outcomes.

### ADMINISTRATIVE ROLE

The administrative role of the managed care pharmacist involves managing the prescription drug benefit. The managed care pharmacist is involved in identifying and meeting the needs of enrolled members by interacting directly with the payers of the drug benefit. The emphasis is on controlling the cost of the drug benefit through various strategies. Administrative activities for the managed care pharmacist include negotiating contracts with pharmaceutical manufacturers, developing pharmacy provider networks, designing the prescription drug benefit, consulting with employers interested in providing a prescription drug benefit, marketing the prescription drug plan, giving sales presentations, drawing up proposals, coordinating the prescription drug benefit, and auditing network pharmacies.

## LEGISLATION AND REGULATIONS FOR MANAGED CARE PHARMACY

There are several legal issues that are related to managed care pharmacy practice. There are several federal and state laws and regulations that pertain to the prescription drug benefit portion of managed care plans. These laws and regulations address the selection of a pharmacy provider, formularies, the regulation of PBM companies, standardized information, and privacy of information.

### ANY WILLING PROVIDER LAW

The Any Willing Provider law allows any pharmacy to participate in a prescription drug benefit plan as long as the pharmacy agrees to the terms and conditions of the plan. It is referred to as an *open pharmacy law* because it requires that these plans be open to all pharmacy providers who are willing to accept the level of reimbursement set by the plan. Third-party plans prefer exclusive contracts with a limited number of pharmacies, referred to as exclusive provider networks. They argue that exclusive contracts keep costs low through discounted fees for the participating pharmacies (in return for increased prescription volume for the pharmacies).

## FREEDOM OF CHOICE LAW

The Freedom of Choice law is an open pharmacy law that focuses on the member rather than on the pharmacy or pharmacist. It allows a member to select the pharmacy of her choice, even a nonparticipating pharmacy, for her pharmacy benefit. The prescription drug plan cannot deny the nonparticipating pharmacy the right to provide the pharmacy benefit as long as the pharmacy agrees to the terms and conditions of the plan, including the rate of reimbursement. Furthermore, the member cannot be penalized financially in any way, for example, by higher co-pays, for her choice.

## PRESCRIPTION DRUG BENEFIT EQUITY ACT

The federal Prescription Drug Benefit Equity Act prohibits a prescription drug plan from providing mail-order prescription drug coverage without also providing non–mail-order prescription drug coverage. This piece of legislation ensures that members are free to obtain their prescription drugs from a participating community pharmacy rather than only through the mail. Also, some states prohibit prescription drug plans from giving their members incentives, such as lower co-pays or larger quantities of medications, to use a mail-order pharmacy rather than a community pharmacy for their prescriptions.

## ANTITRUST LAWS AND EXCLUSIVE PHARMACY CONTRACTS

Antitrust laws prohibit practices that restrain trade and prevent competition. An exclusive contract exists when a pharmacy or a group of pharmacies (e.g., a pharmacy chain) in a particular area contract with a prescription drug plan to be the only provider(s) of the prescription drug benefit for the plan members. Exclusive contracts are generally legal but can be in violation of antitrust laws if the market share of the pharmacy or pharmacies under exclusive contract hurts the competition, possibly forcing other pharmacies in the area out of business. Many small pharmacy chains and independent community pharmacies do not favor exclusive contracts and are advocates of open pharmacy laws.

## ISSUES REGARDING FORMULARIES

There are three areas of legal concern that are related to the development and management of formularies. These are in response to physician and member concerns about the restrictive nature of some formularies. These areas are:

- *Disclosure.* Many states have passed legislation regarding informing the patient about the prescription drug benefit. In particular, pharmacy plans must disclose their policies and procedures pertaining to their drug formulary, along with a copy of the formulary. Disclosure also includes information about the pharmacy and therapeutics committee and any financial arrangements with pharmaceutical manufacturers, such as discounts or rebates.

■ *Exclusion.* A formulary should include drugs that cover most medical conditions. A formulary that does not include available drug therapy for a particular condition may be in breach of contract. Furthermore, some states prohibit a prescription drug plan from excluding a nonformulary drug from coverage that a patient has been taking and is controlled on before joining the plan.

■ *Drug selection.* Under the federal Patient's Bill of Rights Act of 1998, a formulary must have an exception process that allows a physician to prescribe a nonformulary drug and have it covered by the plan. A formulary exception process is a form of consumer protection. A prescription drug plan that requires a physician to prescribe formulary drugs without exception may be liable if the patient is harmed by an alternative formulary drug or by the denial of the nonformulary drug.

## PHARMACY BENEFIT MANAGEMENT REGULATIONS

In recent years, some pharmacy benefit management companies have been acquired by pharmaceutical manufacturers. Pharmacy benefit management companies that are owned by pharmaceutical manufacturers are regulated by the Federal Trade Commission (FTC) to prevent unfair competition with other pharmaceutical manufacturers. These pharmaceutical manufacturer–owned PMB companies may give preferential status to the drug products of their partners on their formularies. This practice represents unfair competition and raises some ethical issues regarding appropriate drug choices for the formulary. Pharmacy benefit management companies must allow other pharmaceutical manufacturers to compete for the inclusion of their drugs on the formulary.

These pharmaceutical manufacturer–owned PBM companies are also regulated by the FDA. The FDA has authority over almost every aspect of a drug, including drug product communication. As with the pharmaceutical manufacturer itself, any communication regarding a drug by a PBM company is subject to FDA approval. This includes statements about a drug in advertising or marketing information given to pharmacy and therapeutics committees in making formulary choices.

## STANDARDIZED PRESCRIPTION DRUG CARD LEGISLATION

Legislation has been introduced and passed in many states regarding standardized prescription drug cards. The prescription drug card is an identification card that is presented at the pharmacy at the time of service. It is used to verify a member's eligibility for the prescription drug benefit and supplies information on the drug benefit, for example, co-payment information. However, many drug cards do not contain all the information needed to process a prescription claim, nor is the information uniform, that is, in the same format from card to card. The results are delays for the patient and less time for the pharmacist to practice pharmaceutical care, since valuable time is spent resolving problems with claims submission.

Standardized prescription drug card legislation requires prescription drug plans to issue standard or uniform prescription drug cards to members. All cards must use the same standard format and include all the information necessary for pharmacists to efficiently process prescription drug claims. The use of standardized prescription drug cards benefits patients, pharmacists, and insurance companies. Patients experience fewer delays and more pharmacist interaction when filling their prescriptions. Pharmacists have fewer insurance hassles and more time for pharmaceutical care activities. Insurance companies benefit from quicker and more efficient claims processing and fewer calls to their help desks.

## STANDARDIZED ELECTRONIC CLAIMS FORMAT LEGISLATION

The federal Health Insurance Portability and Accountability Act of 1996 (HIPAA) requires that a standard electronic format be used for processing prescription drug claims. The goal is to improve the efficiency of electronic claims submission. The result is a decrease in processing costs for the plans and increased time for patient care for pharmacists.

## PRIVACY REGULATIONS

Regulations under the Health Insurance Portability and Accountability Act of 1996 protect the privacy of personal health information in all forms—electronic, paper records, and oral communications—by all health care organizations. This health information includes prescription drug benefit records. These regulations limit the use and release of information, restrict the disclosure of information to the minimum needed for the intended purpose, and establish new requirements for access to records by researchers and others. These regulations allow a PBM company or other managed care organization to use patient data and health information to provide the pharmacy benefit and other activities such as disease management programs, drug utilization review, and outcomes research. Exceptions permit a pharmacy to share prescription information with business associates in order to send health information and promotions to the members. However, this information cannot be given to the member's employer who sponsors the pharmacy benefit plan, who could possibly use it for hiring, firing, promotions, or other uses, without permission from the member. In addition, this information cannot be sold. The PBM company or managed care organization is responsible for protecting the privacy of the information by establishing policies and procedures to prevent the unauthorized use of this information within the organization. The goal of these regulations is to protect personal health information while allowing it to be used to improve patient care.

## THE ROLE OF THE PHARMACY TECHNICIAN IN MANAGED CARE

The role of the pharmacy technician in managed care pharmacy practice is non-traditional. Like the managed care pharmacist, the technician works in a managed care setting outside of a traditional pharmacy and does not perform any dispensing activities. Rather, the pharmacy technician supports the managed care pharmacist in performing administrative and clinical activities. This role calls for a highly trained and motivated technician. The pharmacy technician must possess traditional pharmacy knowledge and skills as well as knowledge and skills that are related to managed care issues, such as:

- A working knowledge of retail pharmacy and prescription claims processing
- A basic knowledge of managed care
- A knowledge of commonly prescribed medications
- An understanding of the legislation and regulations pertaining to managed care pharmacy practice
- Good computer skills
- Excellent communication skills, especially telephone communication skills

The activities and responsibilities of the pharmacy technician in managed care pharmacy practice can be as different and as challenging as those for the managed care pharmacist. The unique aspects of this type of pharmacy practice, in particular, the lack of dispensing activities, may appeal to some pharmacy technicians. Managed care pharmacy practice can be a personally and professionally rewarding pharmacy area in which to work. The role of the pharmacy technician in this area can be divided into three roles: customer service, clerical, and auditing.

## CUSTOMER SERVICE ROLE

All PBM companies have a customer service department or a member services department, also referred to as a help desk. This department receives calls from members, physicians, and pharmacists regarding the prescription drug benefit. These calls may pertain to patient eligibility, prescription drug coverage, formulary exceptions, prescription drug cards, and other issues. The pharmacy technician can act as a customer service or member service representative. The technician in a customer service role serves as the first line of communication with the PBM company. She works under the managed care pharmacist to address member, physician, and dispensing pharmacist concerns and to help maintain satisfaction with the PBM company. The pharmacist is usually available to answer questions beyond the scope of the pharmacy technician's knowledge. Examples of customer service responsibilities for the technician include fielding questions regarding the pharmacy benefit, handling special requests (e.g., coverage for a glucometer), resolving routine member issues or concerns, processing formulary override and prior authorization requests per protocol, and documenting verbal communications properly.

## CLERICAL ROLE

The pharmacy technician in a clerical role supports the managed care pharmacist in activities related to managing the prescription drug benefit as well as activities related to managing drug therapy and performing clinical functions. These responsibilities include collecting data and statistics, preparing and distributing correspondence (such as the formulary and its updates, DUR reports, committee agendas, and meeting reports), maintaining current information on the pharmacy benefit, maintaining drug information references, participating in team meetings or on committees, assisting in the preparation of pharmacy patient educational programs (such as wellness programs), assisting in contracting pharmacy provider networks, contacting pharmaceutical manufacturer sales representatives on behalf of the pharmacist (regarding appointments or contracts), and assisting the pharmacist in any other projects, reviews, mailings, or other matters pertaining to the pharmacy benefit.

### AUDITING ROLE

The pharmacy technician may participate in pharmacy audits. Participating plan pharmacies are periodically audited to ensure that they are complying with the terms of the prescription drug benefit plan. This audit is performed through an on-site visit to the pharmacy. The auditor, sometimes referred to as a pharmacy audit investigator, reviews pharmacy records. Depending on the auditor's findings, a request for a dollar adjustment may be made by the PBM company or managed care organization for questionable claims. The pharmacy technician in this role may participate in or conduct a pharmacy audit or may assist in setting up an audit.

## ■ KEY CONCEPTS

- The prescription drug benefit is prescription drug coverage that is offered as a benefit by employers.
- The types of pharmacy provider networks include the community pharmacy, in-house pharmacy, mail-order pharmacy, and physician dispensing networks.
- Pharmacies are reimbursed for their services through a reimbursement formula that includes the cost of the drug and a dispensing fee.
- Not all drugs are covered under a prescription drug benefit.
- The use of an open, closed, or restricted formulary helps control the cost of the prescription drug benefit; however, there are formulary exception processes that allow access to nonformulary and certain formulary drugs.
- A fixed, percentage, or variable member co-payment helps lower the cost and discourages unnecessary use of the drug benefit.
- There are limits on the amount of prescription drug that can be dispensed at one time, such as quantity, day supply, dollar, number, and time limits.
- The cost of the prescription drug benefit is rising, especially owing to the increase in the use of drugs and the high cost of new drugs.
- Cost containment strategies used to lower the cost of the prescription drug benefit include restrictive pharmacy networks, higher and tiered member co-payments, an aggressive formulary, and mandatory generic substitution.
- Pharmacy benefit management involves managing the cost and the quality of the pharmacy benefit through cost containment, member, and clinical services.
- Managed care pharmacy practice involves clinical and administrative activities performed by a pharmacist in managing the prescription drug benefit.
- There are many legal issues that are related to managed care pharmacy practice and the prescription drug benefit.
- The pharmacy technician has a nondispensing role in managed care pharmacy practice.

## SELF-ASSESSMENT QUESTIONS

### MULTIPLE CHOICE

1. Patients who need a nonformulary drug can be accommodated by:
   a. a lower co-pay
   b. a generic drug
   c. a formulary exception process
   d. a mail-order pharmacy

2. All of the following statements concerning the prescription drug benefit are false except:
   a. a drug benefit is a mandatory part of health care coverage
   b. a drug benefit can include tiered co-pays and can exclude certain drugs
   c. all drug benefit plans are identical
   d. all members must use mail-order pharmacies for their prescriptions

3. Formulary drugs are selected on the basis of all of the following except:
   a. effectiveness
   b. source
   c. safety
   d. cost

4. Which of the following terms refers to a limit on the amount of a prescription drug that can be dispensed at one time?
   a. time limit
   b. day supply limit
   c. dollar limit
   d. drug benefit maximum

5. Which is not a managed care pharmacy service?
   a. disease management programs
   b. drug utilization review
   c. mail-order pharmacy
   d. unit-dose repackaging

6. Standardized prescription cards result in all of the following except:
   a. quick claims processing
   b. increased calls to help desks
   c. decreased problems with claims submission
   d. increased time for patient care

7. Which of the following statements does not apply to therapeutic interchange?
   a. it requires a physician to be included in the decision
   b. it can decrease the cost of the prescription drug benefit
   c. it is guided by a drug formulary
   d. it is a formulary exception process

8. All of the following statements apply to disease management except:
   a. the focus is on managing the patient's disease
   b. drug costs are not the only consideration
   c. acute medical problems are managed in this way
   d. drugs used in disease management protocols are included in the formulary

9. A drug utilization review finding is:
   a. duplicate drug therapy
   b. drug interactions
   c. overuse of a drug
   d. all of the above

10. A pharmacy technician working in a managed care organization may:
   a. participate in a pharmacy audit
   b. process prior authorization requests
   c. answer customer service calls
   d. all of the above

## TRUE/FALSE (CORRECT THE FALSE STATEMENTS)

1. _____ A properly designed and managed formulary is a valuable tool in providing high-quality, cost-effective drug therapy.
2. _____ The use of generic drugs is the most effective pharmacy benefit cost control strategy.
3. _____ Therapeutic equivalent drugs have the same chemical structure but are in a different drug class.
4. _____ Insulin is one of the few injectable drugs that is usually covered under the prescription drug benefit.
5. _____ Pharmacy benefit management involves managing both the cost and the quality of the prescription drug benefit.
6. _____ Member satisfaction is not an important consideration in prescription drug plans.
7. _____ Managed care pharmacy practice is called pharmacy without walls because it does not involve dispensing activities.
8. _____ The administrative role of the managed care pharmacist involves drug therapy management.
9. _____ A managed care organization may give prescription benefit information to a member's employer without the member's consent.
10. _____ Formulary drugs require an exception process to be covered.

## FILL-IN

1. A _____ is a limited list of drugs approved for use in a prescription drug benefit plan.
2. _____ _____ is a process that controls the unnecessary and inappropriate use of certain drugs.
3. A _____ is a group of providers linked through a contract to provide services.
4. The portion of the total cost of a prescription that is paid by the member is the _____.

5. _____ _____ is a coordinated team approach to treating a specific disease.

6. The _____ _____ _____ law is an open pharmacy law that pertains to the member.

7. Reimbursement for a prescription drug is determined by adding a _____ _____ to the cost of the drug.

8. A _____ type of co-payment charges the same dollar amount for any prescription drug dispensed.

9. _____ control has an effect on the use of the prescription drug benefit.

10. A pharmacist who is employed by a pharmacy benefit management company is known as a _____ _____ _____ .

## CRITICAL THINKING

1. What are the advantages and disadvantages of the various cost containment strategies used to lower the cost of the prescription drug benefit?

2. What should be the reimbursement for pharmacists providing pharmaceutical care?

3. What are some reasons that formulary drugs are designated preferred and nonpreferred?

4. Why does the pharmacy benefit need to be managed?

5. How can *structure, process,* and *outcomes* be applied to managed care pharmacy?

## BIBLIOGRAPHY

Abood, R., & Brushwood, D. (2005). *Pharmacy practice and the law* (4th ed.). Sudbury, MA: Jones and Bartlett Publishers, Inc.

Arneson, D., & Hunter, T. (2005). Complying with HIPAA regulations. *Drug Topics, 149*(6), 67–76.

Cahill, J., & Manasse, H. (2005). Medicare therapy management programs: To optimize pharmacy outcomes. *Journal of Managed Care Pharmacy, 11*(2), 179–186.

Culley, E. (2005). Pharmacy benefits management and the Medicare Modernization Act. *Journal of Managed Care Pharmacy, 11*(4), 350–351.

Delate, T., & Henderson, R. (2005). Effect of patient notification of formulary change on formulary adherence. *Journal of Managed Care Pharmacy, 11*(6), 493–498.

Fallik, B. (2005). The Academy of Managed Care Pharmacy's concepts in managed care pharmacy: Prior authorization and the formulary exception process. *Journal of Managed Care Pharmacy, 11*(4), 358–361.

Foxhall, K. (2005). More states have PBMs in their crosshairs. *Drug Topics, 149*(10), 33.

Gebhart, F. (2005). Under mounting pressure, a new breed of PBM is born. *Drug Topics, 149*(17), 34.

McCarthy, R., & Schafermeyer, K. (2004). *Introduction to health care delivery: A primer for pharmacists.* Gaithersburg, MD: Aspen Publishers, Inc.

Navarro, R. (2005). *Managed care pharmacy practice* (2nd ed.). Gaithersburg, MD: Aspen Publishers, Inc.

Olson, B., Malone D., Zachary, W., & Coons, S. (2005). Consumer understanding and satisfaction associated with a 3-tier prescription drug benefit. *Journal of Managed Care Pharmacy, 11*(6), 480–492.

Piturro, M. (2005). The future of PBMs and patient care. *Caring for the Ages, 6*(9), 5–9.

Richard, C. (2005). Deadline for HIPAA security standards approaches. *Pharmacy Today, 11*(2), 28.

Sanofi Aventis Pharmaceuticals. (2006). *Managed care digest series HMO-PPO Digest* 2006. Bridgewater, NJ: Author.

Simonsen, L. (2005). A win-win with freedom of choice. *U.S. Pharmacist, 30*(6), 10.

Sipkoff, M. (2005). PBMs are driving up generic utilization. *Drug Topics Supplement, 149*(15), 145–165.

United States Department of Health and Human Services. Office for Civil Rights—HIPAA. (2005). *Medical privacy—National standards to protect the privacy of personal health information.* [On-line] U.S. Department of Health and Human Services. Available: www.hhs.gov/ocr/hipaa.

## Learning Objectives

Upon completion of this chapter, the student should be able to:

- Explain the concept of mail-order pharmacy.
- Describe the types of mail-order pharmacies and other high-volume pharmacies.
- List the advantages and disadvantages of mail-order pharmacy.
- Describe the elements of a mail-order pharmacy.
- Understand the role of automation in a mail-order pharmacy.
- Describe the prescription-filling process and the typical workflow in a mail-order pharmacy.
- Be familiar with the services of a mail-order pharmacy.
- Understand the legislation and regulations pertaining to mail-order pharmacy.
- Describe the roles of the pharmacist and the pharmacy technician in mail-order pharmacy.

## Key Terms

| | | |
|---|---|---|
| acute medication | maintenance medication | task specialization |
| central fill pharmacy | nonresident pharmacy | workflow |
| Internet pharmacy | rogue site | |
| mail-order pharmacy | specialty mail-order pharmacy | |

## Introduction

Mail-order pharmacy is an important component of the prescription drug market and has been growing for several years. It is offered by the majority of health plans today as an option to the traditional retail pharmacy for obtaining prescriptions. Mail-order pharmacy helps reduce the cost of the prescription drug benefit, offers better access and patient convenience, and ensures quality. Mail-order pharmacy is a unique practice setting for pharmacists and pharmacy technicians. It differs in several ways from traditional retail pharmacy practice. Both pharmacists and pharmacy technicians need to have a broad knowledge of the concept and operation of a mail-order pharmacy in order to work in this type of setting. They also must be familiar with the legislation and regulations that pertain to mail-order pharmacy. This chapter focuses on the mail-order pharmacy and the unique roles of the pharmacist and pharmacy technician in this setting. ■

## OVERVIEW OF MAIL-ORDER PHARMACY

A **mail-order pharmacy** is defined as a pharmacy that dispenses maintenance medications to members through mail delivery. A **maintenance medication** is a medication that is taken on an ongoing basis for a chronic condition such as asthma, depression, high blood pressure, high cholesterol, or diabetes. Mail-order pharmacy is intended to be an option to the traditional community retail pharmacy for obtaining maintenance drugs. However, it is not intended to compete with a retail pharmacy for **acute medications,** which are medications that are taken on an urgent basis for an acute condition such as infection or pain. Owing to the extra time involved in dispensing and mailing a prescription from a mail-order pharmacy, it is not the best source of acute medications.

A mail-order pharmacy is an extremely high-volume pharmacy. It dispenses a large number of prescriptions from a single site. In order to fill large numbers of prescriptions on a daily basis, the mail-order pharmacy has a unique workflow. It also has stricter quality controls than a traditional retail pharmacy as a result of this workflow.

Mail-order pharmacies are considered to be a recent development, but they have been in existence for over 50 years. Mail-order pharmacy was started in the mid-1940s by the U.S. Veterans Administration. In the late 1950s, the American Association of Retired Persons (AARP), a private, not-for-profit organization, began to offer mail-order pharmacy to its members in order to meet two needs. The first need was convenient access to a pharmacy, because many AARP members lived in rural areas where *access* to a pharmacy was limited. The second need was *low-cost* prescriptions, because at that time, many AARP members lived below the poverty line. For-profit managed care organizations started to market mail-order pharmacy to employers in the 1960s. Today, mail-order pharmacies are owned and operated not only by pharmaceutical benefit management companies but also by independent companies and retail pharmacy chains. The majority of employers offer a prescription drug benefit that includes a mail-order pharmacy option. The mail-order pharmacy is used to complement the network of community retail pharmacies. Only a small percentage of members use a mail-order pharmacy exclusively. However, some or most members use it frequently, especially senior citizens.

Mail-order pharmacy use is growing. One reason is that pharmacy benefit plans are encouraging members to use the mail-order option to fill prescriptions for maintenance medications. Mail-order pharmacy use results in cost savings for both the member and the managed care organization. It also offers better access for patients and high-quality prescription service. Mail-order pharmacies have found overall acceptance, and their use is predicted to continue to grow.

## TYPES OF MAIL-ORDER PHARMACIES

There are two types of mail-order pharmacies: the traditional mail-order pharmacy and the specialty mail-order pharmacy. A traditional mail-order pharmacy fills prescriptions for individuals for maintenance medications in general. These prescriptions are usually covered by a single payer, with the patient responsible for any co-payment.

A **specialty mail-order pharmacy** is a mail-order pharmacy that concentrates on specific areas of the prescription drug market. It fills prescriptions for patients with specific chronic diseases, such as cancer, diabetes, rheumatoid arthritis, multiple sclerosis, hepatitis, or infertility, or for patients who have undergone an organ transplant. The medications dispensed are usually injectable drugs, some produced by biotechnology, that are expensive and hard to find in the normal retail community pharmacy. These medications are often referred to as specialty drugs. Due to the fact that their diseases and medication regimens are complicated, these patients may be treated by a number of health care professionals and various health care facilities. Their prescriptions are often covered by multiple payers, such as Medicare, Medicaid, and private insurance, and payment must be coordinated among these sources.

In general, the services provided by a specialty mail-order pharmacy are more demanding than the services provided by a traditional mail-order pharmacy. Billing is more complicated owing to multiple payers, and it involves special processing, pricing, and reporting. There is more interaction with the many health care professionals participating in the patient's care, such as the primary care physician, specialist physicians, other pharmacists, nurses, case managers, and others. The type and amount of information that are needed to process prescriptions are greater. The specialty mail-order pharmacy must assemble, track, and use a large amount of data, for example, from the referring physician, procedures and tests that have been performed, and the health care institutions involved. The computer system must be able to accommodate the different types of information needed. The workflow is often different, and there may be different activities performed than in a traditional mail-order pharmacy. The opportunity for generic and therapeutic substitution is limited in these chronic diseases. Finally, patient monitoring is more intense for the pharmacist.

Two examples of a specialty mail-order pharmacy are Accredo Health, Inc., managed by the PBM Medco Health Solutions, and Pharmacare Specialty Pharmacy, owned and operated by the retail pharmacy chain CVS.

## ADVANTAGES AND DISADVANTAGES OF MAIL-ORDER PHARMACY

There are several advantages to mail-order pharmacy. These include:

- *Cost savings.* The patient can receive a larger supply of medication for a lower cost than in a retail pharmacy. There are also cost savings for the managed care organization. Mail-order pharmacies often receive discounts on their large-volume drug purchases from pharmaceutical manufacturers. Automation also decreases the costs associated with filling prescriptions.

■ *Patient convenience.* Prescriptions can be delivered to the home or office. Delivery saves time and is especially important for patients who are elderly, have disabilities, or live in rural areas. Mail-order pharmacy also offers convenience through different payment options (credit card or direct billing). On-line access also is available.

■ *Unlimited access to a pharmacist.* A pharmacist is available for consultation by way of toll-free telephone lines 24 hours a day, 7 days a week. The pharmacist has access to the patient's records and can answer any questions or concerns a patient may have about his medications.

■ *Improved compliance.* Mail-order pharmacy service encourages compliance by making it easy and convenient for patients to obtain their medications. In addition, mail-order pharmacy tries to improve overall compliance through compliance monitoring and refill reminders.

■ *Improved pharmacy efficiency.* A mail-order pharmacy is a more efficient pharmacy operation than retail pharmacy through its organized workflow and the use of automation.

■ *Decreased dispensing errors.* Despite the large volume of prescriptions dispensed in a mail-order pharmacy, there are fewer dispensing errors than in a traditional retail pharmacy. This accuracy is due to the use of automation, employees performing specialized tasks, and fewer distractions, such as the phone ringing or patients waiting at the prescription counter. There also are very strict quality and safety checks for every prescription filled.

■ *Patient privacy.* A mail-order pharmacy is more private than a traditional retail pharmacy. Patient consultation is over the phone rather than within earshot of other patients. Many people, especially senior citizens, prefer to have a relaxed conversation with a pharmacist in the privacy of their own homes, rather than trying to talk to the pharmacist in a busy retail pharmacy.

■ *Availability of medications.* A mail-order pharmacy is able to stock expensive, infrequently used, and hard-to-find medications that a community pharmacy may find difficult to stock because of high cost and slow turnover.

There are also some disadvantages associated with mail-order pharmacy. These include:

■ *Lack of personal contact.* Mail-order pharmacy does not allow face-to-face contact between a pharmacist and a patient.

■ *Medication waste.* There is the potential for waste if a medication is discontinued. This waste is due to the large amounts or day supplies of medications dispensed through mail order, on the average of a 90-day supply.

■ *Time delays.* Mail-order pharmacy service can result in a delay to the patient in receiving needed medications owing to the nature of the business.

# OTHER HIGH-VOLUME PHARMACIES

There are other high-volume pharmacies that work on the same principles as a mail-order pharmacy: the central fill pharmacy and the Internet pharmacy. Both of these types of high-volume pharmacies are growing in popularity and should be mentioned here.

## CENTRAL FILL PHARMACY

A **central fill pharmacy** is a high-volume pharmacy that centrally fills prescriptions for a number of individual pharmacies. It is usually found in a centralized location, close to the individual pharmacies that it serves in a particular area. A central fill pharmacy is most often used by a retail pharmacy chain to handle prescriptions for its many individual pharmacy locations. Some large long-term care pharmacy corporations also use a central fill operation.

A central fill pharmacy is used primarily to fill prescription refills. Prescription refills are ordered by patients in several ways: by telephone, on-line, or at their local pharmacy prescription counter. The prescriptions are filled, labeled, and packaged at the central fill pharmacy, then they are delivered back to the local pharmacy or to the patient's home. Like a traditional mail-order pharmacy, a central fill pharmacy is highly automated. Because of the increase in the number of prescriptions being written by physicians and the shortage of pharmacists in some areas, central fill pharmacy is growing in use.

In addition to dispensing activities, there are other nonclinical activities that are performed at a central fill pharmacy. These activities include adjudicating claims, resolving problems with claims, calling physicians, and performing drug use review. These are activities that occupy a great deal of the pharmacist's time in a traditional pharmacy operation. By having these activities performed at the central fill pharmacy, the pharmacist at the local pharmacy has more time for clinical and patient care activities, such as patient counseling.

A central fill pharmacy has many advantages. It lowers the cost and increases the efficiency of filling prescriptions through the use of a central site, automation, and high volume. It provides the patient with several options for ordering and receiving prescription refills. It reduces the workload and relieves congestion behind the local pharmacy counter. Finally, it enhances patient care by enabling the local pharmacist to spend more time with the patient and less time preparing refills. In short, a central fill pharmacy combines the efficiency of a mail-order pharmacy with direct contact between the local pharmacist and the patient.

## INTERNET PHARMACY

The Internet has affected almost every industry, including pharmacy. Internet pharmacies are becoming an important component of the prescription drug market and, in fact, are revolutionizing this market. Internet pharmacies, also referred to as on-line pharmacies, are being recognized as a convenient, easy-to-use, cost-effective way for patients to receive their medications.

An **Internet pharmacy** is defined as an established commercial Web site that enables a patient to obtain prescriptions and over-the-counter medications by way of the Internet, usually at reduced prices. It combines prescription dispensing with access to information. Most Internet pharmacies are full service, on-line pharmacies. They provide prescription and nonprescription medications, as well as vitamins, herbals, and health and beauty products. They accept and bill the patient's prescription drug insurance and charge the co-pay to a credit card account. They deliver promptly by way of the mail or overnight delivery and keep delivery costs to a minimum. In addition, Internet pharmacies provide toll-free telephone lines or e-mail to communicate directly with the pharmacy. They also provide medication and disease information, prescription drug price quotes, links to related Web sites, some clinical services such as compliance monitoring, disease state management, and patient education, and patient support services by way of telephone or e-mail. In fact, many prescription drug plans are offering the use of an Internet pharmacy in addition to community and mail-order pharmacies to obtain prescriptions. One of the best-known Internet pharmacies is www.drugstore.com.

The dispensing operation of an Internet pharmacy is a high-volume operation similar to that of a mail-order pharmacy. Like a traditional mail-order pharmacy, an Internet pharmacy is held to the same standards of care as any traditional retail pharmacy. It must comply with all state and federal laws and regulations. It has the same obligation to counsel patients regarding their prescriptions. Most Internet pharmacies have extensive safeguards in place that ensure proper prescription-dispensing practices. These include making sure that all prescriptions are valid, confirming that an actual relationship exists between a physician and a patient, using bar coding and automation to decrease dispensing errors, performing drug utilization review (DUR) before dispensing, and performing quality control checks of every prescription by a pharmacist before shipping. At the minimum, an Internet pharmacy must have a secure Web site, be licensed in the states in which it does business (where the patient lives), and disclose the location of its headquarters.

Although most Internet pharmacy sites are legitimate businesses, there are some illegitimate Internet pharmacy sites, called **rogue sites,** that may endanger the health and safety of patients. Some of these businesses operate outside of the United States. They have inappropriate business and pharmacy practices such as selling unsafe medications (outdated, counterfeit, damaged, or contaminated drugs and drugs unapproved for medical use in the United States) and dispensing medications without a legitimate prescription (without a physical consultation between a physician and a patient). In addition, there have been some consumer concerns regarding patient privacy and delivery time. However, overall, Internet pharmacies provide improved access to medication and medical information for millions of people. This area is becoming popular with consumers, and it is expected to grow.

Relative to Internet pharmacies, it should be mentioned that mail-order pharmacies, large national pharmacy chains, independent community pharmacies, and even drug wholesalers are establishing Web sites to serve their customers better and to increase their market exposure.

## ELEMENTS OF A MAIL-ORDER PHARMACY

There are many elements that make up a mail-order pharmacy. Some of these elements are the same as those found in a traditional retail pharmacy. However, some are unique to a mail-order pharmacy and other high-volume pharmacy operations.

## PERSONNEL

As in any other type of pharmacy, a variety of personnel are needed in the mail-order pharmacy for its efficient operation. Pharmacists, pharmacy technicians, and other support personnel are found in a mail-order pharmacy. Within each type of personnel group are specific job titles. Each job title carries specific duties. The person holding a particular job title is highly proficient in performing his specific job duties.

There are several job titles for pharmacists in a mail-order pharmacy. One type of pharmacist reviews the prescription orders that have been entered into the computer and may be called a *screening pharmacist*. Another pharmacist checks finished prescriptions and may be called a *checking pharmacist*. There are pharmacists who handle phone calls for patients, called *consulting pharmacists*. Finally, there are pharmacists who are involved in clinical services such as DUR, formulary management, disease management, compliance monitoring, and education. Their job title within the mail-order pharmacy is *clinical pharmacist*.

There are also several job titles for pharmacy technicians in a mail-order pharmacy. One type of pharmacy technician interprets the written prescription orders and enters them into the computer and may be referred to as an *order entry* or *item entry technician*. Another technician fills the prescription orders with the appropriate medications and may be called a *filling technician*. There are also pharmacy technicians who make phone calls on behalf of the pharmacist and may be referred to as *support technicians*.

Finally, there are several types of support personnel in a mail-order pharmacy operation. Data entry personnel open the mail to retrieve written prescriptions and to enter basic patient and insurance information into the computer. Billing personnel help with adjudication, prescription reimbursement, and patient billing. Shipping personnel package the finished prescriptions and prepare them for shipping. Customer services personnel, referred to as customer service representatives, answer telephone calls from members for general information about their prescription orders.

The appropriate number of pharmacists, pharmacy technicians, and other personnel in the mail-order pharmacy depends on the volume and size of the mail-order pharmacy operation. It is not uncommon for a mail-order pharmacy to employ dozens, even hundreds, of pharmacists, pharmacy technicians, and support personnel.

## INVENTORY

The drug inventory in a mail-order pharmacy usually differs from the drug inventory found in a traditional retail pharmacy in that it primarily contains medications that are used to treat chronic conditions, that is, maintenance drugs. Owing to the nature of the mail-order pharmacy business, there is little demand for acute medications that need to be taken right away, for example, pain medications, antibiotics, and cough syrups. However, most mail-order pharmacies do stock a small amount of these types of medications for their few patients who take them chronically. Most mail-order pharmacies also carry expensive, infrequently used, or hard-to-find medications that some traditional retail pharmacies may not stock. The mail-order pharmacy tries to maintain a high level of service and member satisfaction by having the appropriate type and amount of inventory on hand.

## PHARMACY DESIGN

The physical design of a mail-order pharmacy is very different from the design of a traditional retail pharmacy. A mail-order pharmacy has a completely different *look*. A mail-order pharmacy is usually quite large, owing to the large volume of prescriptions it fills and the corresponding large numbers of employees. It resembles a warehouse operation more than it resembles a traditional retail pharmacy operation. The most important difference is that a mail-order pharmacy is divided into separate and different work areas, sometimes referred to as workstations. These areas are designed for specific tasks. Each work area is designed to handle a specific step in the prescription-filling process, where only that one step is performed. Table 9–1 lists the specific work areas in a mail-order pharmacy and their corresponding tasks. In addition to the areas in Table 9–1, there are also separate departments designed to handle billing, administration, sales, and marketing.

In general, a mail-order pharmacy is designed to allow a large volume of prescriptions to be dispensed in an organized and efficient manner. The design of the pharmacy also should take into consideration employee safety and comfort, such as adequate space for tasks and good lighting; proper storage conditions for medications, including refrigerated medications and controlled substances; cleanliness and pest control; and security.

**TABLE 9–1**  Specific Work Areas in a Mail-Order Pharmacy

| WORK AREA | SPECIFIC TASK |
| --- | --- |
| Mail room | Prescriptions received |
| Data entry area | Patient and insurance data entered into the computer |
| Order entry area | Prescription data entered into the computer |
| Filling or dispensing area | Prescription orders filled |
| Compounding area | Compounded prescriptions formulated |
| Controlled substances area | Controlled substances stored and prescriptions filled |
| Checking area | Finished prescriptions checked by a pharmacist |
| Shipping area | Checked prescriptions prepared for shipping |
| Inventory receiving area | Drug inventory received |
| Customer service area | Calls received concerning customer service |
| Pharmacist counseling area | Calls received concerning patient counseling |
| Clinical services area | Clinical services performed |

## EQUIPMENT AND SUPPLIES

Traditional pharmacy equipment is found in the mail-order pharmacy and consists of computer hardware and printers, facsimile machines, telephone systems, extemporaneous compounding equipment, and manual counting equipment such as counting trays. There is a variety of specialized equipment found in a mail-order pharmacy. This equipment varies depending on the type of automation used in the mail-order pharmacy.

### Automation

Automation is used in all pharmacy practice areas today, but nowhere is it used more extensively than in the mail-order pharmacy. Automated pharmacy equipment stores, retrieves, counts, packages, and labels medications. All of these activities are repetitive and labor-intensive and are subject to human error. Automation in the mail-order pharmacy reduces the need for manual labor, increases productivity, reduces dispensing errors, increases the security of medications, reduces the stress on employees, streamlines the workflow, minimizes work space, provides documentation, and improves overall quality control. Automation is used in almost every step in the prescription-filling process in the mail-order pharmacy. Specific examples of automation that can be found in a mail-order pharmacy include:

- *Conveyor belts.* These automatically move the prescription order and medication from station to station and keep the production line moving.
- *Robotics.* Robotic arms that operate on vertical and horizontal rails automatically select and retrieve a medication from among hundreds of drug products on storage shelves.
- *Counting machines.* These automatically count out the correct quantity of capsules or tablets and place them into the appropriate-sized prescription vial.
- *Labeling units.* These automatically place the prescription label, containing a bar code, on the prescription vial.
- *Bar code scanning devices.* These automatically identify whether the correct medication has been dispensed by scanning a bar code on the pharmaceutical manufacturer's container.
- *Imaging systems.* These automatically make a digital computerized picture of the written prescription by scanning it into a computer. The copy is then passed through the prescription-filling process instead of the paper copy. Imaging systems also provide a database of color images of tablets and capsules for use by the pharmacist when checking finished prescriptions.

### Computer Software

There is computer software specifically designed for mail-order pharmacy use. The computer software system used in the mail-order pharmacy handles all of the functions needed for the large-volume production of prescriptions. It guides normal prescription-processing functions as well as the operation of automated equipment and shipping. It also assists in customer service, clinical services, and security. Mail-order pharmacy computer software provides a paperless system through the digital imaging of written prescriptions. Most of these software systems today interface with the Internet to receive prescription refill orders.

## TOLL-FREE TELEPHONE LINES

Toll-free telephone lines are a unique and vital component of a mail-order pharmacy operation. They are used to receive both new prescription orders from physicians and refill requests from patients. They also are used for customer service and patient counseling. In addition to regular toll-free lines, there are special toll-free lines, such as integrated voice response (IVR) lines and automated Touch-tone™ lines for refill requests. There also are telecommunication devices (TTDs) or text telephones (TTYs) for people who are deaf or hearing-impaired and foreign-language lines for non–English-speaking patients. The goal of providing toll-free telephone lines is to give the best possible service to patients who use a mail-order pharmacy to obtain their prescriptions.

## MAIL SERVICE

The timely, efficient, and confidential delivery of prescriptions is the hallmark of mail-order pharmacy. There are two components to the mail service: the packaging and preparation of the finished prescriptions for delivery and the delivery service itself.

In general, all types of prescription medication can be shipped, including controlled substances. Controlled substances are permitted to be shipped under the Controlled Substances Act. However, there are special packaging requirements. They must be shipped in a container or with an outside wrapper that does not indicate or identify the nature of the medication inside. Refrigerated medications may also be shipped if properly packaged.

The goal of packaging is to protect and preserve the integrity of a prescription medication during shipment. This is accomplished in a number of ways. Padded or durable plastic mailing envelopes prevent damage in shipping and handling. Bubble wrap is used to protect all types of prescription containers, especially glass. Refrigerated drugs are packaged in insulated containers or with cool packs. Once the proper packaging is selected, the prescription is prepared for delivery; the proper paperwork is included; and the package is routed to the proper shipper or carrier for delivery.

The choice of a shipper or carrier depends on several factors. These include the shipping rates of different carriers, the destination of the prescription(s), the volume or weight of the prescription(s) being mailed, the value of the prescription(s) being mailed, and the ability of the carrier to track the shipment. Delivery services can be arranged through the U.S. Postal Service (USPS), United Parcel Service (UPS), Federal Express (FedEx), or other services. Only the USPS can deliver to post office box numbers in the United States because it has the rights to those addresses. Most mail-order pharmacies will then arrange to deliver prescriptions anywhere the patient desires, including home, work, a vacation address, or post office box. Prescriptions also can be mailed to patients who reside overseas. International delivery is available through most carriers. Delivery can be made to overseas post office box numbers by any carrier because the USPS does not have any jurisdiction over these addresses. However, a valid telephone number must be provided. International delivery requires that the shipment of prescription medications be cleared through customs in the destination country. A certificate of origin, a document that certifies the origin of the shipment, must be completed to clear customs.

The amount of time required for prescription delivery depends on several factors. These include the manner in which the prescription was received, such as the mail, facsimile, telephone, electronically, or on-line; the type of drug being shipped, especially refrigerated, controlled, or expensive medications; whether the medication is in stock, because out-of-stock or special-request medications may need to be ordered; where the prescription is being delivered, such as in state, out of state, overseas, or to a post office box number; and how fast the patient wants or needs the medication. Most mail-order pharmacies usually require several days for routine delivery, although sometimes patients can receive their prescriptions within a few days after their request is received. Oftentimes, prescription refills are mailed out on the same day they are received. Patients have the option of express delivery or next-day delivery at their own expense. Of course, if a patient will be without his medication for reasons beyond his control, most mail-order pharmacies will ship the prescriptions by the next day at the pharmacy's expense. Also, most mail-order pharmacies routinely arrange for express delivery of expensive medications, due to their cost, and refrigerated medications, due to their special packing and shipping requirements.

## THE PRESCRIPTION-FILLING PROCESS IN A MAIL-ORDER PHARMACY

A mail-order pharmacy handles a large volume of prescriptions on a daily basis. Managing this process in an organized and efficient way is accomplished through a controlled workflow. **Workflow** is defined as an organized way of filling prescriptions. It is a repeatable, defined set of activities. Workflow can be applied to any type or size of pharmacy filling any volume of prescriptions, but it is especially important in a high-volume pharmacy such as the mail-order pharmacy. In the mail-order pharmacy, the prescription-filling process is broken down into a number of separate, well-defined, repeatable tasks or steps. These tasks are assigned to appropriate personnel who focus only on the specific task. The tasks or steps take place in the separate work areas or workstations within the mail-order pharmacy. The prescriptions and medications then move or progress from station to station in an assembly line fashion. The entire process takes place by means of automation, such as conveyor belts, robotics, and counting machines. An efficient workflow results in high quality and safety despite the high volumes of prescriptions being filled.

The majority of prescriptions are received in a mail-order pharmacy by mail. A small amount are received by telephone, facsimile machine, electronically, or over the Internet. Prescription processing begins as these prescriptions enter the workflow. The typical workflow in a mail-order pharmacy consists of the following steps:

- *Order entry.* Mail is opened, and basic patient and insurance data are entered into the computer, usually by data entry personnel. These data include safety cap preference, brand or generic preference, allergy and disease state information, shipping preference, and payment information. Prescriptions are then processed into batches and are digitally scanned into the computer or assigned a bar code or both. From this step on, the prescription-filling process is a paperless process. Prescription orders move through the system electronically. The written prescriptions are filed, as in a traditional retail pharmacy.

- *Prescription item entry.* The prescription order is interpreted, and the prescription data are entered into the computer, usually by a pharmacy technician.

- *Screening.* The prescription order is reviewed and analyzed by a pharmacist. The pharmacist verifies that all prescription information has been correctly interpreted and entered into the computer. As in any traditional pharmacy, the pharmacist performs a prospective drug utilization review to ensure that the medication is therapeutically correct, to ensure that the dosage is correct, to identify allergies or drug interactions, and to eliminate duplicate drug therapy. The pharmacist may make a telephone call to a physician to resolve a problem or make a recommendation concerning a prescription. All problems are resolved before a prescription order is forwarded to the next step in the workflow.

- *Adjudication.* The prescription claim is submitted electronically to verify insurance coverage and payment. Successful adjudication of the prescription results in reimbursement for the prescription and the generation of a prescription label.

- *Dispensing.* The appropriate medication is dispensed by a pharmacy technician on the basis of information on the prescription label. Dispensing is accomplished with the help of some type of automation. It involves selecting, counting, labeling, and packaging the medication.

- *Quality assurance check.* The finished prescription is checked by a pharmacist to verify that the correct medication has been dispensed, that the labeling of the prescription is correct, and that all the appropriate educational materials are included with the prescription order. Checking is accomplished by scanning the bar-coded prescription to produce a reference image (from the data bank of reference images for tablets and capsules) and comparing that image with the medication inside the prescription container.

- *Packaging and shipping.* The checked prescription is packaged and prepared for shipment to the patient by packaging personnel.

Most prescription orders move through the workflow without any problems. However, some prescriptions require special attention and are routed out of the regular workflow into special areas for specific tasks. These areas include:

- *Early refill.* A prescription that is presented for filling too early is held in this area and is released for filling on the appropriate date.

- *Adjudication support.* Claims that fail adjudication are routed to this area, where claim details are corrected and another attempt is made at adjudication.

- *Fill on arrival.* A prescription is held in this area until inventory is on hand to fill it. If the inventory is not received within a specified time, or if the medication is back-ordered, the prescription order is split and partially filled with the available inventory.

- *Prescription intervention.* Prescriptions that are candidates for therapeutic substitution or that require the attention of a pharmacist are routed to this area, where a pharmacist consults a physician or resolves the problem.

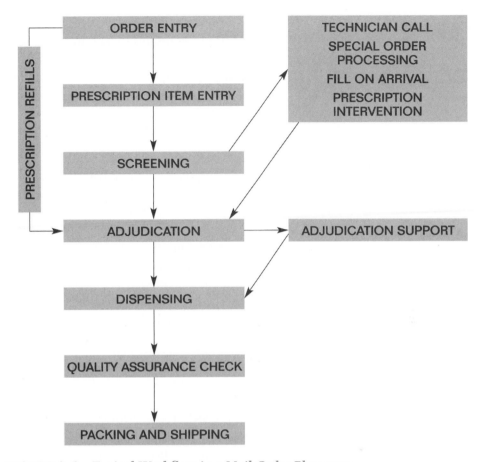

**FIGURE 9–1**    Typical Workflow in a Mail-Order Pharmacy.

- *Technician call.* Prescriptions that are expired or have no refills remaining are routed to this area, where a pharmacy technician calls the patient or calls or faxes the physician's office to obtain authorization, if allowed by state board of pharmacy regulations.

- *Special order processing.* Prescriptions for medications that have to be special ordered, that require special handling, or that require clinical interventions, such as laboratory testing, are handled in this area.

In general, once prescription problems have been resolved in these special areas, the prescriptions are routed back into the proper place in the workflow for completion. Prescription refill requests are routed forward to adjudication, bypassing the first few steps in the workflow. The typical workflow in a mail-order pharmacy is represented by Figure 9–1.

## SERVICES OF A MAIL-ORDER PHARMACY

Traditional mail-order pharmacy service consists of a prescription-dispensing service coupled with a delivery service. In addition to the dispensing and delivery services, however, most mail-order pharmacies offer a variety of other services that enhance patient satisfaction, improve the outcomes of drug therapy, and help reduce drug costs. In fact, there is a new emphasis on these services, as reflected in another term for mail-order pharmacy: *mail service pharmacy*. Many of these services are the same services that are offered in other pharmacy settings. In addition to computerized patient profiles, drug use review, and OBRA-mandated patient counseling, several types of programs can be found in a mail-order pharmacy operation.

### DISEASE MANAGEMENT PROGRAMS

Disease management programs are used to maximize the benefit of drug therapy for chronic diseases associated with high drug costs, such as diabetes, hypertension, and heart disease. First, data from prescription processing are used to identify patients who can benefit from disease management programs. These programs then monitor patients for compliance with their drug therapy, adverse reactions, drug interactions, and the outcomes of their drug therapy. These programs also involve physician education by the pharmacist on all aspects of drug therapy for a particular disease, including recommendations for more appropriate drug therapy. The goal of these disease management programs is to prevent acute episodes of a chronic disease through the best use of the patient's drug therapy.

### DRUG UTILIZATION REVIEW

Drug utilization review (DUR) involves collecting, analyzing, and reporting prescription data generated by filling prescriptions. The mail-order pharmacist evaluates physician prescribing practices to determine the appropriateness of drug therapy. This evaluation may lead to suggestions by the pharmacist to the physician on how to improve drug therapy. An example is identifying a drug that is considered to be potentially inappropriate for use in an elderly patient. The pharmacist would contact the physician to recommend switching the patient to a more appropriate drug choice.

### FORMULARY MANAGEMENT

Formulary management in the mail-order pharmacy setting involves helping physicians and patients adhere to a formulary that has been designed for them. The pharmacist may contact the physician regarding generic or therapeutic substitution in appropriate patients as required by the formulary.

### COMPLIANCE MONITORING

Compliance monitoring identifies patients who do not adhere to their medication regimens or schedules. Prescription refill records are audited to identify patients who fail to refill a chronic medication within an appropriate period of time. These patients are then contacted by telephone or mail as to the importance of taking their medications and managing their disease. Medication-taking behavior surveys and drug regimen reviews are also part of compliance monitoring. Pharmacists sometimes need to contact a prescriber to suggest alternative drug therapy to help simplify a patient's drug regimen, so that it is easier to comply with. An example would be a pharmacist's recommendation for a once-a-day sustained-release form of a medication rather than the immediate-release form that needs to be taken four times a day. The mail-order pharmacist also may contact the patient to make suggestions on how to be more compliant.

## PATIENT EDUCATION

A mail-order pharmacy provides patient education in written form on a variety of topics. A patient package insert, which is printed educational material concerning a particular medication, is sent to the patient with each prescription. This material explains how to take the medication, how to store the medication in the home, what types of symptoms to look for and report concerning side effects and adverse drug reactions, and other information. Patients also may receive other written materials on wellness or healthy living, such as information on nutrition, fitness, and exercise. Patients who are identified as high risk due to high drug use or a chronic disease may receive educational material that may discuss their condition, how to better manage their disease, and the importance of being compliant with their drug regimen. Overall, patient education results in better outcomes of drug therapy.

# LEGISLATION AND REGULATIONS FOR MAIL-ORDER PHARMACY

A mail-order pharmacy is licensed and regulated by the state board of pharmacy in the state in which it is located, referred to as its home state. Most mail-order pharmacies are licensed as "retail" pharmacies because most states do not have a separate license category for mail-order pharmacies. A mail-order pharmacy must comply with all state and federal pharmacy laws and regulations. There are several specific regulations that pertain to mail-order pharmacy, and they are discussed next.

### OMNIBUS BUDGET RECONCILIATION ACT OF 1990

There are two provisions of OBRA 90 that apply to a mail-order pharmacy in a unique way. First, OBRA 90 requires DUR. A mail-order pharmacist performs a prospective DUR before dispensing and delivering each prescription. What is unique to mail-order pharmacy, however, is that in addition to the patient's profile, the pharmacist also has the benefit of looking at the patient's entire prescription claim history to detect problems with drug therapy. Second, OBRA requires patient counseling. In order to satisfy this requirement, a mail-order pharmacy must provide comprehensive written or printed information with all new prescription orders and must extend a written offer to counsel. The counseling requirement of a mail-order pharmacy is unique in that it may be satisfied by toll-free telephone lines, which are usually available 24 hours a day, 7 days a week. Patients may call a pharmacist whenever they have a question or problem with their medications.

### MEDICARE PRESCRIPTION DRUG BENEFIT

The Medicare Prescription Drug Benefit, or Medicare Part D, also applies to the Medicare beneficiary who chooses to use a mail-order pharmacy to dispense his drugs and to the mail-order pharmacy itself. Medicare regulations allow Medicare patients to use a mail-order pharmacy as an alternative to a community retail pharmacy. In most instances, Part D plans offer a 90-day supply of covered medications, often at a reduced co-pay, through mail order.

Any mail-order pharmacy may be a pharmacy provider for a Medicare Part D plan that offers mail-order pharmacy service as long as it agrees to the terms and conditions of the plan under the Any Willing Provider law. As in long-term care and home infusion pharmacy, the cost of mailing prescriptions is incorporated into a higher dispensing fee for the mail-order pharmacy versus a retail community pharmacy. Medication therapy management (MTM) services must also be provided to targeted patients who use a mail-order pharmacy, but their MTM services may come from a local pharmacy provider as well as from a mail-order pharmacist. As in home infusion pharmacy, the law also requires that specialty drugs administered by injection that are not already covered under Medicare Part B be covered under Medicare Part D.

## NONRESIDENT PHARMACY LEGISLATION

In addition to the rules and regulations for in-state mail-order pharmacies, many individual states have passed laws that pertain to out-of-state mail-order pharmacies. An out-of-state mail-order pharmacy is referred to as a nonresident pharmacy. A **nonresident pharmacy** is defined as a pharmacy that is located outside of a particular state that mails, ships, or delivers prescriptions to patients inside that particular state. A nonresident pharmacy must possess a valid pharmacy license from its home state. In addition, some states require that a nonresident mail-order pharmacy obtain a nonresident license in their state. A nonresident pharmacy license is a pharmacy license issued by a particular state to a pharmacy located in another state to provide prescriptions to patients within their state. Instead of this type of additional licensure, some states require that the nonresident mail-order pharmacies register with the state board of pharmacy within the state that they are delivering to or obtain a permit to do business within that state. There are additional requirements for nonresident mail-order pharmacies, and these vary from state to state. Some of these requirements are:

- A nonresident mail-order pharmacy must comply with patient counseling requirements of the state in which the patient is located. Almost all states require an accessible toll-free telephone line and a registered pharmacist for patient counseling. The telephone number must be displayed on the prescription label affixed to the prescription container.

- Most states require that a nonresident mail-order pharmacy keep readily retrievable patient profiles and prescription-dispensing records, especially records of controlled substances dispensed.

- Some states have specific regulations regarding generic substitution. However, these regulations do not supersede the laws and regulations pertaining to generic substitution in the mail-order pharmacy's home state.

- Some states prohibit the advertising of the prescription services of a nonresident mail-order pharmacy that is not licensed, that has not registered, or that has not obtained a permit to do business in that state.

- Some states require that the names of all of the corporate owners, officers, and out-of-state pharmacists who are employed by the nonresident mail-order pharmacy be disclosed to their state board of pharmacy.

- Some states require that the "pharmacist in charge" of a nonresident mail-order pharmacy be licensed in their state by reciprocal agreement or by an equivalency exam.

Ideally, each state board of pharmacy should license and regulate only the mail-order pharmacies within its state. Otherwise, a mail-order pharmacy serving several states could be subject to conflicting and overlapping regulations imposed by several states. Some states have conflicting legislation, and some states have no nonresident pharmacy regulations at all. It remains to be seen whether all states will implement consistent nonresident pharmacy legislation. A mail-order pharmacy, therefore, must be familiar with the nonresident pharmacy legislation in each state in which it does business.

## DRUG ENFORCEMENT AGENCY REGULATIONS

There are DEA regulations that pertain to a mail-order pharmacy in a unique way. As it does for any pharmacy, the DEA requires that controlled substances be kept in a locked cabinet or dispersed throughout the noncontrolled drug stock to prevent their diversion. A mail-order pharmacy usually stocks large quantities of controlled substances. Consequently, additional security is provided, usually in the form of a secure enclosure for controlled substances, such as a vault or cage, an alarm system, and through policies and procedures concerning access to and the handling of controlled substances.

According to the DEA, under federal law there is no limit to the amount of a controlled substance that may be dispensed according to a valid prescription if it is allowed by state law. A mail-order pharmacy typically dispenses larger day supplies of medications than a traditional retail pharmacy. Federal law permits more than a 30-day supply or more than 120 dosage units of a Schedule II controlled substance to be dispensed to ensure that patients have uninterrupted access to these drugs. However, some states have laws pertaining to quantity limits, and some of these state laws are more stringent than the federal law and therefore do not permit large quantities of Schedule II controlled substances to be dispensed by a mail-order pharmacy. A mail-order pharmacy should be familiar with individual state laws regarding quantity limits of Schedule II controlled substances.

## PHARMACY AUTOMATION REGULATIONS

There are currently no consistent pharmacy regulations concerning automation. Many state boards of pharmacy have provisions that do not allow or that limit the use of pharmacy automation. Pharmacy automation regulations are needed to safeguard patients while allowing pharmacies to take advantage of the latest in automation technology. In 1995, the Automation in Pharmacy Initiative, a collaboration of national pharmacy organizations, was established to identify and address the legal barriers to automation in pharmacy in all practice areas. It has worked with the National Association of Boards of Pharmacy (NABP) to review existing or proposed regulations addressing automation in pharmacy, identify areas of concern to state boards of pharmacy, and develop model regulations to address these concerns. The resulting model regulations have prompted many individual state boards of pharmacy to develop more consistent regulations for pharmacy automation, especially robotics, and to allow their appropriate and efficient use.

## TEMPERATURE STANDARDS GOVERNING MAILED PRESCRIPTIONS

There are currently no consistent regulations concerning temperature standards for mailed prescriptions. However, several states have drafted regulations establishing temperature standards for medications that are mailed. There has been concern that temperature and humidity changes can occur during the shipment of prescriptions by mail and that these changes can affect the integrity of the medications. Studies conducted by the USP have shown that some packages of prescription medications can experience temperatures outside of the USP definition of controlled room temperature, as well as spikes in the relative humidity. On the basis of these studies, the USP has proposed guidelines for packaging to maintain temperatures within allowable limits. This proposal, in turn, has influenced state boards of pharmacy to draft similar guidelines. Some states require that temperature and humidity indicators be included with prescriptions sent by mail. Other states require that a written notice be included with mailed prescriptions to alert patients that, under certain conditions, a medication's effectiveness can be affected by exposure to extreme heat or humidity or that a notice be included that provides a toll-free telephone number to answer patients' questions.

## CENTRAL FILL REGULATIONS

The Drug Enforcement Agency (DEA) has recognized the practice of centralized prescription filling by issuing federal regulations that became effective in 2003. These regulations describe legitimate central fill activities and allow the filling of controlled substance prescriptions.

The NABP has also been involved in the issue of centralized prescription filling. Central fill is such a new concept that many state boards of pharmacy restrict the practice. Regulations are needed to safeguard patients while allowing this innovative practice. In 1999, the NABP established the Task Force on Centralized Prescription Filling to develop model regulations that individual state boards of pharmacy may use to develop consistent regulations addressing central fill dispensing. Many states have since developed central fill regulations. Some of these state regulations include:

- A license similar to any other mail-order pharmacy
- A contract or ownership between a central fill pharmacy and the pharmacies that it serves
- The name and address of both pharmacies on the prescription label
- A common electronic file shared between the pharmacies
- Complete and accurate prescription records in both pharmacies
- Patient counseling at the home pharmacy

Rather than restrict centralized prescription filling, state boards of pharmacy are recognizing the increased opportunity for patient care at the home pharmacy that is made possible by central fill.

## INTERNET PHARMACY LEGISLATION

The sale of prescription drugs in the United States over the Internet has been relatively unregulated. Several states have introduced or enacted legislation in an attempt to regulate Internet pharmacies. Some states require that Internet pharmacies abide by the same regulations as traditional "brick and mortar" pharmacies. Some states require that Internet pharmacies comply with the licensure requirements and generic substitution laws of the state in which they are located. Many states are applying the nonresident pharmacy requirements to Internet pharmacies. Other states have introduced legislation that does not explicitly regulate Internet pharmacies but that affects their practice, such as legislation regarding the transmission of controlled substances, the use of Internet pharmacies by insurance companies to provide the drug benefit for its members, and a physician-patient relationship before prescribing.

Likewise, the federal government is attempting to regulate Internet pharmacies through the Federal Trade Commission (FTC) and the FDA. The FTC fights deceptive practices by Internet pharmacies, such as false advertising, and violations of patient privacy. The FDA works to protect patients against unsafe drugs being sold by illegitimate sites.

In recent years, the FDA has clarified the law that states that FDA-approved drugs that are manufactured in the United States and exported to other countries cannot be reimported back into the United States. Internet pharmacies outside of the United States that ship prescription drugs to patients in the United States are violating the law, and the U.S. Customs Service may stop these drugs from entering the country. Furthermore, the FDA has been issuing warning notices electronically to foreign Internet pharmacy sites, informing them that marketing drugs for sale to citizens of the United States is illegal and that violators may be held liable.

Other federal legislation has been recently introduced to regulate Internet pharmacies within the United States. If passed, the Internet Pharmacy Consumer Protection Act will require Internet pharmacies to fully disclose their sites and operations; it will prohibit these pharmacies from dispensing prescriptions based on an on-line questionnaire and will require a legitimate physician-patient relationship; and it will allow a rogue Internet pharmacy site that does not comply with these federal regulations to be shut down.

## VERIFIED INTERNET PHARMACY PRACTICE SITE

A quasi-legal standard for Internet pharmacies is the Verified Internet Pharmacy Practice Site™ program (VIPPS™). The VIPPS™ program was developed by the National Association of Boards of Pharmacy in 1999 to address the safety of pharmacy practice on the Internet. VIPPS™ certification ensures that an on-line pharmacy is legal and that it provides the highest quality and safest prescription drug care. It also is a way to help protect consumers from unscrupulous Internet sites selling prescription drugs.

The VIPPS™ program is a voluntary program for Internet pharmacies. To be VIPPS™ certified, an Internet pharmacy must comply with licensing requirements in its home state and each state in which it dispenses medications to patients. In addition, the Internet pharmacy practice must meet certain criteria, including:

- Verification of the prescriber and patient's identity
- Communication with physicians
- A medication-dispensing process, including DUR
- Compliance with state and federal laws and regulations
- Tracking medications during shipment
- Patient consultation with a pharmacist

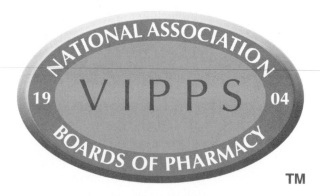

**FIGURE 9–2** Verified Internet Pharmacy Practice Site™ Seal. (Courtesy of the National Association of Boards of Pharmacy and the Verified Internet Pharmacy Practice Sites™ [VIPPS™] Program.)

- Patient confidentiality
- Quality assurance programs for safe dispensing of medications
- Security of prescription orders and patient information

Finally, the Internet pharmacy must pass an on-site visit from a team of VIPPS™ inspectors at the pharmacy headquarters. If VIPPS™ certification is awarded, the Internet pharmacy may display the VIPPS™ seal on its site's home page and may maintain a link from the seal to the VIPPS™ Web site. The VIPPS™ seal is shown in Figure 9–2. Due to the increased use of mail-order pharmacies and the success of the VIPPS™ program in relation to Internet pharmacies, studies are being done to determine if the VIPPS™ program should be applied to mail-order pharmacies.

It should be mentioned here that the VIPPS™ program has been adopted in Canada. However, an Internet pharmacy in Canada that dispenses and ships prescriptions to patients in the United States cannot be VIPPS™ certified because it violates U.S. law.

## THE ROLE OF THE PHARMACIST IN MAIL ORDER

Mail-order pharmacy practice offers a variety of roles for the pharmacist. These can be divided into clinical, dispensing, and administrative roles. In general, a mail-order pharmacist must possess traditional pharmacy knowledge and skills and clinical skills. A mail-order pharmacist also must possess excellent telephone communication and listening skills in order to determine what a patient is trying to communicate or how the patient is feeling, considering the lack of face-to-face contact.

### CLINICAL ROLE

The clinical role of the pharmacist involves providing pharmaceutical care services. In this role, the mail-order pharmacist performs activities that can improve the outcomes of drug therapy. A clinical pharmacist usually works in an area within the mail-order pharmacy that is separate from the dispensing and compounding areas of the pharmacy. Typical clinical activities include participating in disease management programs, performing retrospective DUR, managing the formulary, providing drug information to physicians, monitoring compliance, and counseling patients. Some pharmacists who work in a clinical role in the mail-order pharmacy may even specialize by disease state.

### DISPENSING ROLE

The dispensing role of a mail-order pharmacist involves activities that are related to the dispensing of prescriptions. Owing to the high volume of prescriptions dispensed in a mail-order pharmacy, most dispensing activities are performed by pharmacy technicians and through the use of automation. However, there are a few separate areas within the dispensing process where the pharmacist is utilized, such as in screening prescription orders, making telephone calls to physicians, and checking the finished prescription order.

### ADMINISTRATIVE ROLE

The administrative role of the pharmacist is related to the management of the mail-order pharmacy. This role involves overseeing the day-to-day operations of the mail-order pharmacy. Typical administrative activities include hiring and training pharmacists and pharmacy technicians, overseeing computer system and equipment maintenance, purchasing drugs, developing policies and procedures, maintaining records, and managing the facility.

## THE ROLE OF THE PHARMACY TECHNICIAN IN MAIL ORDER

Pharmacy technicians perform almost all of the dispensing functions involved in filling prescriptions. In the mail-order pharmacy, pharmacy technicians take on more data entry and production tasks than in a traditional retail pharmacy. What makes the role of the pharmacy technician unique is that, owing to the organized workflow in the mail-order pharmacy, the pharmacy technician is usually assigned an individual task to perform. This performing of an individual task is referred to as **task specialization.** There are several advantages to task specialization. By performing one task, the pharmacy technician knows exactly what skills and responsibilities are required for the assigned role. The pharmacy technician can stay focused on that specific task rather than performing many different tasks at the same time, as in a traditional pharmacy. The pharmacy technician also becomes highly proficient in performing the specific task. In general, task specialization provides a more organized and less stressful work environment for the pharmacy technician, and it may appeal to some pharmacy technicians. In some mail-order pharmacies, pharmacy technicians do perform single tasks but rotate to a different work area and task every few hours. Rotating tasks keeps the technician from becoming bored or fatigued and allows him to develop and maintain the skills needed in each work area.

In order to work in a mail-order pharmacy, the pharmacy technician must possess traditional pharmacy knowledge and skills as well as knowledge and skills specific to mail-order pharmacy, such as:

- A working knowledge of a traditional retail pharmacy and the prescription-filling process
- A knowledge of commonly prescribed medications
- A knowledge of the translation and interpretation of prescription orders
- A thorough knowledge of automated pharmacy systems
- An understanding of the legislation and regulations that pertain to mail-order pharmacy
- Excellent computer skills
- Excellent telephone communication skills

The role of the pharmacy technician in a mail-order pharmacy can be divided into three areas: prescription order entry, dispensing, and pharmacist support.

## PRESCRIPTION ORDER ENTRY ROLE

The pharmacy technician in the role of prescription order entry interprets a written prescription order and enters it into the computer. The technician enters the following information directly from the prescription: patient, physician, drug, dosage strength, dosage form, directions for use, acceptability of generic substitution, and refills. Any questions or problems with a prescription order are referred to a pharmacist for resolution. This role is very challenging and involves a higher level of responsibility for the pharmacy technician. Usually, the most highly trained and motivated pharmacy technicians in a mail-order pharmacy are found in this role.

## DISPENSING ROLE

The pharmacy technician in a dispensing role fills the prescription order with the appropriate medication in the appropriate amount. Dispensing involves selecting the proper drug from the inventory, counting or pouring out the appropriate amount of medication, packaging the medication in the proper-sized container, and affixing the prescription label to the container. These tasks can be done manually or through the use of automation. Other duties in this area include ordering medications, receiving and stocking medications, and ordering and restocking pharmacy supplies.

## PHARMACIST SUPPORT ROLE

The pharmacy technician in a pharmacist support role assists the pharmacist with prescriptions that require special attention. One of the most important functions of the technician is to make telephone calls to patients or to physician offices to obtain authorization to fill expired prescriptions or prescriptions with no refills. Other responsibilities can include assisting with special orders, identifying noncompliant patients, training other pharmacy technicians, and maintaining computer systems.

## KEY CONCEPTS

- Mail-order pharmacy is pharmacy that dispenses maintenance medications to members through mail delivery.
- Mail-order pharmacies, central fill pharmacies, and Internet pharmacies are all high-volume pharmacies that are an option to traditional pharmacies for obtaining prescriptions for maintenance drugs.
- Mail-order pharmacy has several advantages, such as cost savings and patient convenience, but also has a few disadvantages, such as lack of personal contact.
- A mail-order pharmacy has many unique elements, especially its design into workstations, its extensive use of automation, and its toll-free telephone lines.
- Automation is used extensively in almost every step of the prescription-filling process in a mail-order pharmacy.
- The prescription-filling process in a mail-order pharmacy is managed through a controlled workflow.
- A mail-order pharmacy offers other services in addition to dispensing prescriptions, including disease management programs, drug utilization review, formulary management, compliance monitoring, and patient education.
- There are several laws and regulations that pertain specifically to a mail-order pharmacy.
- Mail-order pharmacy offers a variety of separate roles for the pharmacist, including dispensing, clinical, and administrative roles, whereas task specialization is a unique feature of the role of the pharmacy technician in a mail-order pharmacy.

## SELF-ASSESSMENT QUESTIONS

**MULTIPLE CHOICE**

1. Workflow involves all of the following except:
   a. defined roles for personnel
   b. distractions
   c. defined work areas
   d. specific tasks

2. Internet pharmacies:
   a. provide access to pharmacists
   b. provide prescription and over-the-counter medications
   c. provide access to drug and medical information
   d. all of the above

3. To receive the VIPPS™ seal, an Internet pharmacy must do all of the following except:
   a. pass an on-site visit from inspectors
   b. have the proper pharmacy licensure

      c. voluntarily apply

      d. not disclose its location

4. Specialty mail-order pharmacy involves all of the following except:

      a. interaction with other health care professionals

      b. complicated billing

      c. limited patient monitoring

      d. increased amounts of information needed for processing prescriptions

5. A disadvantage of mail-order pharmacy is:

      a. 24-hour access to a pharmacist

      b. cost savings

      c. indirect contact between patient and pharmacist

      d. patient privacy

6. Which is not an example of automation used in a mail-order pharmacy?

      a. robotics

      b. bar code scanners

      c. conveyor belts

      d. counting trays

7. An example of a medication that can be mailed is:

      a. a controlled substance

      b. a refrigerated medication

      c. an expensive medication

      d. all of the above

8. Which is not a step in the typical workflow of a mail-order pharmacy?

      a. prescription item entry

      b. adjudication support

      c. dispensing

      d. packaging and shipping

9. Which is not an advantage of task specialization?

      a. ability to do many tasks at the same time

      b. ability to stay focused on the task

      c. increased proficiency in the task

      d. understanding the responsibilities involved in the task

10. Which is not a unique element of a mail-order pharmacy?

      a. toll-free telephone lines

      b. facsimile machines

      c. pharmacy design into workstations

      d. mail service

## TRUE/FALSE (CORRECT THE FALSE STATEMENTS)

1. _____ The majority of prescriptions filled in a mail-order pharmacy are for medications used for chronic conditions.

2. _____ In the centralized filling process, a prescription is ordered through a local pharmacy but filled in a large-volume centrally located pharmacy.

3. _____ Mail-order pharmacies have been in existence for over 50 years.

4. _____ Most prescription drug benefit plans do not offer a mail-order pharmacy option.

5. _____ A high-volume prescription operation that works on the same principles as a mail-order pharmacy is an Internet pharmacy.

6. _____ A mail-order pharmacy is divided into different workstations designed for specific tasks.

7. _____ The majority of prescriptions in a mail-order pharmacy are received by telephone.

8. _____ Pharmacist screening of prescriptions before adjudication is not a part of the prescription-filling process in a mail-order pharmacy.

9. _____ A mail-order pharmacy is licensed and regulated by the state board of pharmacy in its home state.

10. _____ Owing to the large volume of prescriptions dispensed in a mail-order pharmacy, there are more dispensing errors than in a traditional retail pharmacy.

## FILL-IN

1. The voluntary certification process for Internet pharmacy sites is called _____.

2. A _____ mail-order pharmacy fills prescriptions for patients in the general population for maintenance medications.

3. An illegitimate Internet pharmacy is called a _____ site.

4. The organized way of filling prescriptions is called _____.

5. An out-of-state mail-order pharmacy is referred to as a _____ pharmacy.

6. _____ _____ is performing a specific task in the mail-order pharmacy.

7. A pharmacist who reviews prescription orders that have been entered into the computer may be referred to as a _____ pharmacist.

8. An example of a toll-free telephone line for the deaf is a _____.

9. International delivery of prescriptions requires a document to clear customs that is called a _____ _____ _____.

10. The pharmacy technician in a mail-order pharmacy who fills a prescription order may be called a _____ technician.

## CRITICAL THINKING

1. Why are maintenance medications well suited for mail-order pharmacy?

2. Compare and contrast pharmacy operations in a mail-order pharmacy with those in a traditional community retail pharmacy.

3. Apply *structure, process,* and *outcomes* to a mail-order pharmacy.

4. Compare and contrast the duties of a pharmacy technician in a mail-order pharmacy with those in a traditional community retail pharmacy.

5. Should traditional community retail pharmacy feel threatened by the existence of mail-order pharmacy?

## ◼ BIBLIOGRAPHY

Burke, J. (2005). Internet prescribing 2005. *Pharmacy Times, 71*(4), 88.

Cahill, J., & Manasse, H. (2005). Medicare therapy management programs: To optimize pharmacy outcomes. Summary of the executive sessions on medication therapy management programs. *Journal of Managed Care Pharmacy, 11*(2), 179–186.

Carroll, N. (2006). Mail-service pharmacy savings: A conclusion in search of evidence. *Journal of Managed Care Pharmacy, 12*(2), 164–167.

Celia, F. (2005). Chains ponder responses to mandatory mail order. *Drug Topics, 149*(8), 58.

Coster, J. (2005). The Medicare Modernization Act Part 2. *U.S. Pharmacist, 30*(8), 47–50.

Fink, J., III, Vivian, J., & Bernstein, I. (2005). *Pharmacy law digest* (40th ed.). St Louis, MO: Facts and Comparisons.

Jerram, L. (2005). Benefits of automation. *Pharmacy Times, 71*(1), 96, 109.

LoBuono, C. (2005). Mail-order program offers savings and pharmacy choice. *Drug Topics, 149*(4), 33.

Moyer, P. (2005). Some Rxs ordered on-line may lack quality control. *Drug Topics, 149*(7), 26s.

Navarro, R. (2005). *Managed care pharmacy practice* (2nd ed.). Gaithersburg, MD: Aspen Publishers, Inc.

Sax, B. (2005). Pharmacy and technology: Industry leaders meet in automation roundtable. *Pharmacy Times, 71*(1), 90–94.

Smith, M., Wertheimer, A., & Fincham, J. (2005). *Pharmacy and the U.S. health care system* (3rd ed.). Binghamton, NY: Pharmaceutical Products Press.

Stern, D., & Reissman, D. (2006). Specialty pharmacy cost management strategies of private health care payers. *Journal of Managed Care Pharmacy, 12*(9), 736–744.

Ukens, C. (2005). Specialty pharmacy wins spot in Medicare program. *Drug Topics, 149*(3), 42.

Ukens, C. (2005). Here's a new central fill operation you can use. *Drug Topics, 149*(5), 49.

United States Department of Justice. Drug Enforcement Administration. (2005). *Code of Federal Regulations Title 21, Section 1306—Pharmacy.* [On-line] U.S. Department of Justice. Available: www.dea.gov.

United States Pharmacopeial Convention. (2006). *The United States pharmacopeia* (29th ed.) and *The national formulary* (24th ed.). Rockville, MD: Author.

Zanni, G. (2005). Rx reimportation and importation: Panacea or prelude to disaster? *Pharmacy Times, 71*(1), 85–89.

# Nuclear Pharmacy

## Learning Objectives

Upon completion of this chapter, the student should be able to:

- Explain nuclear pharmacy practice.
- Describe a radiopharmaceutical.
- Understand the uses of the most common radiopharmaceuticals.
- Be familiar with adverse reactions and drug interactions associated with radiopharmaceuticals.
- Describe the elements of a nuclear pharmacy.
- Describe the prescription-filling process in a nuclear pharmacy.
- Explain the need for quality control testing.
- Describe the special packaging required for shipping radiopharmaceuticals.
- Understand radiation safety, including radioactive waste disposal.
- Understand the legislation and regulations pertaining to nuclear pharmacy practice.
- Describe the roles of the pharmacist and the pharmacy technician in nuclear pharmacy.

## Key Terms

| | | |
|---|---|---|
| authorized user | elution | radionuclide |
| carrier drug | half-life | radionuclide generator |
| eluant | nuclear pharmacy | radiopharmaceutical |

## Introduction

Nuclear pharmacy is a recognized specialty area of pharmacy. It is a pharmacy practice area that is unfamiliar to many pharmacists and pharmacy technicians. Nuclear pharmacy is possibly the most specialized practice setting for pharmacists and pharmacy technicians. It bears little resemblance to any other pharmacy practice area; it involves the handling of radioactive materials; and it involves some unique sterile compounding. In order to work in a nuclear pharmacy, pharmacists and pharmacy technicians must possess special knowledge and sterile compounding skills. They must be familiar with radiation safety. There are also specific legislation and regulations that pertain to nuclear pharmacy practice. This chapter focuses on the nuclear pharmacy and the unique roles of the pharmacist and pharmacy technician in this recognized specialty area of pharmacy. ∎

## OVERVIEW OF NUCLEAR PHARMACY

A **nuclear pharmacy,** also referred to as a radiopharmacy, is defined as a pharmacy that prepares, stores, and dispenses radiopharmaceuticals. A **radiopharmaceutical** is a radioactive drug that is used for the diagnosis and treatment of disease. Nuclear pharmacy practice involves the compounding and dispensing of radiopharmaceuticals. In fact, nuclear pharmacy is essentially a sterile compounding practice. Nuclear pharmacists and nuclear pharmacy technicians compound prescriptions for a wide range of radiopharmaceuticals on the order of physicians for specific patients. Nuclear pharmacy also promotes the safe and effective use of radioactive drugs.

Nuclear pharmacy has been in existence for over 30 years. The practice of nuclear pharmacy was recognized in 1975 by the American Pharmaceutical Association (APhA) with its creation of the Section on Nuclear Pharmacy. This section developed guidelines for nuclear pharmacy practice, which became the basis for the recognition of nuclear pharmacy as a specialty area of pharmacy by the Board of Pharmaceutical Specialties (BPS). In 1982, nuclear pharmacy became the first formally recognized pharmacy specialty in the world. Nuclear pharmacy has increased in services and in the number of board-certified nuclear pharmacists. Today, there are several hundred nuclear pharmacies in the United States and throughout the world.

There are two types of nuclear pharmacies: institutional nuclear pharmacy and centralized nuclear pharmacy. An institutional nuclear pharmacy is a nuclear pharmacy that operates within a nuclear medicine department in an institution such as a large hospital. A centralized nuclear pharmacy is a nuclear pharmacy that operates out of a centralized site in the community and services a number of customers in different locations within a reasonable distance of the pharmacy. These customers can be hospitals, outpatient diagnostic imaging centers, mobile imaging centers (in rural areas where there is no other facility), and cardiology practices. Examples of centralized nuclear pharmacy companies are Nuclear Pharmacy Services of Cardinal Health, the largest radiopharmacy services provider; Tyco Healthcare/Mallinckrodt Radiopharmacy; and GE Healthcare Nuclear Pharmacies. Before discussing nuclear pharmacy, the pharmacy technician must understand some background information regarding radioactivity.

### RADIOACTIVITY AND RADIONUCLIDES

The atom is the smallest particle of matter. It consists of a nucleus at the center and electrons that rotate around the nucleus (Figure 10–1). The nucleus is

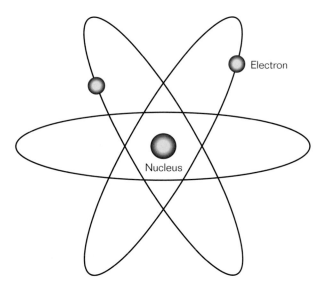

**FIGURE 10–1** The Atom.

composed of protons and neutrons. The composition of the nucleus is some-times referred to as a nuclide. Most nuclides are stable, but certain nuclides have excess internal energy and are said to be unstable. A **radionuclide** is an atom that has an unstable nucleus. It spontaneously disintegrates in an attempt to return to a stable state. This disintegration is referred to as radioactive decay. As a radionuclide decays, it releases its excess internal energy in the form of radiation, and it is said to be radioactive.

There are three types of radiation that can be released by a radionuclide: alpha, beta, and gamma radiation. Alpha radiation is very short-range radiation. These particles move very slowly and travel only a few inches in the air. They can be easily stopped by a sheet of paper or the outer layer of a person's skin. Beta radiation is more penetrating radiation. These particles are more energetic and travel in the air for a few feet. They can be stopped with a sheet of aluminum foil or glass. Gamma radiation is the most penetrating type of radiation. Unlike alpha or beta radiations, which are particles, gamma radiation is in the form of high-energy rays. This type of radiation requires shielding with materials such as concrete, lead, or steel. The type of radiation that is released by a radionuclide will determine the use of the radionuclide. Nuclear medicine uses very small quantities of radionuclides for the diagnosis and treatment of disease.

The rate of radioactive decay for a radionuclide is designated by its **half-life,** which is defined as the time required for one-half of a radionuclide to decay or, stated another way, the time required for a radionuclide to lose one-half of its radioactivity. It is expressed as $t$ and it is unique for each radionuclide. Half-lives can range from a few minutes to several years, depending on the radionuclide. Carbon-14, which is used for archaeological dating, has a half-life of 5,730 years. Technetium-99, which is used in the diagnosis of disease, has a half-life of 6 hours. This means that a given amount of technetium-99 will lose half of its strength in 6 hours, half of its remaining strength in another 6 hours, and so on.

Radioactivity is expressed in units called curies (Ci), where 1 curie (Ci) = 1,000 millicuries (mCi). The international unit of radioactivity is called the becquerel (Bq). Both the curie and the becquerel are derived from the names of early researchers in radioactivity.

Radionuclides are used in medicine for two purposes: the diagnosis and treatment of disease. Radionuclides release radiation within the body that can be detected by instruments to evaluate the structure or function of an organ or system and therefore diagnose disease. For treatment, they are used to destroy cells, such as cancer cells. The two most frequently used radionuclides are technetium and iodine compounds.

Technetium-99 ($^{99}$Tc) was discovered in 1938 by Italian and American scientists and has become the basis for nuclear medicine. It is used in about 80 percent of radioactive drugs. Most technetium is used for diagnosis. It has a short half-life of 6 hours and therefore delivers a very small amount or dose of radiation to the patient, yet it results in very good diagnostic images. It can be easily produced in the nuclear pharmacy by a generator.

There are several iodine compounds used in medicine. Some are used for diagnosis; others are used for treatment. Iodine-131 ($^{131}$I) is commercially available in a solution of 0.9 percent sodium chloride, and it is very volatile. It is for oral administration in a capsule or liquid form. Capsules are compounded from the liquid in the nuclear pharmacy. Iodine-131 has a half-life of 8 days, and, because of this longer half-life, it is used in the treatment of thyroid cancer and hyperthyroidism (overactive thyroid cells). Iodine-123 ($^{123}$I), a slightly different radioactive form of iodine, has a short half-life of 13 hours and is used for the diagnosis of thyroid disease rather than for treatment.

There are numerous other radionuclides used in medicine. These include xenon (a gas used to image the lungs), thallium, gallium, cobalt, chromium, indium, and strontium.

## RADIOPHARMACEUTICALS

A radiopharmaceutical, also referred to as a radioactive drug, is defined as a drug that releases radiation within the body. It is available in many dosage forms, such as oral capsules, "seeds" or pellets (for implanting into the body), oral solutions, sterile injections, and gases. A radiopharmaceutical is compounded and dispensed on the order of a physician, that is, by a prescription, for a particular patient. Radiopharmaceuticals include traditionally compounded radiopharmaceuticals, positron emission tomography (PET) drugs, and radioactive blood elements and antibodies, as well as radionuclide generators and non-radioactive "kits" that are used to prepare radiopharmaceuticals.

A traditionally compounded radiopharmaceutical usually consists of two parts: a radionuclide and a carrier drug. A **carrier drug**, sometimes referred to as a tracer drug, is a pharmaceutical that delivers the radionuclide to the desired area of the body for study or treatment. It is not evenly distributed throughout the body but concentrates in a specific region or organ of the body. Therefore, when a radiopharmaceutical is administered to a patient, it travels to the desired site, where it releases radiation for the intended purpose. Examples of carrier drugs and their sites of action are given in Table 10–1.

Radiopharmaceuticals are used for diagnosing and treating disease. The majority of radiopharmaceuticals, about 90 percent, are used for diagnosis. The radiation that is released within the body can be detected by special instruments, along with computers, to form images of internal structures such as organs, bones, and tissues and to evaluate body functions. Radiopharmaceuticals that are used for diagnosis usually have no pharmacological effect on the internal

**TABLE 10–1**    Common Carrier Drugs

| CARRIER DRUG | SITE OF ACTION |
|---|---|
| MAA (microaggregated albumin) | Lung |
| MDP (medronate) | Bone |
| Choletec (mebrofenin) | Liver |
| Cardiolyte (sestamibi) | Heart |
| Techniscan (mertiatide or MAG 3) | Kidney |

**TABLE 10–2**    Common Radiopharmaceuticals for Diagnosis

| RADIONUCLIDE | CARRIER DRUG | RADIOPHARMACEUTICAL | USE |
|---|---|---|---|
| $^{99m}$Tc | MAA | $^{99m}$Tc-MAA | Lung perfusion study |
| $^{99m}$Tc | MDP | $^{99m}$Tc-MDP | Bone and skeletal imaging |
| $^{99m}$Tc | Mebrofenin | $^{99m}$Tc-mebrofenin | Liver imaging |
| $^{99m}$Tc | Sestamibi | $^{99m}$Tc-sestamibi | Heart perfusion study |
| $^{99m}$Tc | MAG 3 | $^{99m}$Tc-MAG 3 | Kidney function |

structures because they are used in very minute quantities and the radionuclide portions have short half-lives. They are active for only a short period of time, not much longer than the time needed to prepare and transport them and to perform the study. Examples of radiopharmaceuticals for diagnosis and their uses are found in Table 10–2.

Radiopharmaceuticals that are used for treatment have longer half-lives and contain higher doses of radiation than do radiopharmaceuticals used for diagnosis. The higher doses of radiation affect the organ or tissue by destroying cells, for example, cancer cells. An example of a radionuclide used for treatment is iodine-131 ($^{131}$I).

## PET Drugs

Positron emission tomography, or PET, is a method of imaging or diagnosing that uses special radiopharmaceuticals called PET drugs. PET drugs have very short half-lives, usually just minutes. Because of these short half-lives, these drugs cannot be produced in a centralized nuclear pharmacy and transported to the customer. They can be prepared only in an institutional nuclear pharmacy close to the nuclear medicine department, where they will be used within minutes of being prepared. They are prepared by pharmacists, as well as radiochemists, cyclotron operators, and technicians, using a nuclear particle accelerator or cyclotron, an extremely large and expensive piece of equipment.

### Radioactive Blood Elements

Red blood cells, white blood cells, and platelets are some blood elements that can be combined or *labeled* with radionuclides. The resulting radioactive blood elements are used for diagnosis. Radioactive red blood cells are used to detect red blood cell survival rates or to image the spleen. Radioactive white blood cells are used to detect infection. Radioactive platelets are used to detect blood clots. Antibodies (monoclonal) can also be combined with radionuclides to detect tumors and other types of cancers.

Radioactive blood elements are prepared in the nuclear pharmacy, usually in a separate area or room. Blood is considered to be a biological hazard and is handled by the pharmacist, using Universal Precautions. A sample of the patient's blood is separated into its elements (red blood cells, white blood cells, and platelets) and plasma, usually by centrifuge. The desired element is combined with the radionuclide, and the resulting radioactive blood element is resuspended in the plasma. The sample is then returned to the facility and injected back into the patient for the study.

### Adverse Reactions to Radiopharmaceuticals

Most patients tolerate radiopharmaceuticals quite well. Adverse reactions to radiopharmaceuticals are rare because the quantities involved are so small. Most reactions involve sensitivity to the carrier drug rather than to the radionuclide. Adverse reactions to radiopharmaceuticals may include nausea and vomiting, difficulty breathing, coughing, decrease in blood pressure or heart rate, and itching or hives.

### Drug Interactions with Radiopharmaceuticals

Some traditional drugs may interact with radiopharmaceuticals. The traditional drug may alter the distribution of the radiopharmaceutical in the body, causing too much or too little of the radiopharmaceutical to be deposited in the target organ. A traditional drug also can cause a radiopharmaceutical to be deposited in a different organ than was intended. For example, steroid drugs interact with the radiopharmaceutical $^{99m}$Tc-MDP, used in bone imaging, resulting in a decrease in the amount of the radiopharmaceutical in the bone. Meperidine interacts with $^{99m}$Tc-MDP, causing it to be deposited in soft tissue instead of in bone.

## ELEMENTS OF A NUCLEAR PHARMACY

There are many elements that make up a nuclear pharmacy. Most of these elements are specific to a nuclear pharmacy and are not found in any other type of pharmacy practice. These elements are discussed next.

### PERSONNEL

As in any other type of pharmacy, a variety of personnel is needed to operate a nuclear pharmacy in a safe and efficient manner. Pharmacists, pharmacy technicians, drivers, and other support personnel are found in a nuclear pharmacy. A pharmacist who works in a nuclear pharmacy is called a nuclear pharmacist or a radiopharmacist. A nuclear pharmacist is a pharmacist who has specialized training in the handling of radioactive compounds. A pharmacy technician who works in a nuclear pharmacy is referred to as a nuclear pharmacy technician. A nuclear pharmacy technician also has specialized training in the handling of radioactive compounds. Drivers are important to the operation of a centralized nuclear pharmacy. Owing to the hazardous nature of radiopharmaceuticals, a driver must have specialized training in the handling of radioactive compounds and must have a safe driving record. There are also several types of support personnel who contribute to the working of a nuclear pharmacy. These personnel include secretaries, billing personnel, sales representatives, customer service representatives, and housekeeping staff.

## INVENTORY

The drug inventory in a nuclear pharmacy is completely different from that found in any other type of pharmacy. A separate class of drugs is used in the nuclear pharmacy. It consists of radionuclides and carrier drugs, both unique to the preparation of radiopharmaceuticals. Radionuclides are purchased from various manufacturers that specialize in nuclear compounds, such as Mallinckrodt and Bristol-Myers Squibb Medical Imaging. They are prepared by the manufacturer on demand and delivered to the nuclear pharmacy on a daily basis. The carrier drugs can be purchased from almost any drug wholesaler.

The drug inventory in a nuclear pharmacy is very limited. Because radionuclides will decay, little or no inventory is kept on hand in the pharmacy. Radionuclides are *time-sensitive*. They have short half-lives, usually several hours, and will lose a substantial amount of their radioactivity if stored for any period of time. Therefore, radionuclides are ordered daily and only in the amounts that are needed. This tightly controlled inventory is referred to as just-in-time, or JIT, inventory.

## PHARMACY DESIGN

The design of a nuclear pharmacy is very different from the design of any other type of pharmacy. It takes the many unique aspects of radiation handling into consideration. The design of a nuclear pharmacy must:

- Protect the personnel from radiation exposure
- Prevent radioactive contamination of pharmacy work areas and equipment
- Ensure proper ventilation of the pharmacy
- Provide for the safe disposal of radioactive waste
- Limit access into the pharmacy
- Ensure the security of the pharmacy

The nuclear pharmacy environment is well controlled and closely monitored so that personnel are exposed to the very lowest doses of radiation possible. It is clean, orderly, properly lighted, and properly ventilated. A nuclear pharmacy is usually locked, and access is usually restricted to authorized personnel by means of a key or electronic opening device. The nuclear pharmacy is divided into different areas designed to handle specific tasks.

- *Breakdown area.* The area where empty or used containers of radiopharmaceuticals are returned and dismantled for reuse.
- *Order entry area.* The area where prescription orders for radiopharmaceuticals are entered into the computer.

- *Compounding areas.* The areas where radiopharmaceuticals are compounded or prepared. They are also referred to as dispensing areas. Some nuclear pharmacies have separate rooms, rather than separate areas, for the handling of radioactive gases and blood.

- *Quality control area.* The area where quality control tests are performed on compounded radiopharmaceuticals before they are released for packaging and delivery.

- *Packaging area.* The area where finished and tested radiopharmaceuticals are packaged and prepared for delivery.

- *Storage and disposal area.* The area where radioactive waste is kept. This area is actually a storage and decay area where some radioactive compounds are stored while they decay. Once they are no longer radioactive, they are disposed of as ordinary trash.

## EQUIPMENT AND SUPPLIES

Some traditional pharmacy equipment is found in a nuclear pharmacy, such as computer hardware and printers, facsimile machines, telephone systems, laminar airflow hoods, and pharmacy balances. However, there is a wide variety of very specialized equipment found in this practice setting.

- *Fume hood.* A laminar airflow hood adapted for compounding radiopharmaceuticals. It is similar to a vertical laminar airflow hood, except that air is vented to the outside, rather than recirculated into the hood. It uses charcoal filters and has an emissions monitor to detect the amount of radiation being released into the atmosphere. It is used for handling volatile radioactive liquids, such as iodine, and radioactive gases, such as xenon (Figure 10–2).

- *Glove box.* Also a type of laminar airflow hood in which the operator works by inserting her hands through special gloves that allow access to the inside of the hood.

- *Dose calibrator.* An instrument used to measure the radioactivity of a sample of radionuclide during the compounding of a radiopharmaceutical and the preparation of individual doses (Figure 10–3).

- *Geiger-Müller counter.* An instrument that is used to measure low-level radiation of an area. It is also known as a Geiger counter.

- *Dosimeter.* A personal monitoring device that is used to measure the radiation exposure of an individual.

- *Lead-lined refrigerator and freezer.* Used for refrigerated or frozen radioactive compounds.

- *Lead-lined storage boxes.* Used for the storage and decay of radioactive materials and waste.

- *Autoclave.* Used to sterilize materials when needed.

- *Heating equipment.* Such as a hot water bath, a dry heat oven, or an incubator. These are used in compounding radiopharmaceuticals that require heat to combine the carrier drug with the radionuclide.

- *Testing equipment.* Instruments used in performing quality control tests, such as a microscope, gas or liquid chromatograph, and pH meter.

- *Centrifuge.* Used to spin down a sample of whole blood in order to separate it into its elements for combining with a radionuclide.

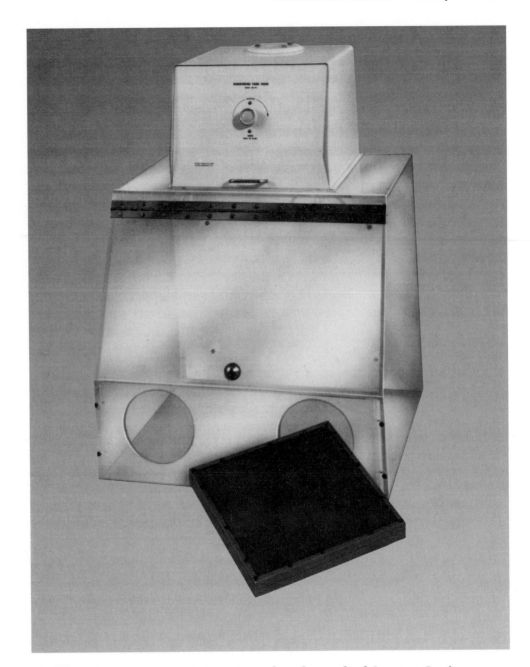

**FIGURE 10–2**    Fume Hood. (Courtesy of Biodex Medical Systems, Inc.)

- *Lead barrier shield.* A shield mounted in front of a countertop, laminar airflow hood, or fume hood. It is used to protect the worker from radioactivity during the compounding of a radiopharmaceutical. The radioactive material is handled behind the shield. Shields consist of a solid lead panel with a sloping leaded glass panel on top that allows the worker to view the work area (Figure 10–4).
- *Deep stainless steel sink.* Used to prevent the splashing of a radioactive compound on a worker during washing.
- *Shower.* Used to remove radioactive contamination from the entire body.
- *Respirator.* Used to protect the worker from inhaling volatile radioactive compounds and radioactive gases.

There are a few traditional pharmacy supplies that are found in a nuclear pharmacy. These include prescription pads, prescription labels, alcohol pads,

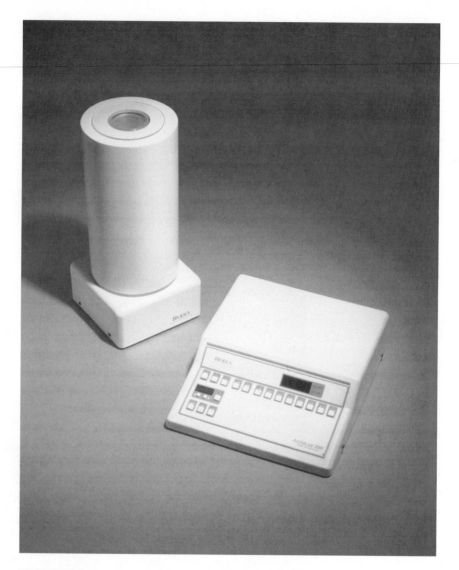

**FIGURE 10–3**    Dose Calibrator. (Courtesy of Biodex Medical Systems, Inc.)

needles and syringes, sharps containers, disposable gowns and gloves, face masks, chemo preparation mats and chemo spill kits (to absorb spills), sterile 0.9 percent sodium chloride injection, and isopropyl alcohol. There are also many special supplies used in a nuclear pharmacy. These include lead aprons, lead-lined gloves, leaded glass protective eyewear, lead or leaded glass syringe shields (Figure 10–5), lead vial shields (Figure 10–6), tongs or long tweezers, ammonia, cushioning material for transport, specialized shipping containers and labels for the shipping containers, and delivery vehicles.

## DELIVERY SERVICE

The safe and timely delivery of radiopharmaceuticals to the customer is critical to a nuclear pharmacy operation, especially a centralized nuclear pharmacy operation. There are several strict requirements for the delivery of a radiopharmaceutical:

- The shipping containers must be wiped down with isopropyl alcohol or ammonia before leaving the pharmacy to remove any external radioactivity.

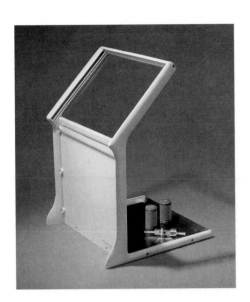

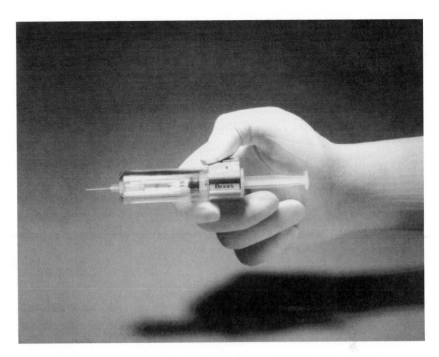

**FIGURE 10–4**    Lead Barrier Shield. (Courtesy of Biodex Medical Systems, Inc.)

**FIGURE 10–5**    Syringe Shield. (Courtesy of Biodex Medical Systems, Inc.)

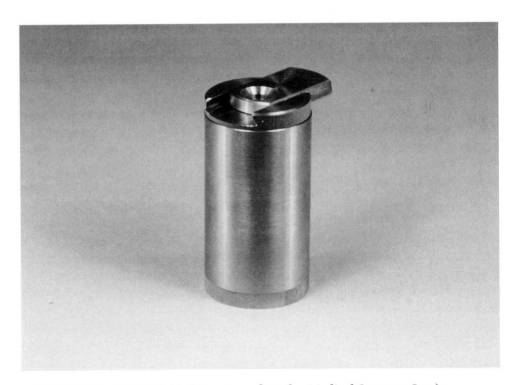

**FIGURE 10–6**    Vial Shield. (Courtesy of Biodex Medical Systems, Inc.)

- A label that denotes radioactive material must be placed on the outside of the shipping container.
- The proper documentation must be included with the shipment of radiopharmaceuticals.

- The shipping containers must be properly loaded and braced inside the delivery vehicle to prevent breaking or spilling in case of an accident.
- The radiopharmaceutical must be delivered directly to the designated area of an institution or facility, usually a nuclear medicine department, and must never be left unattended.

In general, owing to the time-sensitive nature of radiopharmaceuticals, they cannot be delivered over long distances. The industry average is delivery within 100 miles of the centralized nuclear pharmacy, or approximately 2 to 3 hours away. Deliveries are usually made several times a day, and most nuclear pharmacies make deliveries 7 days a week.

## THE PRESCRIPTION-FILLING PROCESS IN A NUCLEAR PHARMACY

A nuclear pharmacy handles potentially dangerous radioactive compounds on a daily basis. Ensuring the safety of the personnel in the pharmacy and the desired radioactivity and sterility of the compounded radiopharmaceuticals requires that prescriptions for radiopharmaceuticals be filled in a strictly controlled manner. The prescription-filling process for a radiopharmaceutical in a nuclear pharmacy consists of several steps.

A prescription for a radiopharmaceutical originates with a radiologist, cardiologist, or other physician at a hospital, a physician's office, or other facility. It can be a written or verbal order, faxed or called in to the nuclear pharmacy. A verbal order for a radiopharmaceutical for diagnosis may be accepted by a nuclear pharmacy technician; a prescription for a radiopharmaceutical for treatment may be accepted only by a licensed nuclear pharmacist or a pharmacist intern. Prescription information must include the patient's name, physician's name, name of the facility where the radiopharmaceutical is to be administered, type of study being done (if for diagnosis), name of the radiopharmaceutical, activity or dose of the radiopharmaceutical, and date *and* time of administration (Figure 10–7). The prescription information is then entered into the computer by a nuclear pharmacist or nuclear pharmacy technician. There is no need to enter the patient's address, phone number, or prescription insurance information because radiopharmaceuticals are usually billed to the facility that performs the study, not to the individual patient. There is currently no third-party prescription coverage for radiopharmaceuticals.

The prescription order is screened and analyzed by the nuclear pharmacist to determine the patient's drug allergies, potential drug interactions, and appropriate dose. The doses of some commonly used radiopharmaceuticals are often standardized. Then a prescription label is generated. The prescription label must contain a prescription number, patient name, radiopharmaceutical, dose, date *and* time of compounding, and the pharmacist's initials. In large nuclear pharmacies, the prescription may be assigned a bar code before the process moves on to the next step.

### RADIOPHARMACEUTICAL COMPOUNDING

In the nuclear pharmacy, compounding refers to the addition or the use of a radioactive compound in the preparation of a radiopharmaceutical. It can be as

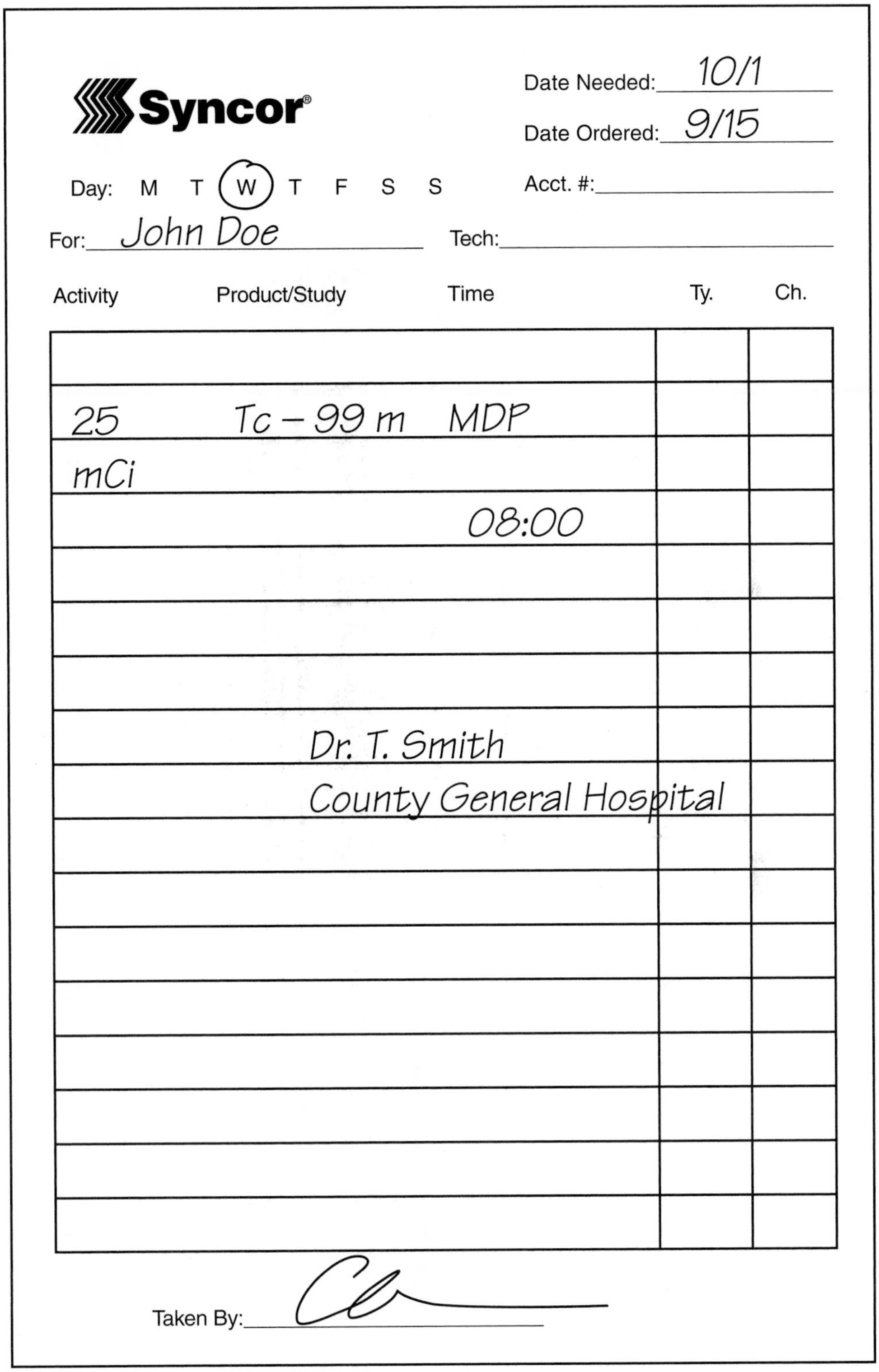

Syncor®

Date Needed: 10/1

Date Ordered: 9/15

Day: M T (W) T F S S

Acct. #:

For: John Doe

Tech:

| Activity | Product/Study | Time | Ty. | Ch. |
|---|---|---|---|---|
| | | | | |
| 25 | Tc – 99 m | MDP | | |
| mCi | | | | |
| | | 08:00 | | |
| | Dr. T. Smith | | | |
| | County General Hospital | | | |

Taken By:

FIGURE 10–7 Sample Prescription for a Radiopharmaceutical.

simple as adding a radionuclide to a commercially available reagent kit or as complex as creating the radionuclide itself. The compounding of radiopharmaceuticals involves, but is not limited to, eluting a radionuclide generator, preparing a batch of radiopharmaceutical from a reagent kit, preparing individual doses of a radiopharmaceutical (making aliquots) from a reagent kit, and conducting quality control tests on radiopharmaceuticals. Compounding may be performed by a nuclear pharmacist or by a nuclear pharmacy technician under the direct supervision of the nuclear pharmacist. Because radionuclides decay quickly, compounding is performed on a daily basis, several times a day, usually within a few hours of administration of the radiopharmaceutical. These compounding activities are discussed next.

### Eluting a Radionuclide Generator

Radionuclides with short half-lives, referred to as *short-lived* radionuclides, can be easily prepared in a nuclear pharmacy through the use of a radionuclide generator. A **radionuclide generator** is defined as a device in which one radionuclide is produced from another radionuclide through the principle of radioactive decay. A *parent* radionuclide with a long half-life is allowed to decay into a *daughter* radionuclide that has a short half-life. The daughter radionuclide is then separated from the parent radionuclide. The process of separating the daughter radionuclide is called **elution,** or eluting the generator. The daughter radionuclide is dissolved in an appropriate solvent and *eluted,* or washed away from the parent radionuclide.

Generators are commercially available from several suppliers. One of the most frequently used generators in nuclear pharmacy is the "moly" generator, or the $^{99}$Mo-$^{99m}$Tc generator. In this generator, molybdenum-99 ($^{99}$Mo), a radionuclide with a half-life of 67 hours, decays into technetium-99 ($^{99m}$Tc), which has a half-life of approximately 6 hours. A schematic diagram of a moly generator is shown in Figure 10–8. It is a closed, sterile, and shielded system.

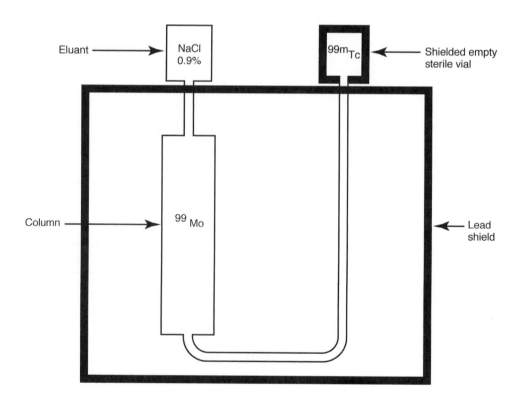

Typical "Moly" Generator

**FIGURE 10–8**   Typical "Moly" Generator.

It consists of an internal column that contains the parent radionuclide, $^{99}$Mo, and two sterile vials. One vial contains the **eluant**, the solvent that washes away the daughter radionuclide, which is a sterile 0.9 percent sodium chloride injection. The other vial is an empty, shielded vial for receiving the daughter radionuclide, $^{99m}$Tc.

The generator is eluted under aseptic conditions. The sterile 0.9 percent sodium chloride is drawn through the column by means of a vacuum. The $^{99m}$Tc dissolves in the sodium chloride, is washed from the column, and is collected into the empty vial, leaving $^{99}$Mo on the column. The $^{99}$Mo continues to generate more $^{99m}$Tc, and the generator can be eluted several more times to yield more $^{99m}$Tc. $^{99m}$Tc is usually eluted daily from the moly generator until the supply of $^{99}$Mo is exhausted. Then the entire generator is replaced.

Generators are relatively small. They are easy to ship to the nuclear pharmacy, and they do not take up much space. Radionuclide generators are also relatively safe and easy to operate by nuclear pharmacists and nuclear pharmacy technicians. It is important to mention that the daughter radionuclides produced from nuclear generators must be labeled and undergo quality control tests before they can be used to prepare radiopharmaceuticals. A commercially available $^{99}$Mo-$^{99m}$Tc generator is shown in Figure 10–9.

### Preparing a Batch of Radiopharmaceutical from a Reagent Kit

The compounding of radiopharmaceuticals in the nuclear pharmacy has been simplified by the introduction of reagent kits, more commonly referred to as "kits." A kit is a commercially available bulk supply of a carrier drug. It contains the carrier drug in a freeze-dried or solution form in a sterile vial. It can be stored for periods of time before being used to prepare the radiopharmaceutical.

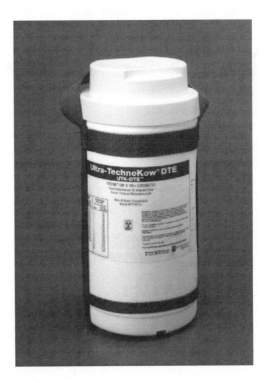

**FIGURE 10–9** $^{99}$Mo-$^{99m}$Tc Generator. (Reprinted with permission of Mallinckrodt, Inc.)

Kits essentially allow a batch of a particular radiopharmaceutical to be made at one time. The radiopharmaceutical is made by simply adding the radionuclide to the kit under aseptic conditions in a laminar airflow hood. The chemical reaction that binds the radionuclide with the carrier drug takes place within the vial. After quality control testing, the resulting quantity of radiopharmaceutical can be used to prepare individual doses based on individual prescriptions.

Kits are accompanied by a package insert that is provided by the manufacturer. It is similar to the package insert for any traditional drug, and it contains important information, such as critical storage temperatures both before and after the addition of the radionuclide and compounding procedures. Most radiopharmaceuticals are available today as kits. The most frequently used kits are for the production of $^{99m}$Tc radiopharmaceuticals.

### Preparing Individual Doses of Radiopharmaceuticals

Individual doses of radiopharmaceuticals are prepared in the nuclear pharmacy in unit-dose syringe form. They are compounded to deliver a prescribed dose of a radionuclide at the time of *administration*, not at the time of compounding. Therefore, the dose of the radiopharmaceutical compounded by the nuclear pharmacist is not the dose prescribed by the physician. The radionuclide begins to decay as soon as it is prepared. A correction must be made for the amount of decay that will occur during the time needed for compounding, delivery to the facility and patient, or other delays. The nuclear pharmacist adds an additional amount, referred to as activity, of the radionuclide to the prescribed dose to allow for this decay. The nuclear pharmacist uses decay tables to calculate the extra activity that needs to be added. These tables list standardized data, called a decay factor, for each individual radionuclide that reflects how fast a particular radionuclide will decay.

A radiopharmaceutical is usually prepared under a laminar airflow hood and behind a lead barrier shield. The nuclear pharmacist or nuclear pharmacy technician wears a laboratory coat and disposable gloves to prevent radiation exposure. Materials are handled using tongs or long tweezers whenever possible. The required volume or radionuclide is drawn up into a sterile shielded syringe by aseptic technique. Sterile 0.9 percent sodium chloride injection is usually used to dilute the very small volumes of radionuclide. Extreme care must be taken when the syringe is being recapped.

The dose or activity of the radionuclide in the syringe is measured with an instrument called a dose calibrator, which is located inside the hood. The syringe is placed inside the chamber or well of the dose calibrator, and the level of activity is displayed on a digital screen. A 10 percent deviation in dose is allowed by the Nuclear Regulatory Commission (NRC). Once the required dose is determined to be in the syringe, it is labeled. The prescription label is usually placed on the outside of the syringe shield, not on the unshielded syringe inside.

Automation has recently been introduced into this phase of radiopharmaceutical preparation. Automated dose drawing machines can fill and cap syringes, measure the activity of the radionuclide, and place finished syringes in shielded containers. Due to the concern with radiation exposure in the nuclear pharmacy, the use of automation can be expected to increase in the future.

## QUALITY CONTROL TESTING

Quality control testing involves the performance of appropriate biological, chemical, and physical tests on radiopharmaceuticals to determine if they are safe to use in humans. Each radiopharmaceutical that is compounded in the nuclear pharmacy must be tested before it can be dispensed. The compounded radiopharmaceutical must be sterile and pyrogen-free, and it must be free of any radionuclide, radiochemical, or chemical impurity. Several types of tests are used. Biological tests are performed to determine the sterility and the presence of pyrogens. These are the same quality control tests used in sterile intravenous compounding. Tests used to detect radionuclide, radiochemical, and chemical impurities are specific to nuclear pharmacy. They are performed using a variety of instruments. A *radionuclide impurity* is defined as the presence of a foreign radionuclide. A typical example is $^{99m}$Tc contaminated with $^{99}$Mo, its parent radionuclide. This type of impurity is detected by different types of radiation detectors. A *radiochemical impurity* is defined as the presence of the radionuclide in a different chemical form. An example is $^{99m}$Tc present as $^{99m}$TcO4, its pertechnate form, in a $^{99m}$Tc-MAA radiopharmaceutical. This type of impurity is due to decomposition or breakdown as a result of changes in temperature or pH, exposure to light, or the type of solvent used. It is detected by a number of methods of chemical analysis. A *chemical impurity* is defined as the presence of a foreign chemical in the radiopharmaceutical. An example is $^{99m}$Tc contaminated with aluminum from the alumina column of a moly generator. This type of impurity also is detected by chemical analysis. Other tests are carried out to ensure the integrity of the radiopharmaceutical, such as the determination of the pH, by using a pH meter, and the particle size, estimated by using a microscope (400 power) and a special grid.

## PACKAGING

Once the compounded radiopharmaceutical has passed all quality control tests, it is packaged for delivery. The individual shielded syringes are first placed in individual lead syringe containers or shields, sometimes referred to as "pigs." A type of tamper-evident covering, such as shrink-wrap, is applied to provide evidence that the dose of the radiopharmaceutical has left the pharmacy intact. The lead syringe containers are then placed inside the shipping container. Many nuclear pharmacies use metal military ammunition boxes, called ammo cans, as shipping containers. These metal boxes are fitted with foam inserts that hold the lead syringe containers and provide bracing (Figure 10–10). Other types of shipping containers include "briefcases" and cardboard boxes. Shipping papers are also placed inside the shipping container before it is closed and secured.

One of the most important steps in packaging is monitoring the shipping container before transport. The shipping container is monitored or *surveyed* for external radiation exposure using a Geiger counter. The exterior of the container also is wiped down with isopropyl alcohol or ammonia to remove any surface radioactive contamination. As a final step, labels that identify the contents of the container are placed on the outside of the shipping container. The appropriate delivery tag also is attached to the container. The shipping containers are then loaded into the delivery vehicle for transport.

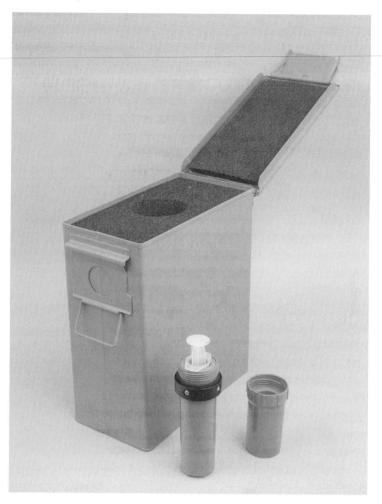

**FIGURE 10–10**  Lead Syringe Container with Foam Insert. (Courtesy of Biodex Medical Systems, Inc.)

## RADIOACTIVE WASTE DISPOSAL

Pharmacy-supplied syringes and vials that contained radiopharmaceuticals or that contain unused doses of radiopharmaceuticals are returned to the nuclear pharmacy. They are returned in the original lead syringe containers and shipping containers in which they were delivered. They are placed in the breakdown area of the nuclear pharmacy and are dismantled. The outside surface of the shipping container is first surveyed for external contamination by means of a Geiger counter. If it is within acceptable limits, the container is then opened, and the radionuclide that was inside is identified. The radioactive waste, if any, is disposed of in the appropriate container, where it is allowed to decay. Each radionuclide has a separate container due to different half-lives. The syringe and vial shields are also surveyed with a Geiger counter. If they are contaminated by radiation, they are wiped down with isopropyl alcohol or ammonia to remove the contamination, or they are taken out of service and allowed to decay until they are no longer radioactive. Finally, the inside of the shipping container is surveyed and wiped down for reuse.

There is quite a variety of radioactive waste generated in the nuclear pharmacy. In addition to returned radiopharmaceutical doses, there are used syringes and needles, empty vials of radiopharmaceuticals or radionuclides, disposable gowns and gloves, alcohol wipes, chemo preparation mats, and chemo spill kits. All of this waste must be safely disposed of. There are several methods for disposing of radioactive waste.

Most radioactive waste is allowed to decay while being stored in a lead-lined box or under other conditions. Only radioactive compounds that have half-lives of less than 65 days are allowed to be held for decay. They are usually held for ten half-lives, after which time they are considered *dead*, or no longer radioactive. Once they are dead, they are disposed of as regular trash or biomedical waste. Radioactive waste that is in solution or liquid form can be disposed of into the sewage system. This disposal method is allowed by the NRC as long as it does not exceed maximum monthly limits. Radioactive gases may be released into the atmosphere as long as they also do not exceed NRC and EPA limits. Finally, radioactive waste that contains radionuclides with long half-lives is transferred to a nuclear waste facility. Here it is either buried or incinerated.

## RADIATION SAFETY

Radiation exposure can cause several ill effects in humans, such as nausea and vomiting, diarrhea, hair loss, burns, and damage to chromosomes. Therefore, radioactive compounds must be properly handled to ensure the safety of personnel. There are three basic principles of radiation safety in order to maintain exposure *as low as reasonably achievable*, or ALARA. These are time, distance, and shielding.

- *Time.* The shorter the exposure to a source of radiation, the lower the dose of radiation. Workers should spend only the time necessary to perform a task near a source of radiation.

- *Distance.* The greater the distance from a source of radiation, the lower the dose of radiation. Workers should stay as far away as possible from a source of radiation. They should use tongs or long tweezers to handle radioactive materials when possible.

- *Shielding.* The better the radiation-absorbing material, the lower the dose of radiation. Shielding is one of the most important protections from radiation. Everything that holds radioactivity or comes into contact with radioactivity should be shielded. Some examples of shielding include lead barrier shields, lead-lined storage boxes, refrigerators and freezers, leaded glass syringe shields, lead vial shields, lead syringe containers, lead bricks, and metal shipping containers. The worker also should wear protective clothing, such as a laboratory coat, lead apron or gown, and a mask, protective eyewear, or respirator if necessary.

The NRC has set guidelines that limit the dose of radiation that a worker may receive. In order to monitor the amount of radiation that a worker may be receiving while working, the worker wears a type of personal radiation monitoring device called a dosimeter. A dosimeter can be in the form of a badge (Figure 10–11) or a ring (Figure 10–12). The radiation-monitoring devices are changed periodically and analyzed to detect the amount of radiation that the worker has received over a period of time.

There are several other radiation safety activities that are regularly performed in the nuclear pharmacy to ensure a safe working environment. These include monitoring the air quality, checking the airflow in fume and laminar airflow hoods, surveying work areas, surveying delivery vehicles, performing instrument checks, and testing wells. Finally, personnel should be familiar with

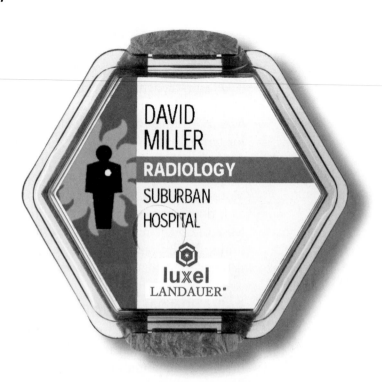

**FIGURE 10–11**    Badge Dosimeter. (Courtesy of LANDAUER, Inc.)

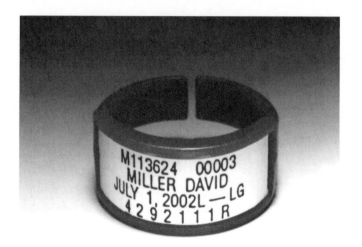

**FIGURE 10–12**    Ring Dosimeter. (Courtesy of LANDAUER, Inc.)

decontamination procedures in case of radiation exposure. These procedures range from handwashing, to removing contaminated clothing, to full body showering.

## LEGISLATION AND REGULATIONS FOR NUCLEAR PHARMACY

A nuclear pharmacy is licensed and regulated by its respective state board of pharmacy. It is usually licensed as a "retail" pharmacy because most states do not have a separate license category for nuclear pharmacies. A nuclear pharmacy must comply with all state and federal pharmacy laws and regulations. As a sterile compounding practice, a nuclear pharmacy must also comply with sterile compounding regulations, which may vary from state to state. However, very few state boards of pharmacy have specific guidelines regarding the practice of nuclear pharmacy. The NABP has developed Model Rules for Nuclear/ Radiologic Pharmacy, which outline some general requirements for pharmacies that prepare radiopharmaceuticals. These rules may help individual state boards of pharmacy develop laws that pertain to nuclear pharmacy.

The use of radiation and radioactive products by any organization is governed by several federal regulatory agencies. A nuclear pharmacy is also regulated by these agencies. Discussion of regulatory agencies follows next.

## OMNIBUS BUDGET RECONCILIATION ACT OF 1990

OBRA 90 mandates patient counseling. This counseling requirement does not apply to nuclear pharmacy practice because radiopharmaceuticals are not dispensed directly to patients, but to physicians and facilities for administration to the patient. However, a nuclear pharmacist may provide counseling and education to physicians, nuclear medicine technologists, and other health care professionals concerning the use of radiopharmaceuticals.

## NUCLEAR REGULATORY COMMISSION REGULATIONS

The NRC regulates the use and disposal of radioactive materials, as well as the safety of radiation workers and the general public. There are several NRC regulations that apply to nuclear pharmacy.

Any facility that handles radioactive compounds must have a license from the NRC (or from a state radiation control branch). This category includes a nuclear pharmacy. The nuclear pharmacy must first hold a traditional pharmacy license from its respective state board of pharmacy. The NRC license lists the name of the nuclear pharmacist manager or the nuclear pharmacist in charge, who is responsible for the operation of the nuclear pharmacy and for compliance with all laws and regulations. It also lists all **authorized users,** personnel who have met specialized requirements for training and experience in the handling of radioactive materials. All qualified nuclear pharmacists and pharmacy technicians would be authorized users. It should be mentioned that some states have requirements of their own that replace or add to those of the NRC.

A nuclear pharmacy must have a separate area for radiation storage and decay. Detailed floor plans that show this area must be submitted to the NRC before an NRC license is approved.

A nuclear pharmacy must keep strict records for the receipt, storage, compounding, disposal, and transport of radioactive materials. Compounding records are required for radionuclide preparation from a generator, called an elution form (Figure 10–13), radiopharmaceutical preparation from kits (Figure 10–14), and radiopharmaceutical unit-dose dispensing (Figure 10–15).

A nuclear pharmacy must be monitored regularly for external radiation exposure and surface radioactive contamination. Radiation exposure is monitored by *surveying* pharmacy areas using a Geiger counter. Compounding areas must be surveyed daily, at the end of each day. Storage areas must be surveyed weekly. Radioactive contamination is monitored by performing a wipe test. A wipe test involves swabbing an area using absorbent paper, then using a type of radiation-detecting equipment to determine the amount of radiation present. Compounding and storage areas must undergo a wipe test weekly.

## NUCLEAR PHARMACY/NUCLEAR MEDICINE
# MOLY GENERATOR ELUTION FORM

Date of Calibration:

Activity:

Manuf. Lot No.:

| DAY | DATE | TIME | ACTIVITY (mCi) | VOLUME (ml) | Mo-99 ($\mu$Ci) | Mo-99/Tc-99m ($\mu$Ci/mCi) A.L. $\geq$ 0.0425 | Al $^{3+}$ | Tc-99m LOT No. | TECH. INITIALS |
|---|---|---|---|---|---|---|---|---|---|
| MONDAY | | | | | | | | | |
| | | | | | | | | | |
| | | | | | | | | | |
| TUESDAY | | | | | | | | | |
| | | | | | | | | | |
| | | | | | | | | | |
| WEDNESDAY | | | | | | | | | |
| | | | | | | | | | |
| | | | | | | | | | |
| THURSDAY | | | | | | | | | |
| | | | | | | | | | |
| | | | | | | | | | |
| FRIDAY | | | | | | | | | |
| | | | | | | | | | |
| | | | | | | | | | |
| SATURDAY | | | | | | | | | |
| | | | | | | | | | |
| | | | | | | | | | |
| SUNDAY | | | | | | | | | |
| | | | | | | | | | |
| | | | | | | | | | |

**FIGURE 10–13** Elution Form. (From Fundamentals of Nuclear Pharmacy (5th ed.), by G. B. Saha, 2005, New York: Springer-Verlag. Used with permission. Courtesy of Gopal B. Saha, Ph.D.)

There are also extensive NRC regulations that deal with radiation exposure limits for personnel, shielding for vials and syringes of radiopharmaceuticals, labeling of radiopharmaceuticals, posting of radiation caution signs in radiation areas, radioactive spills, and errors involving radiopharmaceuticals.

## DEPARTMENT OF TRANSPORTATION REGULATIONS

The U.S. Department of Transportation (DOT) regulates the shipment of hazardous materials through the Federal Hazardous Materials Transportation Law. Radioactive materials are considered hazardous materials. DOT regulations affect the packaging, labeling, and transporting of radioactive materials.

## Tc-99m RADIOPHARMACEUTICAL RECORD

| Date | Time | NP No | Tc-99m Pertechnetate | | | | Kit Data | | | | | Saline | | | Total* Vol. (ml) | Conc. (mCi/ml) | Prep'd By |
|---|---|---|---|---|---|---|---|---|---|---|---|---|---|---|---|---|---|
| | | | Mfr. | Lot No. | Activity (mCi) | Vol. (ml) | Type | Mfr. | Lot No. | Vol. (ml) | Mfr. | Lot No. | Vol. (ml) | | | |
| | | | | | | | | | | | | | | | | |
| | | | | | | | | | | | | | | | | |
| | | | | | | | | | | | | | | | | |
| | | | | | | | | | | | | | | | | |
| | | | | | | | | | | | | | | | | |
| | | | | | | | | | | | | | | | | |
| | | | | | | | | | | | | | | | | |
| | | | | | | | | | | | | | | | | |
| | | | | | | | | | | | | | | | | |
| | | | | | | | | | | | | | | | | |
| | | | | | | | | | | | | | | | | |
| | | | | | | | | | | | | | | | | |
| | | | | | | | | | | | | | | | | |
| | | | | | | | | | | | | | | | | |

**FIGURE 10–14** Radiopharmaceutical Preparation Record. (From Fundamentals of Nuclear Pharmacy (5th ed.), by G. B. Saha, 2005, New York: Springer-Verlag. Used with permission. Courtesy of Gopal B. Saha, Ph.D.)

## RADIOPHARMACEUTICAL RECORD

## UNIT DOSE

| Date | NP No. | Product | Patient's Name | Clinic No. | Study | Calib. Dose | Calib. Time | Activity (Dispensed) | Time of Injection | Initials |
|---|---|---|---|---|---|---|---|---|---|---|
| | | | | | | | | | | |
| | | | | | | | | | | |
| | | | | | | | | | | |
| | | | | | | | | | | |
| | | | | | | | | | | |
| | | | | | | | | | | |
| | | | | | | | | | | |
| | | | | | | | | | | |
| | | | | | | | | | | |
| | | | | | | | | | | |
| | | | | | | | | | | |
| | | | | | | | | | | |
| | | | | | | | | | | |
| | | | | | | | | | | |
| | | | | | | | | | | |
| | | | | | | | | | | |
| | | | | | | | | | | |

**FIGURE 10–15**  Radiopharmaceutical Dispensing Record. (From Fundamentals of Nuclear Pharmacy (5th ed.), by G. B. Saha, 2005, New York: Springer-Verlag. Used with permission. Courtesy of Gopal B. Saha, Ph.D.)

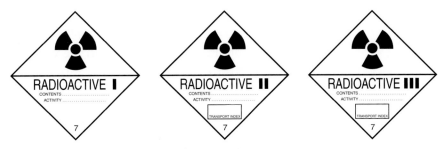

**FIGURE 10–16**　DOT Labels.

According to the DOT, the shipping container for transporting radioactive materials must be able to maintain its integrity and the integrity of the radioactive materials inside during normal transport. For this reason, many nuclear pharmacies use metal military ammunition boxes, which are sturdy and which also provide shielding.

The shipping container must be specifically labeled. There are three categories of labels for radioactive materials, based on the activity of the radioactive material in the container: Radioactive White-I, Radioactive Yellow-II, and Radioactive Yellow-III. Radioactive Yellow-III contains the highest amount of radiation. The majority of radiopharmaceuticals shipped are Radioactive White-I or Radioactive Yellow-II. This label must include the radiation symbol and the words *Caution Radioactive Material*, the name of the radionuclide or its abbreviation, and the quantity of radioactivity at a specified date and time (Figure 10–16).

As part of the labeling, shipping papers must be included *inside* the shipping container. Shipping papers contain information about the radioactive material being shipped and the hazards involved. These papers must include the name of the radionuclide, quantity, form, label category, emergency response phone number and information (for personnel responding to an emergency involving the hazardous material), and the pharmacy's identification. A copy of the shipping papers also must be kept with the driver of the delivery vehicle, and a copy is retained in the pharmacy.

DOT regulations also specify when the delivery vehicle carrying radiopharmaceuticals must be labeled, that is, display a placard. A placard is a much larger version of the label that is placed on the outside of the shipping container. A delivery vehicle must have a placard only if it is transporting Radioactive Yellow-III material. A placard is not required for Radioactive White-I or Radioactive Yellow-II material, the majority of radiopharmaceuticals shipped.

The DOT requires that the shipping containers be blocked and braced inside the delivery vehicle so that they cannot change position during normal transport, which includes turns, curves, potholes, stops, acceleration, and deceleration. Most delivery vehicles are equipped with special dividers, holders for shipping containers, customized sliding racks, cages, and other types of bracing.

Finally, the Department of Transportation requires the proper training of personnel. Any employee involved in the transport and delivery of radiopharmaceuticals must receive specific training in the handling of radioactive materials within the first 90 days of employment, and the training must be updated every 3 years.

## OCCUPATIONAL SAFETY AND HEALTH ADMINISTRATION

The Occupational Safety and Health Administration (OSHA) is concerned with the safety of employees. Both the NRC and OSHA have jurisdiction over the occupational safety and health of employees at NRC-licensed facilities, including a nuclear pharmacy. While the NRC deals with radiation hazards, OSHA deals with nonradioactive hazards in the workplace. There is a coordinated effort between the two agencies to protect pharmacists, pharmacy technicians, and other personnel from possible workplace hazards present in a nuclear pharmacy.

## FOOD AND DRUG ADMINISTRATION REGULATIONS

The Food and Drug Administration (FDA) regulates all drugs used in humans for diagnosis and treatment. The FDA Modernization Act of 1997 (FDAMA) regulates pharmacy compounding. However, the compounding of radiopharmaceuticals has been excluded from this act. As a result, in 2000, the Section on Nuclear Pharmacy Practice, the Academy of Pharmacy Practice and Management of the American Pharmaceutical Association developed Nuclear Pharmacy Guidelines for the Compounding of Radiopharmaceuticals to set up good compounding practices for the compounding of radiopharmaceuticals. These guidelines address all aspects of radiopharmaceutical compounding, including personnel, the nuclear pharmacy environment, quality control, labeling, packaging, and documentation.

## UNITED STATES PHARMACOPEIA STANDARDS

USP Chapter <797> sets standards for the compounding, preparation, and labeling of sterile drug preparations and applies to all practice settings that compound sterile preparations, including a nuclear pharmacy. Radiopharmaceuticals are sterile drug preparations. However, there are unique issues involved in preparing radiopharmaceuticals, such as shielding and quality control testing, and in storing radiopharmaceuticals, such as their short half-lives, that affect compliance with Chapter <797>. For example, Chapter <797> calls for direct visual inspection of compounded sterile products. However, close visual inspection of compounded radiopharmaceuticals is not recommended due to the risk of radiation exposure. Revised standards that specifically address issues unique to nuclear pharmacy may be released in the future.

## ENVIRONMENTAL PROTECTION AGENCY

The Environmental Protection Agency (EPA) regulates the release of radioactive materials into the atmosphere under the federal Clean Air Act. The EPA limits the amount of radionuclides that the public can receive through the air from nuclear laboratories and pharmacies and monitors the effect of radioactive material releases on the public's health. A nuclear pharmacy may release radioactive gases into the atmosphere in amounts approved by the EPA.

## THE ROLE OF THE PHARMACIST IN NUCLEAR PHARMACY

A nuclear pharmacist is a licensed pharmacist who possesses the necessary knowledge and training to work with radioactive compounds. A nuclear pharmacist must first hold a traditional license in her individual state. As of this writing, only the state of Florida requires a separate *radiopharmacist license* in addition to the traditional license. The pharmacist must meet minimum training and experience requirements set by the NRC. These are a minimum of 200 hours of classroom training in nuclear pharmacy and a minimum of 500 hours of experience in handling radiopharmaceuticals in a nuclear pharmacy under the supervision of a qualified nuclear pharmacist.

There are several ways for a pharmacist to receive nuclear training. Most pharmacy schools offer an introductory course in nuclear pharmacy but do not provide all of the training needed. Large centralized nuclear pharmacy companies and several major universities, as well as the U.S. Army, provide nuclear pharmacy training programs.

After meeting these training and experience requirements, the pharmacist is listed as an authorized user of radioactive materials on the license of the pharmacy or hospital. She also may be referred to as an *authorized nuclear pharmacist,* or *ANP.*

A nuclear pharmacist can also seek certification as a Board Certified Nuclear Pharmacist and the initials BCNP from the Board of Pharmaceutical Specialties (BPS). Certification is voluntary and is different from and in addition to the NRC training and experience requirements. Board certification means that the nuclear pharmacist has demonstrated advanced education, experience, knowledge, and skills in nuclear pharmacy beyond what is needed for licensure and to be designated as an authorized user. In addition to a pharmacy degree and current active license, the nuclear pharmacist must have 4,000 hours of training or experience and must pass the Nuclear Pharmacy Specialty Certification exam. Recertification is required every 7 years. Board certification may result in increased respect, a higher salary, and a competitive edge when applying for jobs.

Nuclear pharmacy practice offers several roles for the nuclear pharmacist. They can be divided into clinical, dispensing, and administrative roles.

## CLINICAL ROLE

The clinical role of the nuclear pharmacist involves pharmaceutical care activities. The nuclear pharmacist monitors patient outcomes and provides consultation and education to physicians and other health care professionals concerning the use of radiopharmaceuticals. Some areas that the nuclear pharmacist may consult in include dosing, allergic and adverse reactions, drug-radiopharmaceutical interactions, radiopharmaceutical handling policies and procedures, safety protocols, and interpretation of the laws pertaining to nuclear pharmacy. Other clinical roles for the nuclear pharmacist include research and (new radiopharmaceutical) drug development, participating in clinical investigations using radiopharmaceuticals, consulting for radiopharmaceutical companies or the government, teaching pharmacy students, and involvement in professional nuclear organizations.

## DISPENSING ROLE

The dispensing role of the nuclear pharmacist involves all of the activities relating to the dispensing of a prescription. As in any traditional pharmacy, the nuclear pharmacist obtains medications, screens prescription orders, resolves problems with prescription orders, and checks finished prescriptions. However, nuclear pharmacy is essentially a sterile compounding practice, and it is here that the nuclear pharmacist uses specialized knowledge and compounding skills. The extensive quality control tests performed on compounded radiopharmaceuticals are also a unique activity for the nuclear pharmacist.

## ADMINISTRATIVE ROLE

The administrative role of the nuclear pharmacist is related to the management of a nuclear pharmacy. The nuclear pharmacist who assumes this role is usually designated the pharmacist in charge. She is responsible for all personnel, for all activities performed in the preparation and dispensing of radiopharmaceuticals, and for compliance with all laws and regulations that apply to nuclear pharmacy.

# THE ROLE OF THE PHARMACY TECHNICIAN IN NUCLEAR PHARMACY

The pharmacy technician who works in a nuclear pharmacy is referred to as a nuclear pharmacy technician. A nuclear pharmacy technician performs tasks specific to nuclear pharmacy. Most state boards of pharmacy define a pharmacy technician, the training, and allowable activities in general. However, only a few states have specific regulations concerning nuclear pharmacy technicians.

The nuclear pharmacy technician must have certain qualifications to work in a nuclear pharmacy. The pharmacy technician must complete a nuclear pharmacy technician education and training program. In addition, the pharmacy technician must possess traditional pharmacy knowledge and skills as well as knowledge and skills specific to nuclear pharmacy such as:

- A knowledge of radiopharmaceutical terms, abbreviations, and symbols
- A knowledge of basic radiopharmaceutical calculations
- A knowledge of specific radiopharmaceutical compounding
- A knowledge of quality control testing
- A knowledge of the packaging and labeling requirements for radiopharmaceuticals
- A knowledge of the record-keeping requirements in nuclear pharmacy
- A knowledge of radiation safety
- A knowledge of purchasing and inventory control of radioactive and non-radioactive compounds
- An understanding of the legislation and regulations pertaining to nuclear pharmacy

There are many activities that the nuclear pharmacy technician can perform in the nuclear pharmacy. However, the nuclear pharmacy technician may not perform any task that involves the professional judgment of a nuclear pharmacist. Nuclear pharmacy is a unique practice area that can be challenging yet rewarding for the pharmacy technician. The role of the pharmacy technician in a nuclear pharmacy can be divided into three areas: compounding, pharmacy maintenance, and computer functions.

## RADIOPHARMACEUTICAL COMPOUNDING

There are many activities the nuclear pharmacy technician can perform in the compounding area. These include accepting verbal orders for radiopharmaceuticals for diagnosis, performing basic radiopharmaceutical calculations, eluting a radionuclide generator, drawing up individual unit-doses of radiopharmaceuticals, performing quality control tests on compounded radiopharmaceuticals, labeling radiopharmaceuticals, completing compounding records, and packaging radiopharmaceuticals.

## PHARMACY MAINTENANCE

The nuclear pharmacy technician plays an important role in maintaining a safe and efficient nuclear pharmacy environment. Activities related to nuclear pharmacy maintenance include performing instrument checks, surveying pharmacy areas and delivery vehicles, monitoring air and water quality, completing records for the receipt, storage, disposal, and transport of radioactive materials, maintaining equipment, assisting with radioactive and nonradioactive drug purchasing and inventory control, purchasing and stocking pharmacy supplies, dismantling and preparing supplies for reuse, maintaining storage areas, and disposing of nuclear waste.

## COMPUTER FUNCTIONS

The nuclear pharmacy technician can perform several computer functions in the nuclear pharmacy. The technician can enter prescription information into the computer and generate prescription labels. She can also generate shipping papers and delivery tags. In addition, the technician can assist the pharmacist in clinical and administrative activities by printing reports, drug information requests, and other types of materials.

## KEY CONCEPTS

- Nuclear pharmacy is a highly specialized practice area involving the production of radiopharmaceuticals, drugs that release radiation within the body.
- A radiopharmaceutical is composed of a radionuclide, an atom that releases radiation, and a carrier drug, a pharmaceutical that delivers the radionuclide to the desired area of the body.
- Radiopharmaceuticals are used for the diagnosis and treatment of disease, the two most commonly used radiopharmaceuticals being technetium-99 and iodine-131.
- Radiopharmaceuticals cause few adverse reactions or drug interactions.
- The unique elements of a nuclear pharmacy include the specialized inventory of radionuclides and carrier drugs, the design into separate work areas, the specialized equipment and supplies, and the safe and timely delivery service.
- The prescription-filling process in a nuclear pharmacy involves radioactive compounding and includes eluting a radionuclide generator, preparing a batch of radiopharmaceutical from a reagent kit, and preparing individual doses of a radiopharmaceutical.
- Quality control tests must be performed on every compounded radiopharmaceutical to ensure that it is sterile, pyrogen-free, and pure.
- There are strict packaging requirements for radiopharmaceuticals, which include the use of special shipping containers and bracing.

- The radiation safety principles of time, distance, and shielding are used in nuclear pharmacy practice.
- There are extensive legislation and regulations that pertain to nuclear pharmacy.
- A nuclear pharmacist has extensive training in the handling of radioactive compounds and has several roles in the nuclear pharmacy; the nuclear pharmacy technician must also complete special training in order to perform activities in a nuclear pharmacy.

## SELF-ASSESSMENT QUESTIONS

### MULTIPLE CHOICE

1. Which is not an example of a radiopharmaceutical?
   a. radioactive red blood cells
   b. PET drugs
   c. carrier drugs
   d. $^{99m}$Tc-MAA

2. Compounding radiopharmaceuticals includes:
   a. adding a radionuclide to a kit
   b. eluting a generator
   c. preparing unit-dose syringes
   d. all of the above

3. Quality control tests are used to detect all of the following except:
   a. bacterial contamination
   b. radiochemical impurities
   c. chemical impurities
   d. temperature changes

4. A nuclear pharmacist:
   a. must hold a traditional license
   b. must meet minimum NRC training and experience requirements
   c. must be listed as an authorized user on the license of the nuclear pharmacy
   d. all of the above

5. Which is not an example of specialized equipment used in a nuclear pharmacy?
   a. a Geiger-Müller counter
   b. a vertical laminar airflow hood
   c. a dose calibrator
   d. a barrier shield

6. Packaging for radiopharmaceuticals includes:
   a. lead syringe containers
   b. ammunition cans
   c. foam inserts
   d. all of the above

7. Which statement concerning a radiopharmaceutical is not true?

   a. it has no effect on the body when used for diagnosis
   b. it may interact with traditional medication
   c. it is distributed to all areas of the body
   d. it is available in different dosage forms

8. Which of the following principles is practiced in a nuclear pharmacy to minimize radiation exposure?

   a. time
   b. shielding
   c. distance
   d. all of the above

9. A method of radioactive waste disposal is:

   a. venting into the atmosphere
   b. storage and decay
   c. transfer of the waste to a nuclear waste facility
   d. all of the above

10. Which is not a NRC regulation for a nuclear pharmacy?

   a. placarding the delivery vehicle
   b. a storage and decay area in the nuclear pharmacy
   c. monitoring the pharmacy for radiation exposure and radioactive contamination
   d. radiopharmacy compounding record keeping

## TRUE/FALSE (CORRECT THE FALSE STATEMENTS)

1. _____ There are more rigorous quality control tests involved in the compounding of radiopharmaceuticals than in any other type of compounding.

2. _____ An institutional nuclear pharmacy operates out of a centralized site in the community.

3. _____ The decay of a radionuclide results in the release of radiation.

4. _____ Adverse reactions to radiopharmaceuticals are quite common.

5. _____ The drug inventory in a nuclear pharmacy is similar to the drug inventory in a traditional pharmacy.

6. _____ Lead is an excellent shielding material.

7. _____ A pharmacy technician may accept a verbal order for a radiopharmaceutical for diagnosis or treatment.

8. _____ According to the NRC, a nuclear pharmacy must have a storage and decay area.

9. _____ Nuclear pharmacy is the first specialty area of pharmacy.

10. _____ Radiopharmaceuticals used for treatment contain higher doses of radiation than do radiopharmaceuticals used for diagnosis.

## FILL-IN

1. An atom with an unstable nucleus is called a _____.
2. The most frequently used radionuclide in medicine is _____.

3. The pharmaceutical that delivers the radionuclide to the desired area of the body is called the _____ _____.
4. The laminar airflow hood that is vented to the outside is a _____ _____.
5. The U.S. regulatory agency that is concerned with the shipment of radioactive materials is the _____ _____ _____.
6. The tightly controlled inventory in the nuclear pharmacy is referred to as a _____ inventory.
7. The area of the nuclear pharmacy where used containers for radiopharmaceuticals are returned and dismantled for reuse is called the _____ area.
8. A radionuclide generator works on the principle of _____.
9. The solvent used to separate a daughter radionuclide from the parent radionuclide is referred to as the _____.
10. The time required for one-half of a radionuclide to decay is the _____.

## CRITICAL THINKING

1. What are the advantages and the disadvantages of a centralized nuclear pharmacy compared to an institutional nuclear pharmacy?
2. Compare and contrast pharmacy operations in a nuclear pharmacy with those in a traditional hospital pharmacy.
3. Apply *structure, process,* and *outcomes* to a nuclear pharmacy.
4. Compare and contrast the duties of a pharmacy technician in a nuclear pharmacy with those in a traditional hospital pharmacy.
5. What steps should be taken in the event of a spill of a radiopharmaceutical in a nuclear pharmacy?

## BIBLIOGRAPHY

American Pharmacists Association. Section on Nuclear Pharmacy Practice. Academy of Pharmacy Practice and Management. (2005). *Guidelines for nuclear pharmacy technician training programs.* [On-line] APhA. Available: www.nuclearpharmacy.uams.edu/techs.

American Pharmacists Association. Section on Nuclear Pharmacy Practice. Academy of Pharmacy Practice and Management. (2005). *Nuclear pharmacy guidelines for the compounding of radiopharmaceuticals.* [On-line] APhA. Available: www.nuclearpharmacy.uams.edu/compounding.

Kowalsky, R., & Falen, S. (2004). *Radiopharmaceuticals in nuclear pharmacy and nuclear medicine* (2nd ed.). Washington, DC: American Pharmacists Association.

National Association of Boards of Pharmacy. (2005). *Model rules for nuclear/ radiologic pharmacy.* [On-line] NABP. Available: www.nabp.net.

Nuclear Regulatory Commission. (2005). *DOT regulations applicable to radio- pharmacy shipments.* [On-line] NRC. Available: www.nrc.gov.

Nuclear Regulatory Commission. (2005). *Model procedure for return of radioac- tive wastes from customers.* [On-line] NRC. Available: www.nrc.gov.

Purdue University. Division of Nuclear Pharmacy. (2005). *History of nuclear pharmacy*. [On-line] Purdue University. Available: www.pharmacy.purdue.edu.

Richard, C. (2005). Tests of special interest: More pharmacists earning certifications. *Pharmacy Today, 11*(6), 28.

Saha, G. (2005). *Fundamentals of nuclear pharmacy* (5th ed.). New York: Springer-Verlag.

United States Department of Labor. Occupational Safety and Health Administration. (2006). *Memorandum of understanding between the OSHA and the U.S. Nuclear Regulatory Commission*. [On-line] U.S. Department of Labor. Available: www.osha.gov.

United States Department of Transportation. (2002). *Federal Hazardous Materials Transportation Law*. [On-line] DOT. Available: www.dot.gov.

United States Department of Transportation. (2004). *2004 Emergency response guidebook*. Chicago: Labelmaster.

United States Environmental Protection Agency. (2006). *Clean Air Act*. [On-line] EPA. Available: www.epa.gov.

United States Pharmacopeial Convention. (2006). *The United States pharmacopeia* (29th ed.). and *The national formulary* (24th ed.). Rockville, MD: Author.

University of the Sciences in Philadelphia. (2005). *Remington: The science and practice of pharmacy* (21st ed.). Easton, PA: Mack Publishing Company.

## Learning Objectives

Upon completion of this chapter, the student should be able to:

- Define the hospice concept.
- Describe the characteristics of hospice.
- Define a hospice pharmacy.
- Describe the elements of a hospice pharmacy.
- Describe some of the special services of a hospice pharmacy.
- Understand the legislation and regulations pertaining to hospice pharmacy practice.
- Describe the role of the pharmacist in hospice pharmacy.
- Describe the role of the pharmacy technician in hospice pharmacy.

## Key Terms

| | | |
|---|---|---|
| breakthrough pain | hospice pharmacy | palliative care |
| hospice | pain management | symptom management |

## Introduction

Hospice pharmacy is an area of pharmacy practice that has grown out of the hospice movement. Hospice has gone from an alternative health care option for terminally ill patients to an accepted part of the health care field. Pharmacists have become involved in hospice by providing needed medications and pharmaceutical care services to patients nearing the end of life. In order to work in this area of pharmacy, pharmacists and pharmacy technicians need to understand the hospice concept. They need special knowledge and skills, especially extemporaneous and sterile compounding skills, unique to hospice pharmacy practice. They also must be familiar with the legislation and regulations pertaining to hospice pharmacy. This chapter focuses on hospice pharmacy practice and the unique roles of the pharmacist and pharmacy technician in this area. ■

## OVERVIEW OF HOSPICE

**Hospice** is defined as an organized program of services to meet the physical, emotional, spiritual, and social needs of a patient who is terminally ill. A terminally ill patient is one who has an illness that is likely to result in death within 6 months. Hospice is a concept of care rather than a place of care. It is a special way of caring for these terminally ill patients and their families. Hospice care focuses on the patient's comfort rather than on a cure for the disease. It is appropriate when a cure for a particular disease is no longer possible and when the disease and aggressive treatment cause undue suffering for the patient. Hospice care allows the patient to live the remainder of his life as free from pain and other symptoms as possible. It offers comfort to the patient and his family so that when death does occur, it is painless, peaceful, and dignified. The goals of hospice are to alleviate pain and other symptoms and to make the patient comfortable until his death.

The hospice movement began in London in 1967 when a physician by the name of Cicely Saunders opened St. Christopher's Hospice to provide relief and comfort for dying patients during their last days. Hospice was introduced into the United States in 1974 when the National Cancer Institute funded the Connecticut Hospice in New Haven. Since then, the hospice movement has spread throughout the United States and has grown from a privately funded volunteer movement to a regulated industry, reimbursed by Medicare, Medicaid, and private insurance. Early hospice care was centered around an institution rather than the home. Today, the focus is on care in the patient's own home. Hospice care is growing, and the need for hospice services is expected to increase as the population ages and as diseases such as AIDS and cancer increase.

Hospice care differs from hospital and nursing facility care in several ways. Hospital and nursing facility care involve an interdisciplinary health care team. Hospice care involves the family and volunteers in addition to the interdisciplinary health care team. Hospital and nursing facility care emphasize treatments that cure disease and prolong life. Hospice care focuses on relieving symptoms and providing support in dying. Hospice accepts that death is inevitable. Hospital and nursing facility care tends to isolate the dying patient from family, friends, and his familiar home environment. Hospice care tries to keep the patient in his own warm and safe environment, if possible. Hospice provides many services that are not offered in institutional health care settings.

Hospice care also differs from traditional home care. Home care focuses on the patient's physical needs. Hospice care considers all of the other needs of the patient in addition to his physical needs. In fact, the hospice movement was started as a volunteer movement outside of organized medicine because it was believed that not all of the needs of the dying patient and his family were being met.

Hospice serves all types and ages of patients. Most hospice patients are elderly, but hospice serves young adults and even children. Approximately half of hospice patients are cancer patients. The remainder have diseases other than cancer, such as AIDS, dementia or Alzheimer's disease, congestive heart failure, chronic obstructive lung disease (COLD), multiple sclerosis, or end-stage kidney or liver disease. Average hospice care is for a few months, although it can extend beyond that to several months.

Hospice care is provided by many different types of hospice organizations. About one-half are independent community hospice organizations. The remainder either are hospital-based or are associated with a home health care agency or a nursing facility. These organizations provide a variety of services, which include pain and symptom management, nursing care, personal care services (ADLs and IADLs), emotional support services, spiritual support services, social services in helping with funeral planning, bereavement support services, dietary support services, and pharmacy services. These services are usually available 24 hours a day, 7 days a week. In order for a hospice organization to be reimbursed by Medicare, it must provide medications and medical equipment related to the patient's terminal diagnosis. The hospice organization may provide these medications through its own pharmacy, or it may contract with an outside pharmacy to obtain medications.

Hospice services are provided in a variety of settings. The preferred setting is in the patient's home, and hospice care is most often provided in the home, allowing the patient to remain with family and friends. However, there may be times when it is no longer possible to remain at home, as when the patient's symptoms cannot be controlled at home by routine hospice services. An inpatient hospice facility may provide a safe and comfortable alternative. An inpatient hospice facility is a specially designed facility that offers a homelike setting for the dying patient. Hospice services can also be provided in a hospital or in a nursing facility.

Funding for hospice programs comes from Medicare, Medicaid, and private insurance. In order for a patient to be eligible for hospice care under Medicare, a physician must certify that death is expected within 6 months. Medicare will cover hospice costs until the patient's death for up to 6 months. If the patient stabilizes or improves, as some do, he can be discharged from the hospice program and readmitted if necessary. The rationale for reimbursement of hospice services by all payers is that hospice care replaces expensive hospital care and offers many special services, regardless of where the services are provided.

## CHARACTERISTICS OF HOSPICE

Hospice care has several unique characteristics. First, hospice treats the patient and family together as a unit. It considers the needs of the family as well as those of the dying patient. Families often require intensive emotional and spiritual support to cope with the patient's terminal illness and impending death. Bereavement services are an example of one of the services provided for the family. Bereavement services in the form of personal contact, support groups, and monthly newsletters for up to one year after the patient's death help the family cope with grief and loss.

 Hospice care involves the whole person. It considers not only the patient's physical illness but also the emotional and spiritual aspects of dying. It takes into consideration the patient's physical, emotional, spiritual, and even social needs.

Hospice care is interdisciplinary care. The hospice interdisciplinary team consists of pharmacists, pharmacy technicians, physicians, nurses, social workers, dieticians, clergy, nurse's aides, and specially trained volunteers. Physicians provide the leadership in the patient's care. However, nurses provide most of the patient care and assessment. The pharmacist is an important member of the hospice team and plays a major role in pain and symptom control and other pharmaceutical care activities. Volunteers provide services such as shopping, childcare, patient care, transportation, bereavement support, clerical support, and fund-raising. The hospice team works with the patient and family to develop a plan of care that addresses their physical, emotional, spiritual, and social needs.

Hospice care involves a care planning process. All hospice patients receive a patient assessment by the interdisciplinary team. The assessment includes information on the patient's pain and other symptoms, current treatments and response to those treatments, spiritual concerns, the patient's support system (family), bereavement plans for the family, social status, and the need for respite care, an alternative setting or another level of care. This assessment leads to an individualized plan of care to meet the patient's and family's needs. The patient is reassessed at various intervals, and the plan of care is adjusted as needed. The patient's care is discussed at weekly team meetings. The patient assessment and plan of care are documented in the patient's clinical record and are requirements for Joint Commission accreditation.

Finally, hospice care is palliative care. **Palliative care** is defined as care that treats the symptoms associated with a disease to provide comfort and relieve suffering rather than care that attempts to cure the disease. Hospice care focuses on pain and symptom management. Basically, all medications that relieve discomfort or prevent further complications are continued. Medications and treatments intended to cure the disease are discontinued. Chemotherapy, for example, would not be continued unless it relieved pain by reducing the size of a tumor. Other steps that can be taken to make the dying person more comfortable would be supplying a hospital bed or special mattress or oxygen to relieve respiratory distress.

## OVERVIEW OF HOSPICE PHARMACY

A **hospice pharmacy** is defined as a pharmacy that prepares and dispenses medications, medication-related equipment and supplies, and pharmaceutical care services to hospice patients at home or in institutions. It combines aspects of a traditional community pharmacy with aspects of a home infusion pharmacy, yet a hospice pharmacy has an identity and purpose of its own. The purpose of a hospice pharmacy is to provide medications and pharmaceutical care to the hospice patient in order to enhance the quality of his remaining life.

A hospice pharmacy can be a traditional community pharmacy, where hospice is a part of its business, or it can be a pharmacy that serves only hospice patients. A dedicated hospice pharmacy may be one of three types. It may be a privately owned traditional hospice pharmacy, or it may be part of a national hospice pharmacy organization, such as Hospice Pharmacia, a division of excelleRx, Inc. Both of these types of hospice pharmacies provide hospice pharmacy services to many different hospice organizations. A dedicated hospice pharmacy may also be an internal hospice pharmacy, owned by an individual hospice organization itself and possibly located within an inpatient hospice facility, if the hospice organization operates such a facility.

## ELEMENTS OF A HOSPICE PHARMACY

There are many elements that make up a hospice pharmacy. Most of these elements are the same elements that are found in other areas of pharmacy, such as traditional community pharmacy practice and home infusion pharmacy practice. The most distinctive element of a hospice pharmacy is its inventory.

### PERSONNEL

As in any other type of pharmacy, a variety of personnel is needed to ensure the efficient operation of a hospice pharmacy. These include pharmacists, pharmacy technicians, drivers, and various support personnel.

A pharmacist who works in a hospice pharmacy is referred to as a hospice pharmacist. He ensures that the terminally ill patient receives medications and related equipment and supplies on a timely basis according to the physician's orders. He also provides many pharmaceutical care services to the hospice patient. The hospice pharmacist has specialized knowledge in pain and symptom management and in extemporaneous compounding. The pharmacy technician is an important member of the hospice pharmacy team and assists the hospice pharmacist in all aspects of drug distribution as well as in compounding medications. A driver or delivery service is needed to transfer medications, equipment, and supplies to the patient at home or in an institution. Finally, support personnel, such as billing personnel, administrative personnel, and customer service personnel, perform activities that contribute to the overall operation of the hospice pharmacy.

### INVENTORY

The inventory in a hospice pharmacy is limited and specialized. It differs from the inventory in a traditional community pharmacy in that it does not include all of the medications used for the treatment of diseases. The hospice pharmacy stock also differs in that it includes more types of dosage forms of medications for terminally ill patients who are not able to take oral medications, such as injectables, suppositories, liquids, transdermal patches, and other forms. The inventory consists primarily of medications used in the control of pain and symptoms such as nausea and vomiting, constipation, and anxiety. Examples of these drugs include narcotic and non-narcotic analgesics, antinauseants, laxatives, and antianxiety drugs. It also consists of injectable drugs and intravenous fluids needed to compound IV infusion therapies, such as pain therapy, hydration therapy, and chemotherapy (for palliative use). Some of the drugs stocked in a hospice pharmacy are unique in that they are otherwise hard to find in a traditional retail pharmacy, such as expensive injectables for nausea (ondansetron) and high-dosage strengths of narcotics (MS Contin 200 mg tablets). The inventory in a hospice pharmacy is customized to meet the specific needs of the hospice patients served by the pharmacy.

## PHARMACY DESIGN

The design of a hospice pharmacy most often resembles the design of a traditional community pharmacy, with the addition of a clean room in which to prepare IV infusion therapies. The pharmacy may have a special area set aside for extemporaneous compounding, which is a large part of hospice pharmacy practice.

## EQUIPMENT AND SUPPLIES

The equipment and supplies found in a hospice pharmacy are many of the same that are found in a traditional community pharmacy and a home infusion pharmacy. The equipment and supplies used most frequently in the hospice pharmacy are those for extemporaneous compounding and sterile IV infusion therapies.

## DELIVERY SERVICE

The safe and timely delivery of medications to the hospice patient either at home or in an institution is a very important component of hospice pharmacy service. Deliveries can occur on a daily basis for maintenance medications as well as on a stat basis for emergency medications. Off-hour delivery service is available because a pharmacist and driver are usually on call 24 hours a day, 7 days a week. The hospice pharmacy should make hospice prescription delivery a priority.

# SERVICES OF A HOSPICE PHARMACY

There are several services that are provided to terminally ill patients by a hospice pharmacy. These services can be divided into two areas: clinical services and dispensing services. Clinical services include pain management, symptom management, medication monitoring and drug regimen review, drug information services, formulary development and management, and in-service programs. Dispensing services include medications and related equipment and supplies, specialized extemporaneous compounding, sterile IV infusion compounding (pain, hydration, and chemotherapy), starter kits, and 24-hour on-call coverage. Several of these services are discussed next.

## PAIN MANAGEMENT

**Pain management** is defined as the pharmacologic management of pain. A hospice patient's pain is often undertreated for several reasons. The terminally ill patient may be taking the wrong type of pain medication; he may be taking a dose of medication that is too low to effectively control his pain; or he may be taking pain medication on an as-needed basis only rather than on a continuous basis. A terminally ill patient should not have to suffer pain. The goal of pain management is to control pain and make the patient comfortable. Pain must be aggressively treated. Pain management involves a pain assessment as part of the patient assessment. The pharmacist collaborates with the patient's nurse in recommending a pain medication regimen. He also performs dosage conversions, that is, calculates equianalgesic doses of pain medications, monitors compliance, and helps to manage side effects. Pain medications must generally be given around the clock. They are given to prevent pain from occurring rather than to treat it when it occurs. Pain medications are available in long-acting and short-acting forms. An effective dosage of a long-acting pain medication is used to provide a baseline level of pain relief. Sometimes a patient will experience **breakthrough pain,** which is defined as an episode of acute pain that occurs spontaneously or as a result of some type of stimulus. This pain is immediately addressed using a short-acting pain medication. Frequent follow-up is important to ensure that the patient is receiving adequate doses of long-acting and short-acting pain medications and to monitor the side effects of these medications.

Opioid medications, such as morphine and oxycodone, are the drugs of choice for the treatment of moderate to severe pain, especially in cancer patients. They are very effective, are easy to adjust, and have few serious side effects. They are available in long-acting and short-acting forms. Opioids are not limited to a *maximum* dose, so an effective dose can be found for any kind or severity of pain. For example, it is not uncommon to see doses in hundreds of milligrams of morphine used to keep terminally ill cancer patients comfortable and pain-free. However, some physicians often are afraid to prescribe these drugs, especially in high doses, because of common misconceptions. They believe that these medications can lead to addiction. Addiction is a psychological as well as a physiological dependence on a drug to obtain a psychic effect, which results in compulsive use and harm. Terminally ill patients with pain do not use opioids compulsively but on a regular schedule. They use these drugs for a clear medical purpose—to relieve pain—not a psychological one. Their use of opioids is beneficial, not harmful. Therefore, addiction rarely occurs in patients who take opioids for pain. Other drugs are often used in conjunction with opioids. Examples are nonsteroidal anti-inflammatory drugs (NSAIDs), tricyclic antidepressants (amitriptyline) for neuropathic pain, and dextromethorphan, which increases the analgesic effect of morphine.

Constipation is an expected side effect of opioids. It is treated by the use of laxatives and stool softeners. Other side effects of opioids are sedation, confusion, and nausea. These side effects usually occur at the beginning of opioid use but can be expected to decrease as the patient is stabilized on a particular dose.

In addition to side effects, other problems in pain management are drug interactions and patient compliance. The pharmacist screens for interactions during the prospective drug utilization review. The pharmacist, as well as other members of the hospice team, helps to educate the patient and family concerning the importance of regularly scheduled, around-the-clock administration of pain medications to keep the patient pain-free.

## SYMPTOM MANAGEMENT

**Symptom management** is defined as the pharmacologic management of symptoms. Various symptoms other than pain often arise in the terminally ill patient.

These symptoms are very uncomfortable and can cause fear and confusion for the patient and family. Some of these symptoms are common to the terminal disease or treatment and can be expected to occur. Symptoms include constipation, nausea, vomiting, hiccoughs, difficulty breathing, weakness, fatigue, loss of appetite, weight loss, dry mouth, seizures, anxiety, and depression. Symptoms must be treated as they arise. Again, the goal of symptom management is to control symptoms and make the patient comfortable until his death.

Constipation and nausea are the two most common symptoms that occur and that need to be managed. Constipation is usually the result of pain medications and can be severe. Therefore, a bowel management program is needed for most patients taking pain medications and consists of regular treatment with laxatives and stool softeners. Bulk-type laxatives generally are not used because they can lead to impaction as well as cause nausea. Nausea is often a result of unrelieved pain or constipation. Nausea can be reduced by alleviating these symptoms. Medications used to treat nausea include antinauseants, antihistamines, metoclopramide, and steroids. Symptom management by the pharmacist can include recommending changes in the patient's medication regimen, recommending the addition of a medication or therapy to alleviate a symptom, and educating the patient concerning the importance of compliance with the medication regimen.

## SPECIALIZED COMPOUNDING

Many hospice patients have special medication needs. Some patients are not able to swallow medications or take a medication in a particular dosage form. The physician may order that a medication be administered in a different dosage form by an alternative route of administration, such as the transdermal, sublingual, rectal, inhalation, SQ, or IV route. An example would be ondansetron for nausea and vomiting, which is commercially available only as an oral tablet and injection, being compounded into a suppository as requested by the physician. Some patients may have pain and other symptoms that are difficult to control with individual medications and may need a special medication formulation that incorporates several different drugs. An example would be a formulation for nausea and vomiting containing metoclopramide, diphenhydramine, and dexamethasone compounded into a suppository. These formulations and dosage forms are not commercially available; therefore, hospice pharmacists are asked to make a wide variety of medications, both prescription and nonprescription, for pain and symptom control. The hospice pharmacist specializes in compounding these special formulations and dosage forms. The pharmacist can individualize drug therapy or make a particular medication in the alternative dosage form needed by the patient. These dosage forms can be flavored oral solutions, transdermal gels (such as scopolamine), suppositories, troches, sublingual drops, nasal sprays, inhalation solutions, and SQ or IV cassettes. For example, a pharmacist may make an oral solution for a patient who cannot swallow a tablet or a capsule, a suppository for a patient who is unconscious and cannot swallow an oral dosage form of a medication, or a cassette for SQ infusion for a patient who cannot tolerate an intravenous line. Specialized compounding for hospice patients involves an expertise in compounding. It also requires a "creative" approach to compounding, as the pharmacist may be able to suggest and compound a formulation or dosage form that meets the unique needs of a particular patient. For many of these approaches, there may not be any documentation of safety and effectiveness, and the pharmacist

**TABLE 11–1**   Common Medications Found in a Starter Kit

| MEDICATION | DOSAGE FORM | USE |
| --- | --- | --- |
| Morphine | Oral concentrate, oral tablet, injection | Pain |
| Acetaminophen | Oral tablet, suppository | Pain, fever |
| Prochlorperazine | Oral tablet, injection | Nausea/vomiting |
| Metoclopramide | Oral tablet, injection | Nausea/vomiting |
| Dexamethasone | Oral tablet, injection | Nausea/vomiting |
| Diphenhydramine | Oral capsule, injection | Nausea/vomiting |
| Lorazepam | Oral concentrate, oral tablet, injection | Anxiety |
| Haloperidol | Oral concentrate, oral tablet, injection | Agitation |
| Senna | Oral tablet | Constipation |
| Bisacodyl | Suppository | Constipation |
| Scopolamine | Transdermal gel, patch | Increased secretions |

may need to rely on his professional judgment, expertise, and experience. The hospice pharmacist can help improve the outcomes of drug therapy through specialized compounding and innovative ways of administering drugs.

### STARTER KITS

A starter kit, often referred to as a symptom relief kit, is a group of medications that is provided to a hospice patient by the hospice pharmacy to provide a "start" in treatment for the majority of urgent problems that can develop during the last days or weeks of life. Problems that can arise include pain, fever, nausea, vomiting, anxiety, agitation, increased secretions, and constipation. Having a starter kit in the home ensures that appropriate medications will be immediately available when needed. Starter kits are usually customized for the individual patient and may contain analgesics, medications for nausea and vomiting, antianxiety medications, and laxatives. Table 11–1 lists medications that may be found in a starter kit.

A starter kit is usually dispensed to each new hospice patient on admission to the hospice program and is delivered with the patient's first order of medications. Typically, the kit is sealed and kept in the patient's refrigerator. A starter kit for a hospice patient not at home but in a facility is referred to as an emergency box. It is a separate box, specific for the hospice patient, containing medications different from those in the standard emergency box found in the institution for general patient use.

## LEGISLATION AND REGULATIONS FOR HOSPICE PHARMACY

A hospice pharmacy is licensed and regulated by its individual state board of pharmacy. A hospice pharmacy is usually licensed as a retail pharmacy. It must comply with all state and federal pharmacy laws and regulations, especially those pertaining to extemporaneous and sterile compounding. Currently there are several federal regulations that govern hospice pharmacy practice, and these are discussed next.

## OMNIBUS BUDGET RECONCILIATION ACT OF 1990

OBRA 90 mandates patient counseling. A hospice pharmacist is required to counsel the terminally ill patient or family about the safe and effective use of medications. This counseling may be accomplished by the use of printed information in the form of a computer-generated printout, in addition to consultation over the phone or home visits when necessary.

## DRUG ENFORCEMENT AGENCY REGULATIONS

DEA regulations concerning the faxing and partial filling of Schedule II controlled substance prescriptions especially pertain to a hospice pharmacy. As for a home infusion pharmacy, there is an exception for a hospice pharmacy to the DEA requirement for a written prescription for a Schedule II controlled substance to be administered by *infusion* (IV, SQ, epidural, or intraspinal) to a hospice patient at home or in an inpatient hospice facility. The prescription may be faxed to the hospice pharmacy, and the facsimile copy is considered to be the written prescription. It is not necessary for the original written prescription to be delivered to the hospice pharmacy, either before or after the delivery of the medication to the patient at home or in an institution. The exception is intended to make it easier for a hospice pharmacist to obtain prescriptions for injectable Schedule II controlled substances for hospice patients whose needs may change quickly. As for a long-term care pharmacy, this exception also applies to the dispensing of *oral* dosage forms of Schedule II controlled substances to a hospice patient in an inpatient hospice facility, but not to a hospice patient at home.

As for a long-term care pharmacy, there is an exception for a hospice pharmacy to the DEA requirements for the partial filling of Schedule II controlled substance prescriptions for patients who are terminally ill. The DEA permits prescriptions for Schedule II controlled substances for terminally ill patients to be partially filled under certain conditions: these prescriptions can be filled only for up to 60 days; the total quantity of the medication dispensed through partial filling cannot exceed the original quantity prescribed; and the hospice pharmacist must make the notation "terminally ill patient" on the written prescription. This exception is intended to eliminate the waste of Schedule II controlled substances as a result of the patient's death.

## FOOD AND DRUG ADMINISTRATION REGULATIONS

The FDA Safe Medical Devices Act of 1990 requires that medical devices be tracked. As for a home infusion pharmacy, a hospice pharmacy that dispenses infusion therapies (for pain, hydration, or chemotherapy) and the corresponding infusion pumps must track these infusion pumps through some type of system.

## CMS CONDITIONS OF PARTICIPATION

The Centers for Medicare and Medicaid Services (CMS) has established and updated Conditions of Participation (COP) for hospice programs in order to be reimbursed by Medicare or Medicaid. Several of these conditions relate to hospice pharmacy.

A hospice program must provide necessary medications, supplies, and equipment related to the patient's terminal diagnosis on a 24-hour basis. These may be provided by its own internal hospice pharmacy or through a contract with another pharmacy, referred to as an outside pharmacy. It must use a pharmacist to provide consultation on all aspects of pharmaceutical care for the patient.

A hospice program must develop a plan of care for each patient and perform assessments relating to the patient's response to therapy, including drug therapy, through an interdisciplinary hospice team. The CMS does not explicitly require that a pharmacist be an official member of the hospice team. However, in order to satisfy this condition, most hospice programs have a pharmacist as a member of the interdisciplinary team, or a consultant pharmacist on call.

A hospice program must conduct a regular drug regimen review for each hospice patient. The CMS does not require that this review be performed by a pharmacist; however, the drug regimen review is performed by a pharmacist in most hospice programs.

## UNITED STATES PHARMACOPEIA STANDARDS

USP Chapter <795> sets standards for the compounding, preparation, and labeling of nonsterile drug preparations, and USP Chapter <797> sets standards for the compounding, preparation, and labeling of sterile drug preparations. These chapters apply to all practice settings that compound nonsterile and/or sterile preparations, including a hospice pharmacy. Like a home infusion pharmacy, areas of concern for a hospice pharmacy that compounds sterile drug preparations are beyond-use dating and maintaining the quality of the sterile drug preparation once it leaves the pharmacy. Another area of concern in a hospice pharmacy that performs both nonsterile and sterile compounding is the separation of these two activities. According to USP Chapter <797> standards, sterile compounding may be performed only in a clean room under a laminar airflow hood, and no type of nonsterile compounding may be performed in the same room. A separate compounding area must be maintained for nonsterile compounding.

## JOINT COMMISSION STANDARDS FOR HOSPICE PHARMACY

A quasi-legal standard for hospice is Joint Commission accreditation. A hospice program, which includes its pharmacy service, is accredited under the home care accreditation program. The Joint Commission recognizes the dispensing and pharmaceutical care services provided by a hospice pharmacy to a hospice program and extends accreditation for these services to the hospice. However, Joint Commission accreditation for a hospice pharmacy is different from accreditation for any other type of pharmacy practice in that accreditation is not awarded to the hospice pharmacy but to the hospice organization.

An on-site survey of the hospice pharmacy is performed for those standards that pertain to the preparation and dispensing of medications. It consists of reviews of pharmacy records, interviews with the hospice pharmacy staff, and interviews with patients and families in their homes. In particular, the hospice pharmacy is surveyed on activities such as the timely and accurate delivery of medications; the education of the patient and family about the safe and effective use of medications; the completeness of the medication profile, considering that the patient may take other medications that may not be supplied by the hospice pharmacy; drug recall procedures; and the expiration date labeling of medications.

Pain management standards have been added to the standards for home care. These are relevant to the hospice pharmacist, who is involved in pain management of the hospice patient.

## PHARMACY COMPOUNDING ACCREDITATION BOARD

The Pharmacy Compounding Accreditation Board (PCAB) was established in 2004 by several national pharmacy organizations. Its purpose is to provide voluntary accreditation to pharmacies that compound drug preparations in order to improve the quality and increase the awareness of compounding. Its strict standards are supported by the USP. As with Joint Commission accreditation, PCAB accreditation is sought by compounding pharmacies as a sign of the pharmacy's dedication to quality compounding services.

## THE ROLE OF THE PHARMACIST IN HOSPICE PHARMACY

Hospice pharmacy practice offers several roles for the pharmacist. In fact, hospice pharmacy is one of the most unusual areas of practice for a pharmacist. Hospice pharmacy gives the pharmacist the opportunity to practice pharmaceutical care and engage in some unique extemporaneous and IV compounding. The role of the pharmacist can be divided into clinical, dispensing, and administrative roles. In general, a hospice pharmacist must have good listening skills, be caring, and respect the patient as a person. He must possess excellent and precise compounding skills. A hospice pharmacist must also have excellent communication skills in order to collaborate with other members of the hospice interdisciplinary team.

### CLINICAL ROLE

Most hospice organizations rely on a pharmacist to help provide quality patient care and to help improve the patient's quality of life until death. Hospice pharmacy provides one of the best opportunities for pharmacists to practice pharmaceutical care. One pharmaceutical care activity for the hospice pharmacist is managing the complex medication regimens that many terminally ill patients require. The pharmacist regularly performs a retrospective drug regimen review for each hospice patient, similar to the drug regimen review performed for nursing facility residents, to identify potentially harmful medication combinations. This review is especially important when the patient is taking medications for diagnoses other than his terminal diagnosis. An example would be a terminal cancer patient who has seasonal allergies and who requires antihistamines, decongestants, and nasal steroids to control this condition, as well as other medications to control the pain and symptoms associated with cancer. The pharmacist also is involved in pain and symptom management. On the basis of the patient assessment and drug regimen review, the pharmacist consults with the patient's physician and makes recommendations to change the patient's drug therapy to manage pain and other symptoms better. Many times, small changes can be made that make a big difference in the patient's comfort.

One unique aspect of the clinical role of the pharmacist in hospice is pharmacist-nurse collaboration. Hospice pharmacists mostly interact with hospice nurses, who, in turn, have direct contact with the patient. Often the pharmacist may make home visits along with the nurse to see the patient in his own environment and to be able to better relate to his needs. The pharmacist may assist the nurse in patient assessment and in the creation of the medication portion of the patient's plan of care. The nurse and the pharmacist then monitor the patient, and the pharmacist may make recommendations to adjust medications, medication dosages, or routes of administration when necessary.

Another important activity in the clinical area is education by the pharmacist of health care professionals, patients, and family to ensure appropriate medication use. The pharmacist provides drug information to the hospice team, including the physician, on drug dosages, dosing conversions, drug costs, therapeutic alternatives, generic equivalents, and side effects. The hospice pharmacist also may conduct in-service education for the hospice team on a variety of drug-related topics. The hospice pharmacist provides consultation and education to the patient and his family concerning the medication regimen and the importance of compliance. For example, the pharmacist may explain pain prevention to the patient and his family to help the family administer analgesics according to instructions *before* the patient experiences pain.

There are several other activities that the hospice pharmacist can perform in this role. These activities include attending hospice team meetings, serving on the quality assurance committee of the hospice organization, developing policies and procedures regarding medication use in the hospice program, and participating in research activities or studies within the hospice organization.

## DISPENSING ROLE

A hospice pharmacist dispenses medications to hospice patients that are related to their terminal diagnosis. As in any other type of pharmacy practice, the pharmacist maintains patient medication profiles and performs prospective drug utilization review. The hospice pharmacist is usually available on call 24 hours a day, 7 days a week. The pharmacist in this role may also help develop and manage a formulary for the hospice organization and control medication costs. The most important aspect of the dispensing role, however, is the specialized compounding that the pharmacist performs in hospice pharmacy practice. The pharmacist creates special medication formulations and dosage forms to meet the specific needs of terminally ill patients.

## ADMINISTRATIVE ROLE

The administrative role of the hospice pharmacist is related to the management of the hospice pharmacy. This involves overseeing the day-to-day operations of a hospice pharmacy. Typical administrative activities may include hiring and training pharmacists and pharmacy technicians, overseeing equipment and computer maintenance, purchasing medications and compounding supplies, developing policies and procedures that pertain to hospice pharmacy practice, ensuring compliance with pharmacy laws and regulations and Joint Commission standards, and maintaining records.

## THE ROLE OF THE PHARMACY TECHNICIAN IN HOSPICE PHARMACY

The role of the pharmacy technician in hospice pharmacy is an important one. It is a role that combines activities common to retail pharmacy as well as activities common to home infusion pharmacy. In general, the pharmacy technician in a hospice pharmacy assists the hospice pharmacist in providing medications and pharmaceutical care services to terminally ill patients. The pharmacy technician must posses traditional pharmacy knowledge and skills as well as knowledge and skills specific to hospice pharmacy, such as:

- A basic knowledge of the hospice concept
- A knowledge of commonly prescribed medications for pain and symptom management and their dosage forms
- A knowledge of commonly prescribed infusion therapies for hospice and their corresponding equipment and supplies
- A knowledge of extemporaneous compounding
- A knowledge of sterile compounding
- A knowledge of pharmaceutical calculations
- An understanding of the legislation and regulations pertaining to hospice pharmacy practice
- Excellent communication skills
- Good computer skills

There are many activities that the pharmacy technician can perform in the hospice pharmacy. However, the pharmacy technician may not perform any task that involves the professional judgment of a pharmacist, and the pharmacy technician must work under the direct supervision of a pharmacist, especially when compounding. The role of the pharmacy technician in hospice pharmacy practice can be divided into three areas: dispensing, compounding, and computer functions.

### DISPENSING ROLE

The pharmacy technician in a dispensing role performs activities related to the dispensing of prescriptions for terminally ill patients. These activities are similar to dispensing activities in any traditional retail pharmacy. One unique activity would be assembling starter kits for hospice patients.

### COMPOUNDING ROLE

The pharmacy technician in a compounding role performs activities related to extemporaneous compounding and sterile compounding for terminally ill patients. Again, these compounding activities are similar to compounding activities in any traditional retail pharmacy or home infusion pharmacy. However, the specialized compounding performed in the hospice pharmacy setting is different from that in other pharmacy settings and requires additional training.

## COMPUTER ROLE

The pharmacy technician can perform many computer functions in a hospice pharmacy. These computer functions also are similar to computer functions in other areas of pharmacy. Computer functions that are specific to hospice pharmacy are maintaining patient records, such as the patient assessment, plan of care and pharmacist recommendations, and printing out weekly team meeting reports.

## ■ KEY CONCEPTS

- Hospice is a concept of care for terminally ill patients and their families that focuses on the patient's comfort rather than on a cure for the disease.
- Hospice characteristics include a family unit of care, consideration of the whole person, an interdisciplinary team, a care planning process, and palliative care.
- A hospice pharmacy is a pharmacy that provides medications and pharmaceutical services to the terminally ill patient at home or in an institution in order to enhance the quality of his remaining life.
- The most distinctive element of a hospice pharmacy is its specialized and limited inventory.
- The special services of a hospice pharmacy include pain and symptom management, specialized compounding, and the provision of starter kits.
- There are specific legislation and regulations that pertain to hospice pharmacy practice.
- Hospice pharmacy practice offers a variety of roles for the hospice pharmacist.
- The pharmacy technician performs many tasks in the hospice pharmacy, including specialized compounding.

## ■ SELF-ASSESSMENT QUESTIONS

### MULTIPLE CHOICE

1. The primary purpose of treatment in hospice care is to:
   a. keep the patient sedated
   b. cure the disease
   c. manage symptoms
   d. none of the above

2. Which medications are not found in a starter kit?
   a. antianxiety medications
   b. antibiotics
   c. laxatives
   d. antinauseants

3. A unique characteristic of hospice is:
   a. it involves care planning
   b. it involves the patient's family
   c. it treats the whole patient
   d. all of the above

4. The dispensing service of a hospice pharmacy consists of:
   a. sterile IV infusion compounding
   b. specialized extemporaneous compounding
   c. starter kits
   d. all of the above

5. Hospice organizations do not provide:
   a. burial services
   b. bereavement services
   c. spiritual support services
   d. nursing care

6. Hospice pharmacies do not provide:
   a. pain management
   b. starter kits
   c. mail order
   d. specialized compounding

7. Specialized compounding involves:
   a. alternative dosage forms of medications
   b. custom medication formulations
   c. products that are not commercially available
   d. all of the above

8. Pharmaceutical care activities performed by a hospice pharmacist include all of the following except:
   a. dispensing medications
   b. pain management
   c. symptom management
   d. education of the hospice team

9. Most hospice patients are:
   a. patients with AIDS
   b. in a nursing home
   c. elderly
   d. children

10. The inventory in a hospice pharmacy probably would not include:
    a. cholesterol-lowering medications
    b. laxatives
    c. narcotic analgesics
    d. antinauseants

## TRUE/FALSE (CORRECT THE FALSE STATEMENTS)

1. _____ Palliative care is the focus of hospice care.
2. _____ Joint Commission accreditation can be awarded to a hospice pharmacy.

3. _____ Pain management involves treating pain before it occurs.
4. _____ There are no maximum doses for opioids.
5. _____ A terminally ill patient is a patient whose illness will result in death within 6 months.
6. _____ Specialized extemporaneous compounding produces products and dosage forms for individualized patient care.
7. _____ A hospice pharmacy may partially fill prescriptions for Schedule II controlled substances for terminally ill patients.
8. _____ Volunteers are members of the interdisciplinary hospice team.
9. _____ Hospice uses aggressive treatment to cure disease.
10. _____ Opioids rarely cause addiction in patients who take them for pain.

## FILL-IN

1. An episode of acute pain that can occur spontaneously is referred to as _____ pain.
2. _____ are the drug class of choice for treating pain.
3. The pharmacologic management of patients with pain is called _____ _____ .
4. A symptom-relief kit is called a _____ _____ .
5. _____ is a program of services to meet all the needs of a terminally ill patient.
6. The majority of hospice patients have a diagnosis of _____.
7. A medical institution that provides a homelike setting for a terminally ill patient is an _____ _____ _____ .
8. The most distinctive element of a hospice pharmacy is its _____.
9. _____ and nausea are the two most common symptoms to manage in the terminally ill patient.
10. _____ is a psychological dependence on a drug to obtain a psychic effect.

## CRITICAL THINKING

1. Compare and contrast pharmacy operations in a hospice pharmacy with those in a traditional community retail pharmacy and a home infusion pharmacy.
2. Apply *structure*, *process*, and *outcomes* to a hospice pharmacy.
3. Compare and contrast extemporaneous compounding performed in a hospice pharmacy with that performed in a traditional community retail pharmacy.
4. Compare and contrast the DEA final rule for the transmission of a Schedule II controlled substance prescription by facsimile in a hospice pharmacy with that in a traditional community retail pharmacy.
5. Compare and contrast the duties of a pharmacy technician in a hospice pharmacy with those in a traditional community retail pharmacy and home infusion pharmacy.

## BIBLIOGRAPHY

American Pharmacists Association. (2005). *Palliative and end-of-life care.* Washington, DC: Author.

Centers for Medicare and Medicaid Services. (2006). *Conditions of participation and conditions for coverage: Hospice.* [On-line] CMS. Available: www.cms.gov.

Fonseca, S. (2006). The dying process. *International Journal of Pharmaceutical Compounding, 10*(2), 103–106.

Joint Commission on Accreditation of Healthcare Organizations. (2006). *2006–2007 Comprehensive accreditation manual for home care.* Oakbrook Terrace, IL: Author.

Joint Commission on Accreditation of Healthcare Organizations. (2006). *2006–2007 Standards manual for pharmacy dispensing, clinical/consultant pharmacist, long-term care pharmacy, and freestanding ambulatory infusion services.* Oakbrook Terrace, IL: Author.

Jones, M. (2006). Hospice from a compounding pharmacist's perspective. *International Journal of Pharmaceutical Compounding, 10*(2), 89–94.

Kuntz, R. (2006). The story of hospice. *International Journal of Pharmaceutical Compounding, 10*(2), 100–102.

National Hospice and Palliative Care Organization. (2006). *Hospice facts and figures.* [On-line] NHPCO. Available: www.nhpco.org.

Petrin, R. (2006). Hospice symptom relief kit: An update. *International Journal of Pharmaceutical Compounding, 10*(4), 288–290.

United States Department of Justice. Drug Enforcement Administration. (2006). *Code of Federal Regulations Title 21, Section 1306—Pharmacy.* [On-line] U.S. Department of Justice. Available: www.dea.gov.

United States Pharmacopeial Convention. (2006). *The United States pharmacopeia* (29th ed.), and *The national formulary* (24th ed.). Rockville, MD. Author.

Vance, D. (2006). Hydromorphone-compound it! *Geriatric Pharmacy Report, 7*(1), 14.

## Learning Objectives

Upon completion of this chapter, the student should be able to:

- Define federal pharmacy.
- Describe pharmacy services in the military.
- Compare and contrast the differences in pharmacy services among the three branches of the military.
- Explain the divisions and purposes of the Public Health Service.
- Describe pharmacy services in the Indian Health Service.
- Describe pharmacy services in the Department of Veterans Affairs

## Key Terms

federal pharmacist
federal pharmacy

medical readiness

military pharmacist

## Introduction

Federal pharmacy is the area of pharmacy that began the most far-reaching change in pharmacy practice: the provision of pharmaceutical care. Many pharmaceutical care services were first provided by pharmacists in the federal government. Even today, federal pharmacy involves pharmacy practice at a higher level than is possible in civilian pharmacy. Pharmacy technicians also have a higher level of responsibility within federal pharmacy practice. This chapter focuses on federal pharmacy, its different sectors, and the roles of the pharmacist and pharmacy technician in this area of pharmacy practice. ■

## OVERVIEW OF FEDERAL PHARMACY

**Federal pharmacy** is defined as the practice of pharmacy within the federal government, and a **federal pharmacist** is a licensed pharmacist who works within the federal government. Federal pharmacy plays an important role in the federal health care system. More important, federal pharmacy has had an impact on the profession of pharmacy in the civilian, or private, sector. Federal pharmacists have been providing pharmaceutical care for decades, as opposed to the private sector, where pharmaceutical care has been recently adopted as the standard of pharmacy practice. The pharmaceutical care provided in federal pharmacy can be described as innovative. In fact, nowhere is pharmacy practice as innovative as in the federal sector, where pharmacists perform a higher level of clinical services and engage in many nontraditional pharmacist activities, such as primary care activities and prescribing medications. Pharmacy technicians in the federal sector, referred to as federal pharmacy technicians, have also been given more responsibilities than their civilian counterparts and perform many nontraditional pharmacy technician activities, such as unsupervised dispensing and patient counseling in certain settings. The reason for the expanded roles of the federal pharmacist and federal pharmacy technician is that federal pharmacy is not under the jurisdiction of the states. Individual state boards of pharmacy limitations on the activities of the pharmacist and pharmacy technician do not apply in the federal sector. For example, there are no pharmacist-to-pharmacy technician ratios that exist in federal pharmacy as they do within some states, so a federal pharmacist may supervise large numbers of pharmacy technicians in a federal pharmacy. Advanced pharmacy technology and automation have also been used in federal pharmacy for years before being used in civilian pharmacy practice. Thus, advances in pharmacy practice in the private sector have come out of the federal sector.

Federal pharmacy includes pharmacy services in the military, the Public Health Service, and the Department of Veterans Affairs. Pharmacy services in each of these areas are different and unique. There are many unique opportunities for pharmacists and pharmacy technicians in federal pharmacy. In general, practice in federal pharmacy initially involves a lower salary than in the private sector. However, the federal government provides extensive benefits such as retirement benefits, health insurance, generous vacations and sick leave, housing, and others.

## OVERVIEW OF PHARMACY SERVICES IN THE MILITARY

The Department of Defense (DOD) oversees the health care services for all three branches of the military: the U.S. Army, the U.S. Navy (which includes the Marines), and the U.S. Air Force. Each branch of the military has its own network of services, health care facilities, and personnel.

Pharmacy services in the military consist of providing medications, medical equipment and supplies, and pharmaceutical care for active duty military personnel and their families throughout the world. **Military pharmacists** are pharmacists who practice in the U.S. Army, U.S. Navy, or U.S. Air Force. They can be found in military hospitals and clinics, on military bases both in the United States and abroad, and with troops deployed or stationed throughout the world. Military pharmacists provide medications and pharmaceutical care, including health promotion and disease prevention, to members of the military and their families during peacetime. Military pharmacists also provide medications, related equipment and supplies, and pharmaceutical care during conflicts, humanitarian aid missions, and disasters such as natural disasters, industrial breakdowns, and ecological disasters. Military pharmacists are an important part of the military health care team. The pharmacist's knowledge and ability to deliver needed medications and pharmaceutical care are the key to achieving positive outcomes.

Military pharmacists can be civilians or commissioned officers. Civilian pharmacists work for the government within the military but do not join as active service members. Commissioned officers are active members of the military and hold the rank of an officer. They can advance in rank up to and including the highest rank in their respective branch of the military. In the army and navy, pharmacists are officers in the Medical Service Corps, and in the air force, they are officers in the Biomedical Service Corps. Therefore, in addition to being highly trained health care professionals, they are also officers in the military. In addition to pharmacy knowledge and skills, they also must possess other qualities such as leadership, honor and integrity, and military skills.

Military pharmacy technicians can be civilians or enlisted members of the military. As an enlisted member of the military, a pharmacy technician is a noncommissioned officer and may advance through the enlisted ranks up to a certain level. It should be noted that the majority of pharmacists and pharmacy technicians in all three branches of the military are active members of the military and are supported by a small number of civilian pharmacists and pharmacy technicians.

Pharmacists and pharmacy technicians who enter the military must usually complete some type of basic training. Pharmacists, as commissioned officers, receive some type of military indoctrination training, where they learn leadership skills, military policies and procedures, and military law. Pharmacy technicians, as enlisted members of the military, usually attend 6 weeks of basic training in what is called "boot camp," where they learn military regulations, military dress, drills, weapons handling, and first aid. It also involves high-level physical training. Pharmacy technicians then receive extensive classroom training in pharmacy practice in schools specifically dedicated to their training in each branch of the military. The army, navy, and air force all differ in the length and type of pharmacy technician training programs they provide. However, as a result of this training, military pharmacy technicians are highly competent. The majority of military pharmacy technicians become certified. Some military pharmacy technicians even go on to attend pharmacy school. Civilian pharmacy technicians who work in the military do not undergo any basic training, nor do they receive extensive pharmacy technician training. They receive on-the-job training only. In general, they are not given the level of responsibility that military technicians have.

Military pharmacists practicing in military facilities have the same responsibilities as pharmacists in the private sector. They are responsible for overseeing the dispensing operation of the pharmacy as well as for providing pharmaceutical care services. Military pharmacists may also perform nontraditional pharmacist activities, depending on the facility and the branch of the military. Military pharmacy technicians are primarily involved in dispensing activities but may also perform nontraditional pharmacy technician activities, depending on the facility and the branch of the military in which they are enlisted. Military pharmacy practice uses a larger number of pharmacy technicians in relation to pharmacists than civilian pharmacy practice to perform dispensing activities. In addition, military pharmacy uses the latest in automation and technology. By using a solid foundation of highly competent pharmacy technicians, automation, and technology, military pharmacists have moved away from the dispensing of medications.

Probably the greatest difference between military pharmacists and pharmacy technicians and their civilian counterparts, in both the federal and private sectors, is that military pharmacists and pharmacy technicians are trained in medical readiness. **Medical readiness** is defined as being prepared for any medical emergency as a result of a wartime or peacetime military mission. The goals of medical readiness are to reduce suffering, injuries, and loss of life and to preserve military strength by returning injured personnel to duty as soon as possible. Medical readiness involves continuous training in which military personnel, including pharmacists and pharmacy technicians, participate in field training exercises that are designed to simulate combat operations. In particular, pharmacists and pharmacy technicians are exposed to situations and equipment that are different from those found in a traditional pharmacy and that prepare them for the challenges they may face during an actual crisis. Military pharmacists and pharmacy technicians play an active role during an emergency. They may be deployed, or sent out, to military positions anywhere in the world at any time. They are prepared to provide a limited formulary of necessary medications, including sterile IV medications, and pharmaceutical care at a moment's notice out in the field. They are responsible for maintaining adequate supplies of these medications as well as medical supplies and equipment, which may consist of portable laminar airflow hoods and computer systems. These activities involve procurement, storage, distribution, and disposal operations. In order to perform these roles, military pharmacists must have special knowledge regarding the treatment of battlefield injuries and disease. In particular, they must be knowledgeable in the fields of emergency medicine, pain management, infectious disease, and medical countermeasures for nuclear, biological, and chemical weapons. Pharmacy technicians likewise must be knowledgeable about pharmacy operations in these situations. It should be mentioned that civilian pharmacy technicians working in the military are never deployed to military positions but remain in traditional military facilities to maintain pharmacy services.

Pharmacy practice is different and unique in each branch of the military because each branch of the military is different and unique. All three branches share the same mission or purpose of pharmacy, but they differ in how and where pharmacy services are provided. Therefore, pharmacy services in the U.S. Army, U.S. Navy, and U.S. Air Force are discussed separately.

## PHARMACY SERVICES IN THE U.S. ARMY

Pharmaceutical services in the U.S. Army began at the time when our nation was born, with the establishment of the first U.S. Army Hospital and the appointment of an *apothecary* to compound and dispense medications. Through the years, army pharmacy has evolved from supplying medications to providing clinical pharmacy services. Today, army pharmacists provide pharmaceutical care to patients and assume responsibility for the outcomes of drug therapy. Pharmacy technicians also have played an important role in army pharmacy through the years. Military pharmacy technicians have essentially run large pharmacies in army hospitals. Today, army pharmacy technicians assume a high level of responsibility for medication dispensing.

The primary mission of army pharmacy is to provide cost-efficient, quality pharmacy services in support of readiness and other missions of the army. In peacetime, army pharmacists provide services to maintain the health of army personnel and their families. In wartime, army pharmacists provide services to wounded army servicemen and women. Pharmacy services are provided in two types of army medical facilities: fixed medical treatment facilities and field units. A fixed army medical treatment facility may be an ambulatory clinic, a hospital, or a large army medical center in the United States or abroad. It provides medical and pharmaceutical services to active military and their families in peacetime. A field unit provides medical and pharmacy services in a remote location. There are three types of field units. A battalion aid station is a small mobile unit located closest to the action. It is mobile in that it can be deployed and assembled in individual units called *boxes* in any location at any time. This unit is usually staffed by army medics, who can be pharmacy technicians. They perform triage care. A combat support hospital is a larger mobile unit located farther away from the action. It is staffed by pharmacists, pharmacy technicians, and medics and provides medical and pharmacy services needed to stabilize injured personnel. A field hospital is a large, stationary, semipermanent medical facility that provides a full range of services, such as operating rooms, a laboratory, x-ray machines, and a separate pharmacy. Both army pharmacists and army pharmacy technicians will be deployed to a field hospital, because it is a large facility with a separate and distinct pharmacy.

Pharmacy services in a fixed army medical treatment facility are similar to pharmacy services in a civilian hospital or outpatient clinic. An inpatient army pharmacy provides dispensing services and pharmaceutical care services and uses the latest in technology and automation, especially robotics. Some inpatient pharmacies also provide specialized clinical pharmacy services, such as oncology pharmacy, nuclear pharmacy, and nutrition support pharmacy, as well as advanced research and educational activities. In addition, all army hospitals and large medical centers include high-volume outpatient or ambulatory pharmacies that fill thousands of prescriptions each day. Army pharmacists practicing in this setting have direct patient care roles. Pharmacy technicians assume responsibility for most of the distributive functions.

Pharmacy services in a field hospital are very different from pharmacy services in a traditional hospital pharmacy department. An army field hospital pharmacy operates 24 hours a day in a hostile environment and provides pharmacy services for large numbers of casualties. It provides medications, including sterile IV products, based on a limited formulary. The pharmacy department does not have a traditional laminar airflow hood in which to prepare sterile IV products. Instead, it has a portable laminar airflow hood or a stainless steel table located in a low-traffic area of the pharmacy and walled off from the rest of the pharmacy. The pharmacy usually has air conditioning or heat and a portable refrigerator for the proper storage of medications. Drug information is often required quickly, so there are sources of information available to the pharmacist in the form of reference books and computer information. These are a few of the differences in pharmacy practice that pharmacists and pharmacy technicians experience in the field hospital.

The army provides many unique and specialized roles for pharmacists. Army pharmacists serve in a variety of executive, administrative, primary care, clinical, research, managed care, teaching, and dispensing positions. Army pharmacists manage all aspects of medication use and pharmaceutical care in an army medical facility. Army pharmacists provide primary care activities and care planning as a member of the interdisciplinary health care team. An army pharmacist can oversee clinical research programs and the use of investigational drugs. Army pharmacists perform pharmacy benefit management activities such as conducting pharmacoeconomic studies, developing and managing a formulary, and contracting with pharmaceutical companies to ensure a well-designed pharmacy benefit for army service members and their families. Army pharmacists also provide instruction in pharmacy, therapeutics, and pharmacology to pharmacy technicians and other health care personnel. A very important and unique role of an army pharmacist is that of overseeing medications, drug distribution systems, and biological products such as vaccines for deployment to field sites, as well as actual pharmacist deployment and utilization in field settings.

The army also provides many unique and specialized roles for the pharmacy technician. Army pharmacy technicians are highly respected paraprofessionals. They have a much broader scope of practice than civilian pharmacy technicians have. The army pharmacy technician performs dispensing functions in inpatient and outpatient settings, such as interpreting, labeling, and filling prescriptions for patients under the supervision of a pharmacist. In remote army field units, army pharmacy technicians perform a unique role. They are allowed by army regulations to maintain the pharmacy and to dispense medications from a very limited formulary without the direct supervision of a pharmacist; that is, the pharmacist is not involved in the dispensing process. Other unique roles for an army pharmacy technician are training other pharmacy technicians, assisting pharmacists with all aspects of pharmacy management, and participating in in-service education.

Army pharmacy technicians are highly trained. The Army Medical Department (AMEDD) trains army pharmacy technicians at the AMEDD Center and School at Fort Sam Houston, Texas. A demanding 19-week program accredited by the American Society of Health-System Pharmacists teaches pharmacy technicians the duties and responsibilities needed to support army pharmacy services in peacetime and in war. In particular, it provides training in sterile product preparation, aseptic technique, medication dispensing, and supply procedures, as well as training in the protocols and regulations involved in army pharmacy practice. During this program, pharmacy technicians are also cross-trained as army medics to perform activities in other areas of medical care, such as transporting wounded soldiers, bandaging wounds, and performing triage, as required during a time of crisis.

## PHARMACY SERVICES IN THE U.S. NAVY

Pharmaceutical services in the U.S. Navy began when early navy regulations defined a navy pharmacist as an attendant to the medical officer on a ship or at a navy yard who has pharmacy duties. For a short time, the navy even operated its own manufacturing facility, called the Naval Laboratory, to produce medications administered to navy personnel. Since then, navy pharmacists and pharmacy technicians have played a role in medical care on navy ships and in other unique navy settings.

The primary mission of navy pharmacy is to provide cost-efficient, quality pharmacy services in support of medical readiness for naval and marine forces (the Marines are part of the U.S. Navy). Pharmacy services are provided in three types of navy medical facilities: fixed medical treatment facilities, tent-based fleet hospitals, and shipboard facilities. A fixed navy medical treatment facility may be a major teaching hospital or an outpatient branch medical clinic in the United States or abroad. It provides medical and pharmaceutical services to active military and their families. A tent-based fleet hospital is a mobile land-based hospital similar to an army field hospital that can be deployed and assembled anywhere in the world as needed. A fleet hospital can range from a small, 50-bed facility to a large, 500-bed facility. The larger fleet hospital is staffed by navy pharmacists and navy pharmacy technicians. It usually accompanies marine combat units. A shipboard facility is a sea-based clinic that provides medical and pharmaceutical services to sailors aboard ship. Small navy ships have a small medical clinic on board that dispenses medications. It is staffed by a medical corpsman, who can be a pharmacy technician. Large navy ships have a larger medical clinic on board that dispenses medications. It is also staffed by a medical corpsman, who can be a pharmacy technician. The U.S. Navy also operates two 1,000-bed hospital ships: the USNS *Mercy* (Figure 12–1), stationed in San Diego, California, and the USNS *Comfort,* stationed in Baltimore, Maryland. These two ships are designed to support navy and army land operations by providing emergency medical care for the U.S. Armed Forces. Both are fully equipped with operating rooms, a laboratory, a radiology department including a CT scan, an oxygen-producing plant, and a large full-service pharmacy. The pharmacy is staffed by navy pharmacists and navy pharmacy technicians. These ships are held in readiness and can be deployed within several days.

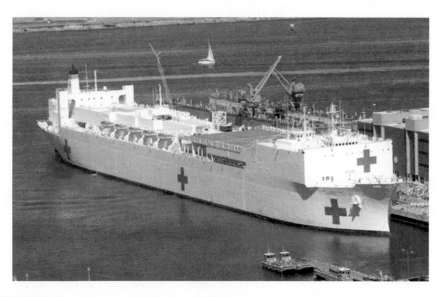

**FIGURE 12–1** USNS *Mercy* Hospital Ship.

Pharmacy services in a fixed medical treatment facility are similar to pharmacy services in a civilian hospital or outpatient clinic. Navy inpatient pharmacies provide medication-dispensing services and pharmaceutical care services and use the latest in technology and automation. Some inpatient pharmacies in larger hospitals provide clinical pharmacy services, such as nuclear pharmacy, oncology pharmacy, and nutrition support pharmacy. Navy hospitals also include high-volume outpatient pharmacies that dispense thousands of prescriptions each day. Pharmacy services in a navy tent-based fleet hospital are similar to pharmacy services in an army field hospital.

The most distinctive pharmacy services are provided aboard all navy ships, with the exception of the two navy hospital ships. Pharmacy services aboard ship are different from pharmacy services in a traditional hospital pharmacy in that they mainly involve the dispensing of medications without the supervision of a pharmacist. In contrast, pharmacy services aboard a hospital ship are similar to pharmacy services in a traditional hospital pharmacy in that pharmaceutical care services by pharmacists are also provided in addition to medication-dispensing services. The pharmacy aboard a hospital ship operates 24 hours a day and provides pharmacy services for large numbers of casualties.

The navy provides many unique and specialized roles for pharmacists. Navy pharmacists serve in a number of executive, administrative, primary care, clinical, research, teaching, and dispensing positions. In particular, navy pharmacists perform primary care activities through their management of special clinics, such as family medicine clinics, internal medicine clinics, anticoagulation clinics, pain management clinics, and asthma clinics. Navy pharmacists have prescribing authority in these clinic situations to continue therapies, although not to initiate therapies.

The navy also provides many unique and specialized roles for the pharmacy technician. Like army pharmacy technicians, navy pharmacy technicians have a much broader scope of practice than civilian pharmacy technicians have. Navy pharmacy technicians perform dispensing functions in inpatient and outpatient settings under the supervision of a pharmacist. They also perform a unique role in small fleet hospitals and aboard ships. They are allowed by navy regulations to maintain the pharmacy and to dispense medications from a limited formulary without the direct supervision of a pharmacist.

Navy pharmacy technicians are very highly trained. *Prospective* navy pharmacy technicians attend Hospital Corpsman School for 14 weeks, where they receive cross-training for all medical fields and become general-duty corpsmen. Prospective navy pharmacy technicians must then apply to Pharmacy Technician School. The Navy Pharmacy Technician School is located at the Naval School of Health Sciences in Portsmouth, Virginia. There, they attend a demanding 23-week program accredited by the American Society of Health-System Pharmacists that provides in-depth training needed to support navy pharmacy services in peacetime and in war, on land, or at sea. As a result, navy pharmacy technicians receive very comprehensive medical and pharmacy training.

## PHARMACY SERVICES IN THE U.S. AIR FORCE

Pharmaceutical services in the U.S. Air Force have been recognized for only a little more than 35 years. The primary mission of air force pharmacy is to provide cost-efficient, quality pharmacy services in support of medical readiness of our air force. As in the other branches of the military, air force pharmacy provides services to maintain the health of air force personnel and their families as well as to assist in the care of wounded air force servicemen and women. Pharmacy services are provided in two types of air force medical facilities: fixed medical treatment facilities and expeditionary medical deployment systems. A fixed air force medical treatment facility may be an outpatient clinic or a hospital. The majority of fixed air force medical facilities are outpatient clinics, both in the United States and abroad. There are only a few inpatient hospitals operated by the air force. An expeditionary medical deployment system (EMEDS), formerly referred to as an air transportable hospital, is a mobile facility similar to an army field hospital that can be deployed by air anywhere in the world when needed. It is assembled in small individual units of 15 beds, each called a *module,* up to the required size, along with other necessary modules, such as a pharmacy module. Smaller systems are staffed only by pharmacy technicians, whereas pharmacists and pharmacy technicians are deployed with larger systems. The air force also operates an aeromedical evacuation unit, which is a worldwide network of aircraft and professionals for the medical evacuation of members of any branch of the military.

Pharmacy services in a fixed air force medical treatment facility are similar to pharmacy services in a civilian hospital or clinic. Air force inpatient hospitals provide medication-dispensing services and pharmaceutical care services and use the latest in technology and automation. Air force hospitals also have high-volume outpatient pharmacies that dispense thousands of prescriptions each day. Pharmacy services within an expeditionary medical deployment system are similar to pharmacy services in an army field hospital or a navy tent-based fleet hospital.

The air force provides unique and specialized roles for pharmacists. Air force pharmacists are involved in a variety of executive, administrative, primary care, clinical, research, and dispensing positions. In particular, air force pharmacists tend to have career-broadening roles, that is, roles outside of pharmacy, for example, as squadron leaders or heads of departments other than pharmacy.

The air force also provides unique and specialized roles for the pharmacy technician. Like army and navy pharmacy technicians, air force pharmacy technicians have a much broader scope of practice than civilian pharmacy technicians have. They perform dispensing functions in inpatient and outpatient settings under the supervision of a pharmacist. Air force pharmacy technicians perform a unique role in small expeditionary medical deployment systems. They are allowed by air force regulations to maintain the pharmacy and to dispense medications from a limited formulary without the direct supervision of a pharmacist.

Air force pharmacy technicians receive very specialized pharmacy technician training. Air force pharmacy technicians are trained in an ASHP-accredited 16-week program at the Air Force School of Healthcare Sciences at Sheppard Air Force Base, Texas, where they receive training to support air force pharmacy services in peacetime and in war. The air force training program for pharmacy technicians is shorter than the army and navy's pharmacy technician training programs. Air force pharmacy technicians are trained to be *specialists;* that is, they are trained to perform only pharmacy technician activities. Army and navy technicians, on the other hand, are trained to perform other medical activities in addition to pharmacy technician activities, and thus their training is longer. However, after their training program, air force pharmacy technicians proceed on a career development track. They continue their education and training to attain higher skill levels in pharmacy practice and work toward an associate degree in pharmacy technology. Air force technicians also receive management training on various levels.

## PHARMACY SERVICES IN THE PUBLIC HEALTH SERVICE

Public health deals with the health needs of a population or community. Public health programs focus on health promotion and disease prevention. The U.S. Public Health Service (PHS) is part of the Department of Health and Human Services (DHHS) and is the oldest and principal health care agency of the federal government. Its mission is to protect and advance the health of the American people. It is composed of several divisions or agencies, each having a separate purpose. These divisions are:

- Agency for Health Care Research and Quality—provides research on health care services
- Agency for Toxic Substances and Disease Registry—protects the public from hazardous wastes and substances
- Centers for Disease Control and Prevention (CDC)—tracks, controls, and helps eradicate communicable diseases
- Substance Abuse and Mental Health Services Administration—prevents and treats drug and alcohol abuse and mental illness
- Health Resources and Services Administration—ensures the availability of health care services to underserved populations
- National Institutes of Health (NIH)—provide disease and investigational drug research
- Food and Drug Administration (FDA)—ensures the safety and effectiveness of foods, drugs, cosmetics, radioactive products, and medical devices
- Indian Health Service (IHS)—provides health care services to Native Americans

All of these divisions provide employment opportunities and roles for pharmacists. Pharmacists in the Public Health Service may be civilians or commissioned officers in the Commissioned Corps of the Public Health Service. Public Health Service pharmacists are found in all divisions of the PHS in addition to non-PHS organizations, such as the U.S. Coast Guard, the Department of Homeland Security, the U.S. Citizenship and Immigration Service, and the Federal Bureau of Prisons. Pharmacy technicians are found only in the Indian Health Service, and are all civilians.

Public health pharmacy practice involves the application of clinical pharmacy to the general population. Pharmacists employed in the Public Health Service provide pharmaceutical care to a wide variety of patients and in a wide variety of settings. Public Health Service pharmacists manage programs, provide leadership, and perform research in many of the Public Health Service divisions. However, nowhere are pharmacists more involved in innovative pharmaceutical care than in the Indian Health Service.

## PHARMACY SERVICES IN THE INDIAN HEALTH SERVICE

The IHS is the division of the Public Health Service that provides health care to Native Americans, that is, American Indians and native Alaskans living primarily in the southwestern United States and in Alaska. Health care is guaranteed to these Americans through treaties signed between various Native American tribes and the U.S. government. The goal of the IHS is to provide the best possible health care by working as an interdisciplinary health care team. The IHS provides primary care and pharmacy services in its own ambulatory clinics and hospitals.

IHS pharmacy practice is based on standards of care that were developed specifically for this type of pharmacy practice. These pharmacy practice standards include ensuring that the drug therapy is appropriate for the patient, ensuring that the patient thoroughly understands her medications, ensuring that medications are available to the patient, providing drug information and consultation to other health care professionals, providing health promotion and disease prevention activities using drugs, and managing the patient's drug therapy.

Pharmacy services in an IHS hospital are similar to pharmacy services in a civilian hospital. An inpatient IHS pharmacy provides dispensing services and pharmaceutical care services. It uses unit-dose and IV admixture systems as well as advanced technology and automation. All IHS hospitals include an outpatient pharmacy. Pharmacy services in an IHS clinic center around the dispensing of medications and patient education. Counseling services by the pharmacist are so important that a unique feature of all IHS facilities is private pharmacy counseling rooms.

The IHS provides unique and special roles for the pharmacist. In fact, pharmacy practice in the IHS is the most advanced and specialized of all of the different types of federal pharmacy practice. As an important member of the interdisciplinary health care team, an IHS pharmacist has many roles. The least important of these roles is dispensing. IHS pharmacists are mostly involved in direct patient care activities. One important activity is participating in hospital patient rounds with physicians and nurses. Another activity is one that IHS pharmacists have been providing for decades—patient counseling. This face-to-face patient counseling takes place in both inpatient and outpatient setting, and can be challenging because of language and cultural barriers. However, the IHS pharmacist is well trained in interactive communication techniques and makes sure that the patient understands her condition; treatment, including medications; and follow-up. Pharmacists also have access to the patient's entire electronic health record, including laboratory results, immunizations, and past medical history. [Patient counseling is considered so important that all IHS facilities have private patient counseling rooms for this purpose.] Pharmacist counseling in the IHS has been so successful that patient counseling training programs for pharmacy schools have been based on IHS counseling techniques. Another very important activity is monitoring drug therapy. American Indians are prone to a variety of chronic illnesses, especially diabetes, hypertension, and high cholesterol. Pharmacists monitor drug therapy through various chronic disease management clinics, such as hyperlipidemia, diabetes, hypertension, asthma, smoking cessation, and anticoagulation clinics. The pharmacist monitors patient compliance, side effects, and adverse drug reactions; orders laboratory tests; makes changes in drug therapy; and provides patient education.

The most distinctive role of the pharmacist in the IHS is providing primary care in the ambulatory clinic setting. IHS pharmacists began to provide primary care for patients in remote rural areas in the 1960s. In 1996, the IHS formally expanded the scope of practice for pharmacists to include diagnosis and prescribing. Today an IHS pharmacist with specialized training, referred to as a clinical pharmacy specialist, can perform basic physical assessments (blood pressure, pulse, height, weight, and finger stick blood glucose measurement), take patient medical and drug histories, and interpret laboratory data. These pharmacist practitioners can diagnose and treat certain acute illnesses and manage certain chronic illnesses according to protocols without physician supervision. The pharmacist has the authority to prescribe medications as well as order laboratory tests. IHS pharmacists work under a federal program and are not subject to state pharmacy laws and regulations. This position allows them to legally assume activities not traditionally performed by pharmacists. These activities are considered the most innovative pharmaceutical care activities that are performed in any type of pharmacy practice today.

The IHS also provides unique and special roles for the pharmacy technician. These roles involve the dispensing of prescriptions previously performed by the pharmacist. The pharmacy technician enters prescription orders into the computer, generates prescription labels, and fills the prescriptions under the supervision of an IHS pharmacist. One unique feature of prescription dispensing in the IHS is that all prescriptions are filled directly from the patient's electronic health record. All of the patient's care is documented in a single electronic record that is accessible to the pharmacist and the pharmacy technician. There is no need for prescription blanks.

## PHARMACY SERVICES IN THE DEPARTMENT OF VETERANS AFFAIRS

The Department of Veterans Affairs provides health care, through the Veterans Health Administration (VHA), to millions of Americans who have served their country. Previously, the VHA provided health care through hundreds of hospitals, ambulatory clinics, and nursing homes. Today, these facilities have been restructured into 21 veterans integrated service networks (VISNs) ranging in size from five to twelve medical facilities within a community or geographical area. These clinical networks stress primary and ambulatory care. The VA health care system is the largest health care system in the United States.

Pharmacy services in a VA hospital are similar to pharmacy services in a civilian hospital. An inpatient VA pharmacy provides medication-dispensing services and pharmaceutical care services and uses the latest in technology and automation. VA hospitals also have a high-volume outpatient pharmacy that fills thousands of prescriptions each day. Pharmacy services in ambulatory clinics involve the dispensing of medications and patient counseling. Many of the pharmacies found in these clinics have been redesigned into open pharmacies with counseling areas to enhance the contact between the pharmacist and the patient.

The VHA has used mail order to provide prescription medications to eligible veterans since the 1960s. Today, the VA processes the majority of its outpatient prescriptions through the mail and is one of the largest mail-order pharmacy operation in the United States. Until the early 1990s, each local VA medical facility pharmacy provided mail-order pharmacy service. In 1993, the VHA consolidated its mail-order pharmacy operations into the Consolidated Mail Outpatient Pharmacy (CMOP) system. Seven large VA mail-order pharmacies called CMOPs operate throughout the country. Local VA medical facility pharmacies act as the center of patient care. The pharmacy within the local facility processes new prescriptions and refill requests. The patient receives the first few doses of a new prescription at the local VA pharmacy, with the remainder of the prescription and any refills being filled by mail order. Prescription information is transmitted electronically to a consolidated mail outpatient pharmacy, where the prescriptions are filled, dispensed, and mailed to the patient's home. This system has several advantages. It decreases prescription dispensing at the local facility, and it allows the pharmacist more time for direct patient care. Large volumes of prescriptions can be filled at a central site with the efficiency that is characteristic of mail-order pharmacy.

The VHA also has its own pharmacy benefit management system. The VA established the Pharmacy Benefits Management Strategic Healthcare Group in 1995 to ensure the appropriate use of medications and to control the cost of providing high-quality pharmacy services to veterans. These goals are accomplished by managing the VA pharmacy benefit in many of the same ways that any civilian drug benefit is managed, especially through the use of a formulary. The VHA has used a formulary for years to improve patient care and reduce costs. Before the development of veterans integrated service networks, each VA medical facility developed and managed its own formulary. Each VISN has a formulary for use in all of its medical facilities. In addition, in 1997, the VHA developed a national formulary with input from the 21 VISNs, which is a list of drugs common to the VISN formularies.

The VHA employs only civilian pharmacists and pharmacy technicians, unlike other federal sectors, where the majority of pharmacists and technicians are members of the military, supplemented by some civilian pharmacists and technicians. Legislation has established career ladders for VA pharmacists with corresponding salary increases. VA pharmacists move up the ladder as they acquire increased training and clinical skills.

The VHA provides unique and specialized roles for the pharmacist. VA pharmacists have moved away from the traditional dispensing role to being part of the primary care team. The VHA delivers primary care through a primary care services system. This system uses a primary care team in which a pharmacist and other health care professionals work together to coordinate patient care. The pharmacist helps ensure the appropriate use of medications, monitor patient compliance, identify drug-related problems, and develop a plan of care for patients. VA pharmacists participate in specialized clinical pharmacy programs in nuclear pharmacy, psychiatry, infectious diseases, geriatrics, nutrition support, oncology, and bone marrow transplantation. VA pharmacists also manage ambulatory clinics. In 1995, pharmacists with specialized training were given the authority to prescribe medications in VA medical facilities. VA pharmacists also work under a federal program that allows them to perform nontraditional pharmacist activities. Other roles for pharmacists within the VA are in disease management clinics, research (the VHA is one of the largest research organizations in the United States), and pharmacy benefit management.

The VHA also offers unique and specialized roles for pharmacy technicians. These roles involve dispensing functions under the supervision of pharmacists. The VA offers more advanced roles for pharmacy technicians who are certified, such as providing patient education and screening laboratory values for the pharmacist. The VA also offers mail-order pharmacy roles for pharmacy technicians at their mail-order facilities.

## ■ KEY CONCEPTS

- Federal pharmacy is the practice of pharmacy within the federal government, where many pharmaceutical care services were first provided.
- Military pharmacists and pharmacy technicians are trained in medical as well as military readiness; in addition, federal pharmacy technicians are given more responsibility and perform more nontraditional pharmacy technician activities, such as unsupervised dispensing and patient counseling in certain settings, than civilian pharmacy technicians.
- Each branch of the military presents unique settings for pharmacy practice, such as in mobile field hospitals and on ships.
- The Public Health Service provides several different practice opportunities for pharmacists within its various divisions.
- The most innovative pharmaceutical care activities performed in any area of pharmacy practice are found in the Indian Health Service, where pharmacists provide primary care and have prescriptive authority.
- The Veterans Health Administration operates one of the largest mail-order pharmacy operations in the United States as well as its own PBM system, and its pharmacists are members of a primary care team that coordinates care.

## ■ SELF-ASSESSMENT QUESTIONS

### MULTIPLE CHOICE

1. All of the following describe mail-order pharmacy service in the Veterans Administration except:
   a. a consolidated mail outpatient pharmacy is the site of mail-order pharmacy operations
   b. the local VA medical center pharmacy is the site of pharmaceutical care
   c. the local VA medical center pharmacy is the site of all prescription processing
   d. it does not involve patient counseling

2.  Which of the following applies to pharmacy practice in the Indian Health Service?
    a. private pharmacy counseling rooms
    b. prescriptions filled directly from a patient's electronic record
    c. primary care provided by a pharmacist
    d. all of the above

3.  Which of the following is a health care setting?
    a. a Veterans Administration hospital
    b. an army field hospital
    c. an Indian Health Service ambulatory clinic
    d. all of the above

4.  An enlisted military pharmacy technician:
    a. is a civilian
    b. is a commissioned officer
    c. is a highly competent pharmacy technician
    d. cannot be deployed to a remote field site

5.  All of the following pertain to pharmacy practice in the Veterans Health Administration except:
    a. a career ladder for pharmacists
    b. a career ladder for pharmacy technicians
    c. a national formulary
    d. a pharmacy benefit management system

6.  All of the following are challenges of pharmacy practice in the field except:
    a. resupplying medications
    b. an area for preparing sterile intravenous medications
    c. the same equipment available as in a civilian pharmacy
    d. must be able to operate any time of day

7.  Public health pharmacy does not include:
    a. the U.S. Navy
    b. the Indian Health Service
    c. the Food and Drug Administration
    d. the Centers for Disease Control and Prevention

8.  A pharmacy technician in the Indian Health Service does not:
    a. enter prescription orders into the computer
    b. counsel patients
    c. generate prescription labels
    d. access the patient's electronic record

9.  A pharmacist in the Indian Health Service does not:
    a. perform patient assessments
    b. interpret laboratory data
    c. perform minor surgery
    d. manage chronic medical problems

10. Which is not a navy pharmacy practice site?
    a. a tent-based fleet hospital
    b. a hospital ship

c. a mobile field hospital

d. a navy hospital

## TRUE/FALSE (CORRECT THE FALSE STATEMENTS)

1. _____ Military pharmacy technicians have been given less responsibility than their civilian counterparts.

2. _____ Navy pharmacy technicians have a unique role in maintaining a pharmacy in a small fleet hospital or on a ship without the direct supervision of a pharmacist.

3. _____ Medical readiness training is an important difference between military and civilian pharmacy technicians.

4. _____ One of the largest mail-order pharmacy operations is within the U.S. government.

5. _____ A military pharmacy may not employ civilian pharmacists and pharmacy technicians.

6. _____ A unique physical feature of Indian Health Service medical facilities is private patient counseling rooms.

7. _____ Air force pharmacy technicians are specialist pharmacy technicians.

8. _____ Pharmacy technicians are found in all agencies of the Public Health Service.

9. _____ Pharmacists in the Veterans Health Service have the authority to prescribe medications.

10. _____ Military pharmacy technicians may be deployed.

## FILL-IN

1. A type of army hospital that provides medical and pharmaceutical services in remote locations is referred to as a _____ _____.

2. Pharmacy technicians, as enlisted members of the military, usually undergo six weeks of _____ _____ before receiving training in pharmacy practice.

3. The phrase _____ _____ means being medically prepared for any type of military wartime or peacetime mission.

4. The most distinctive and advanced federal pharmacy practice is in the _____ _____ _____.

5. A pharmacy technician who is employed by the government is referred to as a _____ pharmacy technician.

6. Another name for an air force air transportable hospital is an _____ _____ _____ _____.

7. The Veterans Health Administration has restructured its many health care facilities into _____.

8. The agency of the Public Health Service that provides disease and investigational drug research is the _____ _____ _____ _____.

9. The unique feature of prescription orders for patients in the Indian Health Service is that they are written on the patient's _____ _____.

10. At one time, the U.S. Navy operated a manufacturing facility called the _____ _____ to produce its own medications.

## CRITICAL THINKING

1. Compare and contrast outpatient pharmacy practice within the Indian Health Service with that in a traditional community retail pharmacy.
2. Apply *structure, process,* and *outcomes* to outpatient pharmacy practice within the Indian Health System.
3. Compare and contrast the duties of a pharmacy technician in the Indian Health Service with those in a traditional community retail pharmacy.
4. How can the patient counseling provided by pharmacists within the Indian Health Service be adapted and applied to traditional community retail pharmacy practice?
5. How does the Veterans Health Administration mail-order pharmacy operation resemble a central fill pharmacy operation?

## BIBLIOGRAPHY

Berry, D. (2004). Inside federal pharmacy. *Pharmacy Today, 10*(4), 18.

Kerr, B., et al. (2004). Navy pharmacy offers diverse practice opportunities. *Pharmacy Today, 10*(11), 19–21.

Philpott, T. (2005, Spring). Pharmacists wanted. *Today's Officer,* 17.

Reynolds, B. (2006). Outstanding federal pharmacists recognized. *Pharmacy Today, 12*(3), 16–25.

Sax, B. (2006). Army pharmacists serve more than soldiers. *Pharmacy Today, 12*(4), 19.

Sax, B. (2006). Meeting the challenge of Air Force pharmacy. *Pharmacy Today, 12*(3), 16–25.

Sax, B. (2006). Navy pharmacy fosters responsibility, patient interaction. *Pharmacy Today, 12*(7), 15.

Sax, B. (2006). Pharmacists stretch professional skills at sea. *Pharmacy Today, 12*(8), 20.

Thomas, J. (2006). USPHS pharmacy category celebrates 75th anniversary. *Pharmacy Today, 12*(1), 12.

Ukens, C. (2005). JCAHO tightens military technician regulations. *Drug Topics, 149*(7), 29.

U.S. Air Force Pharmacy. (2006). *Air Force pharmacy.* [On-line]. Available: www.af-pharmacists.org.

U.S. Army Pharmacy. (2006). *Army pharmacy.* [On-line]. Available: www.medicalservicecorps.amedd.army.mil/67e/.

U.S. Department of Health and Human Services. (2006). *Indian Health Service. IHS pharmacy program.* [On-line] HIS. Available: www.pharmacy.ihs.gov.

U.S. Public Health Service. (2006). *Commissioned corps. Pharmacist.* [On-line] USPHS. Available: www.usphs.gov.

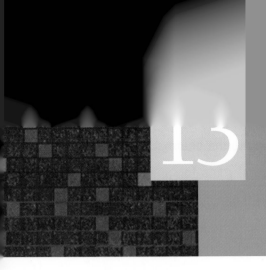

# 15 Industry

## Learning Objectives

Upon completion of this chapter, the student should be able to:

- Discuss the pharmaceutical industry in general.
- Describe the drug approval process.
- Describe the drug manufacturing process.
- Describe the drug marketing process.
- Discuss the generic pharmaceutical industry.
- Discuss pharmaceutical biotechnology and generic pharmaceutical biotechnology.
- Understand the legislation and regulations pertaining to the pharmaceutical industry.
- Describe pharmaceutical industry roles for the pharmacist and the pharmacy technician.

## Key Terms

abbreviated new drug application (ANDA)

adulterated drug

biologics license application (BLA)

biotechnology

biotechnology drug

direct-to-consumer (DTC) advertising

drug sample

good manufacturing practices (GMPs)

investigational new drug application (INDA)

master batch record

misbranding

new drug application (NDA)

orphan drug

pedigree law

unapproved use

## Introduction

The pharmaceutical industry is the cornerstone of modern pharmacy. Much of pharmacy and medical practice depends on the drugs discovered and marketed by this industry. For this reason alone, pharmacists and pharmacy technicians should have an understanding of the pharmaceutical industry and of the changes occurring in this industry. Pharmacists and pharmacy technicians need to know how drugs reach the market. They also should be familiar with the legislation and regulations pertaining to the pharmaceutical industry. The pharmaceutical industry presents several roles for pharmacists and a few employment opportunities for pharmacy technicians. This chapter focuses on the pharmaceutical industry and the unique roles of the pharmacist and the pharmacy technician in this area. ∎

## OVERVIEW OF THE PHARMACEUTICAL INDUSTRY

The pharmaceutical industry has produced new and better drug treatments that have improved the quality of life. People today are healthier and are living longer because of the drugs produced by the pharmaceutical industry. Drugs play an important role in the health care system. We have seen that drugs can help prevent surgery and the need for hospitalization. They can cure and prevent disease. Drugs help reduce overall health care costs.

The pharmaceutical industry has been growing at a remarkable rate. This growth is due to extensive research and development, the hallmark of the pharmaceutical industry. Research and development is extremely expensive and involves great financial risk for a pharmaceutical manufacturer. Independent data from the Pharmaceutical Research and Manufacturers of America, the organization that represents pharmaceutical manufacturers, state that it costs approximately $800 million for a pharmaceutical manufacturer to develop a single new drug. However, despite the high cost of drug research and development, and the role of managed care in health care, pharmaceutical manufacturers have managed to continue to produce new drugs and to realize profits.

The pharmaceutical industry has undergone a major consolidation in the past several years with the acquisition and merger of pharmaceutical manufacturers. Pharmaceutical manufacturers have acquired or merged with other pharmaceutical companies, domestic or foreign, biotechnology companies, and research organizations to form massive pharmaceutical companies. These acquisitions and mergers are due to the high cost of research and development and the lack of new products in some companies. Acquisitions and mergers can result in adequate funding for research and development, marketing expertise, an expanded sales force, and access to new drug products. These can result in efficiency, higher profits, and expanded services.

## THE DRUG APPROVAL PROCESS

Before a new drug can be manufactured and marketed in the United States, it must be approved by the FDA as being safe and effective for a particular use. This approval involves extensive time, testing, and expense on the part of the pharmaceutical company. The FDA drug approval process in the United States is recognized as being the most rigorous in the world. On average, it takes 12 to 15 years and $800 million for a new drug to reach the market. Only 5 compounds in approximately 10,000 that undergo preclinical testing go on to clinical trials. Of those five, only one drug that is tested on humans is finally approved for sale. The other four are discarded with no return on investment (PhRMA, 2005).

The first step in bringing a new drug to market is to identify a new drug. Identifying a new drug product involves discovering some type of pharmacologic activity. Scientists within a pharmaceutical company, governmental agency, academic institution, or other type of organization try to identify a potential new drug in several ways: through random screening of chemical or biological compounds, through a targeted screening of compounds, using a theory they may have, or through some type of technology. Drug discovery is unique and sometimes accidental, and thus there is no standard process for identifying a potential new drug.

Once a chemical compound or biological compound has been identified as having activity, a formulation and a manufacturing process are developed so that the potential new drug product can be made on a small scale. These prototype samples then proceed through the steps in the FDA drug approval process. These steps are:

- *Preclinical trials.* Preclinical trials involve testing a new drug in the laboratory and on animals to identify the drug's physical, chemical, biochemical, and pharmaceutical properties. This type of testing also determines if the drug is reasonably safe for humans and if it exhibits pharmacologic activity that justifies further development.

- *Investigational new drug application.* An **investigational new drug application**, or **INDA**, is submitted to the FDA to begin the testing of a new drug on humans. It is a request for authorization to administer the drug to humans, as well as to transport the investigational drug across state lines. An INDA contains the data obtained from preclinical testing as well as the manufacturing procedures for the new drug. Human trials may begin 30 days after an INDA is filed, unless it is not approved by the FDA.

- *Clinical trials.* Clinical trials involve testing the new drug on humans to determine the safety and effectiveness of the drug. Clinical trials are conducted in three phases. *Phase I* clinical trials usually involve a small number of healthy volunteers who do not have the disease or medical condition that the drug is intended to treat. This phase determines the pharmacologic actions, a *safe* dose, and the absorption, distribution, metabolism, and excretion of the new drug. *Phase II* clinical trials involve testing in several hundred patient volunteers who have the disease or medical condition that the drug is intended to treat. This phase studies the *effectiveness* of the drug for its particular use as well as side effects and risks associated with the drug. *Phase III* clinical trials are larger trials that involve hundreds or thousands of patient volunteers. This phase verifies the effectiveness of the drug and the incidence of side effects and adverse reactions.

- *New drug application.* A **new drug application**, or **NDA**, is submitted to the FDA to request approval for marketing the new drug. It contains the results of clinical trials that demonstrate the safety and effectiveness of the new drug as well as pharmacokinetic data and proposed labeling for the new drug.

- *Approval.* The NDA is reviewed by the FDA and a decision is made whether to approve the drug. The FDA will approve an NDA if clinical trials demonstrate that the new drug is safe and effective and that it will be manufactured in such a way as to ensure its identity, strength, quality, and purity. By law, the FDA has 6 months in which to review the NDA and approve the drug. After approval, the drug can be prescribed by physicians.

- *Postmarketing studies.* Postmarketing studies, referred to as *Phase IV* clinical trials, are studies conducted during the general use of the drug following approval by the FDA. They are performed to monitor the long-term effects of the drug and to detect adverse effects or other problems that were not discovered during clinical trials owing to the limited number of patients who were involved. These studies are mandatory for the manufacturer of the drug but are also performed on a voluntary basis by other agencies. This safety monitoring continues for the life of the drug, and periodic reports must be sent to the FDA. Legislation may be enacted in coming years to establish a center within the FDA itself to conduct postmarketing review of approved drugs.

A new drug is awarded a patent for 17 years from the date that the patent is awarded or 20 years from the date that the patent is applied for, whichever is greater. A pharmaceutical company usually applies for a patent as soon as it recognizes that a drug has promising activity. However, because it takes up to 10 years for development, testing, and approval, most drug patents provide only several years of market value. When the patent expires, other pharmaceutical manufacturers, namely generic drug companies, are free to market the drug. Legislation may be enacted in coming years that will make changes to the existing patent laws.

The drug approval process in the United States as established by the FDA is very strict. As a result, many new drugs are first marketed in other countries. Many countries do not have a counterpart to the FDA and have many more drugs in their market than we have in the United States. Many of these drugs have not been proven to be effective. On the other hand, some countries approve a drug only on the FDA's approval of the new drug in the United States.

## THE DRUG MANUFACTURING PROCESS

The drug manufacturing process is the process by which a bulk raw material is made into an active drug product in a specified dosage form. It is a process that is highly monitored and regulated in order to produce a safe and effective drug product. It involves several steps that progress from pharmaceutical processing to testing and finally packaging. Pharmaceutical processing involves milling or grinding, mixing, emulsifying, compressing, filtering, drying, sterilizing, and other physical processes in order to arrive at the final dosage form, such as a tablet, capsule, sustained-release dosage form, liquid, suspension, emulsion, suppository, aerosol, powder, cream, ointment, transdermal patch, or sterile product. Samples of the finished dosage form are then tested to determine whether they meet USP standards for drug identity, strength, quality, and purity. The final packaging and labeling of the drug product are conducted according to USP standards.

The drug manufacturing process is based on current **good manufacturing practices**, or **GMPs**, established by FDA regulations. Good manufacturing practices set minimum standards for the manufacturing of drugs. They describe the methods, equipment, facilities, and controls required to produce these drugs. GMPs require that equipment and facilities be properly designed, maintained, and cleaned; that personnel and management be well trained; that a quality control program be in place; and that all standard operating procedures, or SOPs, be written and approved. As a result, drugs that are manufactured according to GMPs can be expected to be safe, pure, the correct strength, and properly labeled. GMPs were introduced in the 1960s and revised in the 1970s and fall under FDA regulations. GMPs continue to change and be revised, which is why they are referred to as *current* GMPs. Failure of a pharmaceutical manufacturer to comply with GMPs can result in regulatory action.

Record keeping is the basis of compliance with GMPs. Specific records must be kept during the entire drug manufacturing process. The **master batch record** is a set of specifications for manufacturing a new drug. This document details the steps necessary to make the drug product on a commercial scale; the testing required; the specifications for the finished product; and the packaging, handling, and labeling for the new drug. A production batch record is a complete and accurate record of what was done during the manufacturing of an individual batch or lot of a drug. The production batch record must be completed and reviewed before the batch of drug can be released. Other records include testing records and equipment use and maintenance records.

## THE DRUG MARKETING PROCESS

The drug marketing process by a pharmaceutical manufacturer is necessary in order to produce sales of a drug and to realize a profit. Drugs are marketed through a marketing cycle that is composed of several different phases: introduction, growth maturity, market saturation, and market decline. The introductory marketing phase involves the introduction of the new drug onto the market accompanied by heavy advertising. This advertising is necessary if the new drug is to capture the attention of physicians, pharmacists, managed care organizations, and consumers. The growth maturity phase involves the steady growth in sales of the new drug as it becomes more frequently prescribed by physicians and included in managed care formularies. The market saturation phase refers to the point in the marketing cycle when the drug reaches a maximum level of use. Finally, the market decline phase occurs as the drug is replaced by newer drug products. During each phase of the marketing life cycle, the drug is actively promoted, but in different ways.

One of the most important considerations in marketing is the choice of a brand name or trade name for a new drug. Pharmaceutical manufacturers develop a name that will be acceptable to health care professionals and patients and that is not likely to sound like or look like another drug name. The manufacturer creates a name so that the drug product is easily recognized and will not be mistaken for or confused with another drug.

The marketing of a drug also involves establishing a price for the drug. The price of a drug is based on several factors. These factors include the uniqueness of the drug, competition from other pharmaceutical manufacturers, the drug's research and development costs, generic competition, and cost containment pressures from managed care organizations.

Marketing strategies include detailing, sampling, advertising in professional journals, direct mailings, educational programs, and direct-to-consumer advertising. Detailing, now referred to as field selling, involves the use of a professional sales force of pharmaceutical sales representatives to promote the sale of a drug. Sampling involves the provision of samples of the new drug to physicians. However, today, the most visible type of marketing is direct-to-consumer advertising. **Direct-to-consumer advertising**, or **DTC advertising**, of prescription drugs is the promotion of a new drug product directly to patients, instead of to health care professionals. Pharmaceutical manufacturers advertise to patients by means of television, radio, magazine, and newspaper advertisements and the Internet. The FDA regulates DTC advertising and requires that drug manufacturers provide a brief summary of information relating to the effectiveness, side effects, and contraindications for any prescription drug advertised. In addition, the Pharmaceutical Research and Manufacturers of America (PhRMA), which represents the country's leading pharmaceutical research and biotech companies, has established voluntary guidelines for DTC advertising. Many drug manufacturers have adopted these guidelines for the honest and complete disclosure of information. The ultimate intent of DTC advertising should be to improve health outcomes by promoting communication between the patient and his physician. However, it is interesting to note that prescription drugs that are advertised directly to patients are the best-selling drugs on the market.

Marketing also involves effective drug distribution. Drugs are distributed by pharmaceutical manufacturers through direct distribution and indirect distribution methods. Direct distribution involves the direct sale of a drug to the outlet for the drug, such as a pharmacy retailer, hospital, or government agency. Indirect distribution involves the sale of a drug to an intermediary between the drug manufacturer and the outlet for the drug. This intermediary is the drug wholesaler. A wholesaler purchases drugs from the pharmaceutical manufacturer and then resells them to a pharmacy or hospital. Wholesalers are the largest channel for drug distribution. An intermediary can also be any other high-volume drug purchaser, such as a chain pharmacy warehouse, a mail-order pharmacy organization, a pharmacy network in a managed care organization, a drug repackager, a group purchasing organization, or an independent buying group. A drug repackager is a company that buys drugs in bulk, both brand name and generic, and then repackages them in small units and sells them to dispensing physicians, HMOs, hospitals, or other outlets. Group purchasing organizations and independent buying groups are similar to one another. A group purchasing organization is composed of high-volume drug purchasers. An independent buying group is usually composed of individual community pharmacies or state pharmacy organizations. Both organizations attempt to buy drugs in volume and to negotiate better prices or discounts from the pharmaceutical manufacturer or from a wholesaler.

## THE GENERIC PHARMACEUTICAL INDUSTRY

The generic drug industry has had a tremendous impact on our health care system. It has contributed to lowering the cost of health care by providing American consumers access to high-quality drugs at low cost. Generic drugs provide a safe and effective alternative to brand-name drugs, and generic drugs save consumers, state and federal governments, and third-party insurance payers millions of dollars each year.

The generic drug industry also has had an impact on the name-brand pharmaceutical industry. Generic drugs create competition for brand-name drugs. This competition has provided the incentive for brand-name pharmaceutical manufacturers to continue drug research and development so that new patented drugs ensure continued profits.

The generic drug industry began in the 1960s. In 1962, the National Research Council of the National Academy of Sciences, through their Drug Efficacy Study Implementation program, reviewed thousands of drugs manufactured before 1962 for safety and effectiveness. After this review, generic drug manufacturers were able to file an application for approval to manufacture generic versions of those drugs that had been determined to be safe and effective without having to conduct additional studies. In 1984, the Drug Price Competition and Patent Term Restoration Act, also called the Waxman-Hatch Act, established a system for the rapid review and approval of generic drugs. It permitted generic drug manufacturers to submit an **abbreviated new drug application**, or **ANDA**, instead of a new drug application, or NDA, for generic versions of drugs marketed *after* 1962. Before this law, ANDAs were available only for generic versions of brand-name drugs approved by the FDA *before* 1962. This act propelled the generic drug industry forward.

Today, the generic drug industry represents over 50 percent of prescriptions filled each year, and that percentage is expected to rise. The growth of the generic drug industry today is due to several factors. Cost is an important factor, and, in fact, the cost of a generic drug can be anywhere from 20 percent to 75 percent less than the brand-name version. Another reason for the growth of the generic drug industry is the emphasis on generic substitution by managed care organizations. The majority of managed care organizations today require generic substitution whenever possible. This requirement has led to an increase in the use of generics, especially in the period following the expiration of a patent on a brand-name drug. A third reason for the growth of the generic drug industry is our aging population. Older individuals have many chronic conditions and take multiple medications. Finally, the generic drug market is expanding as the patents on hundreds of popular and frequently prescribed brand-name drugs expire.

The drug approval process for generic equivalents of brand-name drug products is a short process, as established by the Drug Price Competition and Patent Term Restoration Act of 1984. Generic drugs are approved by the Office of Generic Drugs, Center for Drug Evaluation and Research of the FDA. An ANDA must be submitted to the FDA. The ANDA requires only information regarding the manufacturing process for the drug and bioequivalency data. Generic drugs are not required to undergo extensive clinical trials that have already been performed in the development of the original, brand-name drug. Instead, to be approved by the FDA, generic drugs must demonstrate that they are bioequivalent and therapeutically equivalent to the brand-name drug. A generic drug is considered to be *bioequivalent* to the brand-name drug if it delivers the same amount of active ingredient into the patient's bloodstream in the same amount of time as the brand-name drug. Bioequivalency is established by administering the brand-name and generic versions of a drug to patients and by measuring and comparing the rate and extent of absorption of the drug. A generic drug is considered to be a *therapeutic equivalent* if it contains the same active ingredient in the same amount, has the same dosage form and route of administration, and works the same way in the body as the brand-name drug. Thus, if the FDA approves a generic drug as bioequivalent and therapeutically equivalent to a brand-name drug, the generic will provide the same intended clinical effect.

The generic drug industry does not engage in direct-to-consumer advertising or detailing to physicians to sell generic drugs. Awareness of generic drugs comes from physicians and pharmacists as well as from consumer education programs. However, one of the most recent developments in the generic drug industry has been the sampling of generic drugs. Brand pharmaceutical manufacturers have traditionally provided samples of their drugs for physicians to use in their patients. However, a prescription for one of these brand-name drugs is very expensive. Sampling of generic drugs provides physicians with awareness and access to generic drugs and results in prescriptions being written for less expensive drugs that in most instances are just as effective as brand-name drugs.

The generic pharmaceutical industry is highly competitive within itself. Generic pharmaceutical companies try to be the first company approved by the FDA to manufacture a particular generic product so that they can market the drug earlier and capture a larger share of the generic drug market. According to the Waxman-Hatch Act, the first generic drug manufacturer that submits an ANDA for a particular brand-name drug is entitled to 180 days of exclusive marketing of the generic version before any other generic company can start to market the drug.

There is, however, a generic competitive marketing technique used by some brand-name pharmaceutical manufacturers. Under FDA regulations, drug manufacturers are allowed or authorized to contract with other companies to market their products. Brand-name pharmaceutical manufacturers often make their own generic versions of brand-name drugs whose patents are about to expire. They then contract with a generic company to sell their generic version in exchange for royalty payments. These generic products are referred to as "authorized generics." In essence, authorized generics are brand-name drugs labeled as generic drugs. The manufacturer does not have to submit an ANDA because it already holds a NDA for its approved brand-name version of the drug. Furthermore, authorized generics do not have to abide by the 180-day exclusive marketing provision granted to the first generic on the market by the Waxman-Hatch Act. Therefore, an authorized generic can be released on the same day that another generic drug manufacturer brings its generic to the market, competing with it. Some generic drug manufacturers see this practice as a threat to competition. Several brand-name pharmaceutical manufacturers have also created their own generic companies or subsidiaries to manufacture authorized generics.

## PHARMACEUTICAL BIOTECHNOLOGY

**Biotechnology** is defined as the use of biology and technology to solve problems concerning living organisms. This biology in particular involves the use of cells and their building blocks. Pharmaceutical biotechnology is the application of biology to the development of drugs. It involves producing drugs from living cells such as bacteria, yeast, or human cells. It results in the creation of naturally occurring drug products that produce specific biological changes in the body. These drugs are called **biotechnology drugs**, or biopharmaceuticals.

Biotechnology began in the 1950s with the discovery of deoxyribonucleic acid, or DNA, the building block of cells. DNA contains all the genetic information for a living organism in the form of genes, each of which directs the production of a specific protein in the body. In the 1980s, scientists discovered that they could manufacture DNA by what is called recombinant DNA technology. Recombinant DNA technology involves combining DNA from different sources to produce a new DNA product with a different function. In 1982, human insulin was the first drug to be produced from biotechnology using recombinant technology. It was made by inserting the human gene that directs the production of insulin into a harmless bacterial cell *(Escherichia coli)*. Insulin could then be produced in large amounts under controlled conditions within the bacterial cell. Another example of the use of biotechnology is monoclonal antibodies, single pure types of antibodies created in the laboratory, that can be directed to bind to and destroy specific types of cells in the body, for example, cancer cells.

Today, advances in the biotechnology field are having an effect on drug discovery and development. New methods of biotechnology are increasing the number and types of drugs that can be produced to prevent, detect, treat, and cure disease. Biotechnology drugs have been approved by the FDA to treat cancer, anemia, growth hormone deficiency, diabetes, cystic fibrosis, and hepatitis, and many more biotechnology drugs are in development to treat diseases such as AIDS, Parkinson's disease, respiratory diseases, multiple sclerosis, osteoporosis, and infertility. Approximately one-half of the biotechnology drugs being tested today are for the treatment of cancer.

The approval process for a biotechnology drug is similar to that for any other type of new drug. After a new biotechnology drug is identified, it is produced in the laboratory in sufficient quantities for study. Preclinical trials involving laboratory and animal testing determine if the drug has biological activity in the body. After an INDA has been submitted to the FDA, clinical trials with humans begin. A **biologics license application**, or **BLA**, is then submitted to the FDA for marketing approval. Biotechnology drugs are reviewed by the FDA's Center for Biologics Evaluation and Research. After the FDA has approved the application, the biotechnology drug can be prescribed by physicians. Postmarketing studies are performed to evaluate long-term effects.

Biotechnology drugs today offer effective treatments for many serious diseases and improve the quality of life for patients. However, they are much more expensive than oral drugs, approximately 10 times the cost. Their high costs are using up an increasingly larger portion of the health care dollar.

## GENERIC BIOTECHNOLOGY

Generic biotechnology drugs, also referred to as generic biopharmaceuticals or biogenerics, are the generic versions of brand-name biopharmaceutical drugs. As the patents of many brand-name biotechnology drugs expire, the opportunity exists for generic biotechnology companies to produce safe, effective, and affordable versions of these drugs. Generic biotechnology companies have the same technology that allows the generic biotechnology drug to be manufactured in the same manner as the name-brand drug. Furthermore, they adhere to the same standards and principles of manufacturing, or GMPs, as the brand-name companies. Generic competition has the potential to lower the costs of expensive biotechnology drugs.

At the present time, however, there is no federal legislation that establishes a definitive and effective process for the approval of generic biotechnology drugs. The existing law for the approval of generic drugs, the Drug Price Competition and Patent Restoration Act of 1984, was passed before most biotechnology drugs existed. Biotechnology drugs were not included under this law, with the exception of the simplest biotechnology drugs in existence at that time, human insulin and human growth hormone, which were approved as drugs under the new drug application (NDA) process, not the biologics license application (BLA) process.

Biotechnology drugs are regulated under the Public Health Service Act (PHSA), which is not part of the Drug Price Competition and Patent Restoration Act. The PHSA does not have a generic biotechnology drug approval process based on an abbreviated biologics license application. The issue is how to ensure the bioequivalence of drugs produced by biotechnology without extensive clinical testing. Biotechnology drugs are manufactured using unique and complex technology, and small changes in the manufacturing process can result in unpredictable changes in the drug and unpredictable effects in the body. The law does not define any methods to determine bioequivalence; therefore, the FDA cannot approve generic biotechnology drugs unless the generic biotechnology company reproduces the clinical studies associated with the drug. The Generic Pharmaceutical Association (GPhA) is working with lawmakers to create legislation that will allow the introduction of FDA-approved, affordable biotechnology drugs.

## LEGISLATION AND REGULATIONS FOR THE PHARMACEUTICAL INDUSTRY

There are several state and federal laws and regulations that pertain to the pharmaceutical industry. Specific laws govern the manufacturing, marketing, and distribution of drugs. These laws are intended to protect the health of the American people by ensuring that drug products in the United States are safe and effective and that they meet the highest standards of quality and purity. These laws have also helped to encourage the research and development of new drugs and contain costs by increasing the availability of generic drugs. Several of these laws are discussed in the sections that follow.

### PURE FOOD AND DRUG ACT

The Pure Food and Drug Act was passed by Congress in 1906. This law prohibited the shipment of adulterated drugs in interstate commerce. An **adulterated drug** is defined as a drug that is not pure. This law meant that foods and drugs had to meet standards for purity as a condition of marketing. The act also prohibited **misbranding**, that is, false and misleading information concerning a drug. It required that the ingredients of a drug be accurately stated on the package label. It also recognized the U.S. Pharmacopoeia (USP) and the National Formulary (NF) as official summaries of legal drug standards. The FDA was created in 1927 to oversee this law.

## FEDERAL FOOD, DRUG, AND COSMETIC ACT

The Federal Food, Drug, and Cosmetic Act was passed by Congress in 1938. This law required pharmaceutical manufacturers to demonstrate to the FDA that a drug was safe to use. Any new drug now required a new drug application to be submitted to the FDA. It was the beginning of the drug approval process. An amendment to this law, the Durham-Humphrey Amendment of 1951, made the distinction between prescription and nonprescription drugs. Prescription drugs were determined to be unsafe to use except under the supervision of a physician, whereas nonprescription drugs were determined to be safe to use without medical supervision. This amendment was passed to ensure that certain drugs, namely prescription drugs, were used safely. Congress passed another amendment to this law that required pharmaceutical manufacturers to prove not only that a drug was safe but also that it was *effective*. The Kefauver-Harris Amendment of 1962 added the requirement that a new drug be effective as well as safe. Pharmaceutical companies now had to demonstrate a drug's effectiveness to the FDA before it could be marketed. The amendment also led to a review of drugs that were marketed between 1938 and 1962. This review resulted in the removal from the market of drugs that could not be proved to be both safe and effective.

## ORPHAN DRUG ACT

The Orphan Drug Act of 1983 was developed to promote the research and development of drugs for rare diseases. An **orphan drug** is defined as a drug that treats a disease that affects fewer than 200,000 people. This law provides financial incentives for pharmaceutical manufacturers to develop drugs that may not be profitable owing to the high cost of research and development and the small number of people who need them. These financial incentives are in the form of tax breaks and a 7-year monopoly on orphan drug sales. As a result of this law, several hundred new drugs for rare diseases have been brought to market.

## DRUG PRICE COMPETITION AND PATENT TERM RESTORATION ACT

A law that boosted the pharmaceutical industry, both the generic and brand-name drug industries, was the Drug Price Competition and Patent Term Restoration Act of 1984, also called the Waxman-Hatch Act. It shortened the drug approval process for generic versions of previously approved brand-name drugs approved after 1962. This act resulted in increased market share for generics and greater access to them for patients.

This act also boosted the brand pharmaceutical industry by extending patent protection for certain brand-name pharmaceutical products. Pharmaceutical manufacturers were given a period of up to 5 additional years of patent protection for brand-name drugs, including antibiotics, that contain a new chemical entity, to compensate for time lost during the FDA review process. It also granted up to 3 additional years of patent protection for drug products that do not contain a new chemical entity but involve a new formulation, dosing schedule, route of administration, or additional use, to compensate for the time spent during clinical testing. The extended patent is capped at 14 years from the date of FDA approval. This extension was granted as an incentive for the pharmaceutical manufacturing industry to continue to develop new drugs.

Extended drug patent protection is also being considered under another piece of recent legislation that would extend the patents for drugs developed for bioterrorism attacks.

## PRESCRIPTION DRUG MARKETING ACT

The Prescription Drug Marketing Act of 1988 was passed to protect Americans from drugs that may be misbranded or adulterated during shipping and handling by regulating the activities of drug wholesalers. It established federal standards for the storage, distribution, record keeping, security, and disposal of drugs. In particular, it requires a drug wholesaler to be licensed by the state where it does business.

Under this act, many states have prescription drug **pedigree laws**, legislation that requires wholesalers to track a drug's movement through the supply chain due to the threat of counterfeit drugs. This tracking involves the movement of the drug from the manufacturer, through the wholesaler, to the pharmacy; that is, it identifies a drug's sellers and buyers. Electronic technology including bar codes or radio frequency identification tags, as well as paper records, provides this kind of tracking. A radio frequency identification tag, or RFID, is an electronic strip placed under the drug package label that contains the drug product code and the manufacturer identification number.

This law also imposes tight control over the distribution of drug samples. A **drug sample** is defined as a prescription drug that is not intended to be sold but is provided by the pharmaceutical manufacturer without charge as a way to promote the use of the drug. The law prohibits the sale, purchase, or trade of drug samples. They may be provided to a physician or an institutional pharmacy only on the written request of a physician. Pharmaceutical manufacturers must track drug samples by obtaining a receipt for their delivery, maintaining drug sample distribution records, and reporting a *significant* loss of samples to the FDA.

## VERIFIED-ACCREDITED WHOLESALE DISTRIBUTORS

A quasi-legal standard for drug wholesalers is the Verified-Accredited Wholesale Distributors™ program (VAWD™). The VAWD™ program was developed by the National Association of Boards of Pharmacy in 2004 to protect the public from the threat of counterfeit drugs. VAWD™ designation assures that a wholesaler has a legitimate license and operation and that it uses adequate security in distributing drugs from manufacturers to pharmacies and other institutions.

The VAWD™ program is a voluntary program for drug wholesalers. In order to be accredited, the wholesaler must comply with its state's licensing requirements. In addition, the drug wholesaler must meet certain criteria, including license verification, a background check, a review of its operating procedures, and an on-site inspection. If VAWD™ accreditation is awarded, the drug wholesaler may display the VAWD™ seal on its site's home page and may maintain a link to the VAWD™ Web site. The VAWD™ seal is shown in Figure 13–1.

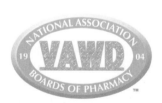

**FIGURE 13–1** Verified-Accredited Wholesale Distributors™ Seal. (Courtesy of the National Association of Boards of Pharmacy and the Verified-Accredited Wholesale Distributors (VAWD™) Program.)

## PRESCRIPTION DRUG USER FEE ACT

The Prescription Drug User Fee Act of 1992 requires that a pharmaceutical manufacturer pay the FDA a fee that the agency uses to hasten the review process for new drugs. Previously, only tax revenues paid for new drug reviews. Under this law, the pharmaceutical industry provides the funding to hire more reviewers in exchange for more timely drug reviews. Any NDA submitted along with a fee must be reviewed and acted on by the FDA within 12 months. As a result, new drug applications have been reviewed and approved within shorter periods of time.

## GENERIC DRUG ENFORCEMENT ACT

The Generic Drug Enforcement Act of 1992 forbids an individual or company that has been convicted of crimes related to the development, approval, or regulation of a drug from participating in the pharmaceutical industry. Under the law, a convicted individual is prohibited from working for a pharmaceutical company in any capacity, and a convicted company is prohibited from submitting applications for drug approvals. This law affects brand pharmaceutical companies as well as generic pharmaceutical companies. It is called the *Generic* Drug Enforcement Act because Congress passed the law after the discovery in 1989 of corruption in the generic drug industry, such as falsifying data and bribing FDA employees who reviewed drug applications.

## GENERAL AGREEMENT ON TARIFFS AND TRADE

A piece of legislation that benefits brand-name pharmaceutical manufacturers was passed by Congress in 1994. The General Agreement on Tariffs and Trade (GATT) changed the rules on patents by allowing companies to keep their patents for an additional period of time. It changed the patent term for all patents filed after June 8, 1995, from 17 years from the date that a patent is awarded to 20 years from the date that a patent is applied for, if that date resulted in a longer patent term. As a result, brand-name drug companies have an additional period of time, over 3 years in some cases, to realize profits from their drugs. However, this change has resulted in a delay in marketing generic versions of drugs, thus costing patients and insurance companies millions of extra dollars.

## FOOD AND DRUG ADMINISTRATION MODERNIZATION ACT

The Food and Drug Administration Modernization Act of 1997 contains several provisions that pertain to the pharmaceutical industry. First, this piece of legislation grants an additional 6 months of exclusive marketing for brand-name drugs in exchange for conducting pediatric studies. The purpose of this provision is to encourage pharmaceutical companies to develop labeling for the use of their products in pediatric patients. Another provision of this law allows pharmaceutical manufacturers to provide information about the unapproved use of a drug. An **unapproved use**, also referred to as an off-label use, is defined as the use of a drug for a disease or a condition that it has not been approved to treat. This law allows the manufacturer to distribute journal articles concerning scientific studies on an unapproved use of one of their products provided that the manufacturer files a supplemental application for the unapproved use to the FDA within a specific period of time. This law also allows pharmaceutical manufacturers to provide economic information about the value of their drug products to formulary committees, managed care organizations, and other high-volume purchasers of drugs. The purpose of this provision is to provide adequate and dependable information about the economic consequences of using a particular drug in order to help drug purchasers make better purchasing decisions. This economic information cannot be provided to individual physicians or patients because it could affect prescribing choices.

In addition to federal laws and regulations, the pharmaceutical industry itself has developed its own guidelines to ensure quality in the manufacturing and marketing processes.

## THE ROLE OF THE PHARMACIST IN THE PHARMACEUTICAL INDUSTRY

The pharmaceutical industry offers several roles for the pharmacist. The role of the pharmacist can be divided into several different areas: sales and marketing, research and development, and manufacturing and quality control. In addition, pharmacists may be employed in other areas such as purchasing, finance, clinical coordination, public affairs, drug information, regulatory affairs, outcomes research and pharmacoeconomics, management, and administration. Some of these areas involve laboratory activities, whereas others involve administrative activities. There are no traditional dispensing roles for pharmacists in the pharmaceutical industry. In general, a pharmacist who works in the pharmaceutical industry must possess traditional pharmacy knowledge and skills as well as business and sales skills, laboratory skills, and excellent communication skills. A career for a pharmacist in the pharmaceutical industry usually starts at an entry-level position in a certain area. As a pharmacist gains pharmaceutical industry knowledge and experience as well as additional education, he may move to a higher job level.

### SALES AND MARKETING

The majority of pharmacists employed in the pharmaceutical industry are in sales and marketing positions. Marketing is focused on the promotion of a drug. It is related to sales in that it develops the programs and materials that are used in sales. Marketing activities include researching the marketplace to determine health care and business trends, physician prescribing habits, and distribution systems; determining drug pricing; creating educational and promotional programs; consulting with professional and trade representatives; and monitoring product sales. Pharmacists are found in all areas of marketing. Pharmaceutical sales, however, attract the largest number of pharmacists.

### Pharmaceutical Sales Representative

A pharmaceutical sales representative is also referred to as a health care representative, professional service representative, or, more commonly, drug rep.

A pharmaceutical sales representative calls on physicians, pharmacists, and other health professionals within an assigned geographical area to educate them concerning the company's drug products and to promote their sale. The goal is to provide the health care professional with accurate and balanced information on a drug product, including its approved use, advantages, and possible side effects. A pharmaceutical sales representative is highly trained to be an expert in his particular drug products. Pharmacists who come into this position already have extensive knowledge of drug products, pharmacology, pharmacokinetics, human physiology, and disease states, as well as knowledge concerning competitor drug products. Being a pharmacist also helps in establishing a relationship with other health care professionals. Specific activities for a pharmaceutical sales representative are contacting customers on a regular basis, providing customer service, negotiating prices and contracts with customers, meeting established sales quotas, submitting sales reports, and controlling expenses within a given budget.

## RESEARCH AND DEVELOPMENT

Research and development involves the discovery and product development of new drugs as well as of new dosages and new dosage forms of older drugs. Research and development are closely linked and extend from the isolation of an active compound in the laboratory to testing on animals and humans. Pharmaceutical research involves identifying chemical compounds that have some identifiable pharmacologic activity and that can be potentially developed into a marketable drug product. Pharmaceutical research activities include performing and overseeing laboratory and animal testing. Pharmaceutical development involves formulating an appropriate dosage form for a new drug product on the basis of the physical and chemical properties of the active compound. The goal is to find a dosage form that guarantees the stability and effectiveness of the drug. Pharmaceutical development activities for a pharmacist include supervising the premanufacturing and analysis of a drug product and developing and writing up a master batch record. Research and development activities are usually performed by pharmacists with many years of experience or an advanced degree.

## MANUFACTURING AND QUALITY CONTROL

Manufacturing and quality control involve the total process of transforming a raw material into a finished drug product on a large scale. A pharmacist found in a manufacturing role oversees the facility, equipment, and personnel involved in the manufacturing process of a drug. The pharmacist in this role oversees manufacturing procedures and the operation of manufacturing equipment by manufacturing technicians and ensures that GMPs are followed. Quality control involves the testing of a drug to ensure that it meets quality standards. A drug must meet standards for potency, purity, quality, and stability as well as standards for packaging and labeling before it can be released for sale. The pharmacist in this role oversees all quality control testing procedures, reviews equipment qualifications, reviews batch records, and performs quality assurance inspections.

## THE ROLE OF THE PHARMACY TECHNICIAN IN THE PHARMACEUTICAL INDUSTRY

The pharmaceutical industry offers relatively few roles for the pharmacy technician. There are no traditional dispensing roles for pharmacy technicians in the pharmaceutical industry. Pharmaceutical industry roles involve manufacturing, laboratory, and quality control activities associated with the production of drugs. Technicians in these areas may be referred to as manufacturing technicians, laboratory technicians, and quality control technicians. Manufacturing technicians formulate and manufacture drug products by operating various types of machinery specific to drug manufacturing, such as large mixers and blenders, tablet presses, tablet-coating machines, and capsule-filling machines. Laboratory technicians perform chemical analyses of drug products using various types of laboratory equipment. Quality control technicians are involved in taking samples, performing various quality control tests, and inspecting the packaging and labeling of the finished drug product. A pharmacy technician working in the pharmaceutical industry should have a thorough knowledge of manufacturing processes, including aseptic manufacturing processes, manufacturing and testing equipment, good manufacturing practices, and FDA regulations.

## KEY CONCEPTS

- The pharmaceutical industry has had a positive impact on the health care system, and pharmaceutical research and development is responsible for the growth of the pharmaceutical industry.
- The FDA drug approval process involves several steps and guarantees that drugs produced in the United States are safe and effective.
- The drug manufacturing process is based on current good manufacturing practices.
- An aggressive drug marketing process is necessary to produce sales of a drug and to realize profits.
- The generic pharmaceutical industry has had an impact on health care costs and on the brand-name pharmaceutical industry.
- Pharmaceutical biotechnology has resulted in drug products that treat a variety of conditions that are more natural and specific in the body.
- There are extensive legislation and regulations that pertain to the pharmaceutical industry.
- Roles for the pharmacist in the pharmaceutical industry include sales and marketing, research and development, and manufacturing and quality control; pharmacy technicians can be found in manufacturing, laboratory, and quality control roles in the pharmaceutical industry.

## SELF-ASSESSMENT QUESTIONS

### MULTIPLE CHOICE

1. Within the pharmaceutical industry, pharmacists would not be found in:
   a. marketing
   b. regulatory affairs
   c. packaging and shipping
   d. research

2. Pharmaceutical sales representatives do not:
   a. provide kickbacks to customers
   b. promote and sell the company's products
   c. maintain effective relationships with health professionals
   d. provide customer service

3. Which statement regarding the marketing of a drug is not true?
   a. marketing follows a cycle
   b. marketing includes determining a price for the drug
   c. marketing includes determining a trade name for the drug
   d. detailing is not a marketing strategy

4. A benefit of the pharmaceutical industry is:
   a. many diseases are prevented from occurring through drugs
   b. overall health care costs are saved through drugs
   c. the quality of life is improved for millions of people through drugs
   d. all of the above

5. Which of the following clinical trials involves testing on humans?
   a. Phase I
   b. Phase II
   c. Phase III
   d. all of the above

6. The Waxman-Hatch Act:
   a. shortened the approval process for generic drugs
   b. extended patent protection for brand-name drugs
   c. benefited the generic drug industry
   d. all of the above

7. In order for a generic drug to be approved by the FDA, the one condition that does not have to be met is:
   a. undergoing clinical trials
   b. having the same route of administration as the brand-name drug
   c. having the same intended clinical effect as the brand-name drug
   d. being bioequivalent to the brand-name drug

8. Good manufacturing practices include all of the following except:
   a. proper equipment and facilities
   b. a quality control program
   c. a pharmacy license
   d. written standard operating procedures

9.  An example of pharmaceutical processing in the manufacturing process is:

    a. mixing
    b. milling
    c. emulsifying
    d. all of the above

10. The piece of legislation that was created to ensure the safety *and* effectiveness of drugs was:

    a. the Pure Food and Drug Act
    b. the Federal Food, Drug, and Cosmetic Act
    c. the Durham-Humphrey Amendment
    d. the Kefauver-Harris Amendment

## TRUE/FALSE (CORRECT THE FALSE STATEMENTS)

1.  _____ The advertisement of drugs directly to patients is called direct-to-consumer advertising.
2.  _____ The law that established the drug approval process and the submission of a new drug application was the Federal Food, Drug, and Cosmetic Act.
3.  _____ Before a new drug can be marketed, it must be approved by the FDA.
4.  _____ A new drug application is submitted to the FDA to request authorization to begin testing a new drug in humans.
5.  _____ Once a drug's patent has expired, a generic version of the drug can be made.
6.  _____ Direct distribution involves the sale of a drug to an intermediary.
7.  _____ The generic drug industry has contributed to decreasing the cost of health care.
8.  _____ There are no traditional dispensing roles for pharmacists and pharmacy technicians in the pharmaceutical industry.
9.  _____ The majority of pharmacists found in the pharmaceutical industry are employed as pharmaceutical sales representatives.
10. _____ Pharmaceutical manufacturers cannot provide information on the unapproved use of a drug.

## FILL-IN

1.  A drug that is used to treat a rare disease is referred to as an _____ _____.
2.  _____ involves the use of a professional sales force to promote the sale of drugs.
3.  An _____ _____ _____ _____ is submitted to the FDA for the approval of a generic drug rather than an NDA.
4.  A generic drug that contains the same active ingredient in the same amount, has the same dosage form and route of administration, and works the same way in the body as a brand-name drug is said to be a _____ _____.

5. The application of biology to the development of drugs is called
   _____ _____.

6. A drug that is not pure is referred to as an _____ drug.

7. The use of a drug for a disease or a condition that it has not been
   approved to treat is referred to as an _____ _____.

8. The set of specifications for the manufacture of a drug is the _____
   _____ _____.

9. The law that strictly controls drug sampling is the _____
   _____ _____ _____.

10. The regulations that describe the methods, equipment, facilities, and
    controls required to produce a drug are _____ _____
    _____.

## CRITICAL THINKING

1. What is the significance of a patent for a drug?
2. When is a pharmaceutical equivalent not a therapeutic equivalent?
3. How are biotechnology drugs influencing our health care system?
4. How will generic biotechnology drugs affect our health care system?
5. Should drugs go through such vigorous testing as they do in the United
   States under the FDA?

## ■ BIBLIOGRAPHY

Blank, D. (2005). State pedigree laws running into some barriers. *Drug Topics,*
   *149*(13), 37.

Buzzeo, R. (2005). Drug counterfeiting: A rising public health concern. *Drug*
   *Topics, 149*(8), 19.

Cassel, D. (2006). Generic biologics: One step closer to reality. *Drug Topics*
   *Generics Supplement, 150*(15), 12s–14s.

Celia, F. (2005). States move to comply with drug pedigree laws. *Drug Topics,*
   *149*(11), 52.

Faden, M. (2006). Authorized generics: Good or bad? *Pharmacy Times, 72*(7), 40.

Fink, J., Vivian, J., & Bernstein, I. (Eds.). (2005). *Pharmacy law digest*
   (40th ed.). St. Louis, MO: Facts and Comparisons.

Frederick, J. (2005, Summer). Safety concerns prompt nationwide spread of
   drug pedigree rules. *Drug Store News,* 43.

Frederick, J. (2006, Winter). Medicaid, biodefense battles rattle generic drug
   makers. *Drug Store News Continuing Education Quarterly, 25,* 44.

Gebhart, F. (2005). Generic biologics face questions on the horizon. *Drug*
   *Topics, 149*(16), 18.

Hong, S., Shepherd, M., Scoones, D., & Wan, T. (2005). Product-line extensions and pricing strategies of brand-name drugs facing patent expiration.
   *Journal of Managed Care Pharmacy, 11*(9), 746–754.

Hussar, D. (2005). Counterfeit meds: Urgent action needed. *Drug Topics,*
   *149*(22), 56.

Jaeger, K. (2005). Patent extensions harming health care? *Generic Pharmacy*
   *Report, 6*(2), 12–13.

Jaeger, K. (2006). FDA needs to support generic biologics. *Pharmacy Times, 72*(6), 40.

Jaeger, K. (2006). Keeping an eye on the future of generics. *Generic Pharmacy Report, 7*(1), 9.

Kelly, K. (2005). Off-label uses of medication. *Pharmacy Times, 71*(4), 33.

Lamb, E. (2005). Authorized generics: Unfair competition or a good thing for patients? *Pharmacy Today, 11*(11), 32.

Levy, S. (2006). Generic industry on cusp of new growth spurt. *Drug Topics, 150*(6), 12.

Levy, S. (2006). How will Rx pedigree law affect you? *Drug Topics, 150*(13), 10.

Lica, L. (2005). Wholesalers take a stand for uniform national licensure. *Drug Topics, 149*(21), 48.

Pharmaceutical Research and Manufacturers of America. (2005). *What goes into the cost of prescription drugs . . . and other questions about your medicine.* [On-line] PhRMA. Available: www.phrma.org.

Reynolds, B. (2005). DTC advertising defended, critiqued at FDA public hearing. *Pharmacy Today, 11*(12), 22–24.

Sipkoff, M. (2005). Battle over authorized generics grows increasingly heated. *Drug Topics, 149*(7), 16s–18s.

Sipkoff, M. (2005). Biogenerics at the gate waiting for the FDA to act. *Drug Topics, 149*(15), 11s–12s.

Sipkoff, M. (2006). Industry bracing for FTC study on authorized generics. *Drug Topics Generics Supplement, 150*(15), 19s–20s.

Ukens, C. (2005). Caught in the middle. *Drug Topics, 149*(22), 24–31.

University of the Sciences in Philadelphia. (2005). *Remington: The science and practice of pharmacy* (21st ed.). Easton, PA: Mack Publishing Company.

Vecchione, A. (2006). FDA: Many barriers remain on generic biologics. *Drug Topics, 150*(14), 32.

# 14    Telepharmacy

## Learning Objectives

Upon completion of this chapter, the student should be able to:

- Define telepharmacy.
- Give reasons for the emergence of telepharmacy.
- List the advantages and disadvantages of telepharmacy.
- Describe the types of telepharmacy models.
- Describe the elements of a traditional telepharmacy.
- Describe the prescription-filling process in a traditional telepharmacy.
- Understand the legislation and regulations pertaining to telepharmacy.
- Describe the roles of the pharmacist and the pharmacy technician in a traditional telepharmacy.

## Key Terms

| | | |
|---|---|---|
| base pharmacy | remote pharmacy | remote telepharmacy |
| base site | remote site | telepharmacy |

## Introduction

Telepharmacy is a new area of pharmacy practice that has grown out of the nationwide shortage of pharmacists and the lack of pharmacy services in remote areas. A traditional telepharmacy is a retail pharmacy practice that differs in a unique way from a traditional community retail pharmacy practice, that is, in the physical absence of the pharmacist in the dispensing pharmacy. Yet, this pharmacy practice uses the same quality standards used in traditional community retail pharmacy practice, including drug utilization review, pharmacist prescription verification, and patient counseling. In this area of pharmacy, the pharmacy technician plays an important role; that is, she has a higher level of responsibility in operating the pharmacy without the pharmacist. In order to work in this area of pharmacy, the pharmacist and technician must possess the knowledge and skills required in a traditional community retail pharmacy practice as well as telecommunication and information technology skills. They must also be familiar with the emerging legislation and regulations governing this pharmacy practice area. This chapter focuses on the remote telepharmacy and the unique roles of the pharmacist and technician in this area. ▪

## OVERVIEW OF TELEPHARMACY

**Telepharmacy** is defined as the provision of pharmaceutical care through the use of telecommunication and information technology to patients at a distance (NABP, 2006). It has been referred to as "virtual pharmacy" or "drugs dispensed from a distance." Telepharmacy involves the dispensing of prescriptions and clinical pharmacy services at a location without the physical presence of a pharmacist. It involves the use of two sites: a remote site and a base site. A **remote site** is the site at which prescriptions are dispensed. In the telephaarmacy model where the remote site is an actual pharmacy, this remote site is referred to as a **remote pharmacy.** A remote pharmacy is defined as a pharmacy site at which prescriptions are dispensed in the absence of a pharmacist. The remote pharmacy is also referred to as **a remote telepharmacy.**

A **base site** is the site at which a supervising pharmacist is located. In telepharmacy models where the base site is an actual pharmacy, this base site is referred to as a **base pharmacy.** A base pharmacy, also referred to as a control pharmacy, central pharmacy, or parent pharmacy, is defined as the pharmacy at which a supervising pharmacist is located. It is further defined as a pharmacy authorized to operate a remote site by means of computer, video, and audio links.

Telepharmacy also involves the use of telecommunication and information technology to link the remote site to the base site. In a telepharmacy practice, a prescription is dispensed at a remote site, usually by means of an automated dispensing machine, on the instructions of a pharmacist at a base site. The entire system is under the full control of the pharmacist. The pharmacist activates and controls the automated dispensing machine located at the remote site. The pharmacist supervises the preparation of the prescription by way of an Internet connection, a video camera, and an audio link. This same video and audio link is used to provide face-to-face counseling to the patient at the remote site by the pharmacist at the base site. To summarize, telepharmacy is a unique and innovative way to deliver pharmacy services to patients.

There are several reasons that telepharmacy has emerged as a practice area of pharmacy. There is a nationwide shortage of pharmacists, which makes it difficult to staff pharmacies, especially in small communities. There is also a lack of pharmacies in some remote or sparsely populated areas of the country because there is not enough prescription volume to support a traditional retail pharmacy business. Telepharmacy is a way to provide pharmacy services to an area without a pharmacist or traditional retail pharmacy.

Another reason for the growth of telepharmacy is an increase in the elderly population and their increased need for medications. Many residents living in remote or sparsely populated areas are elderly. They are unable to travel to a distant pharmacy or to utilize a mail-order pharmacy to meet their medication needs. Telepharmacy is a way to service these elderly patients.

There is a need for pharmacy services in various areas of outpatient care that are difficult to serve, areas in which pharmacy services are an extension of this care. These areas include rural health clinics, physician offices, emergency care centers, surgical centers, long-term care facilities, and correctional facilities. Telepharmacy is being used in these types of settings in rural areas in several states. It has also been implemented by several federal agencies, including the Department of Veterans Affairs, the Department of Defense, the Immigration and Naturalization Service, and the Indian Health Service.

Finally, telepharmacy is being used to provide overnight pharmacy services at small or rural community hospitals that do not have a pharmacist on duty 24 hours a day. It involves a licensed pharmacist providing services from a base hospital pharmacy site to a remote hospital site. Telepharmacy is being used to comply with new Joint Commission hospital standards that ban nonpharmacy personnel from accessing the hospital pharmacy at night and prohibit medication ordering and dispensing without pharmacist oversight. The practice of telepharmacy assures Joint Commission–approved after-hours dispensing of medications and clinical services to the hospital.

Telepharmacy has several advantages for the patient. The most important advantage is access to pharmacy services in rural and remote areas. It allows patients to obtain prescriptions in areas that do not have a pharmacist and in towns that are too small to support a traditional retail pharmacy. Another advantage is patient convenience. Patients do not have to drive a considerable distance to a traditional pharmacy to obtain their medications. Telepharmacy also allows pharmacy care to be provided in a personal and private setting, with real-time face-to-face communication with a pharmacist. In the hospital setting, telepharmacy reduces medication errors. There are several advantages for the telepharmacy practice itself. Telepharmacy enables one pharmacist to serve several remote sites at the same time without the expense of having a pharmacist at each site. A remote pharmacy also does not have the high overhead costs of a traditional pharmacy due to several factors, such as its smaller size, limited inventory, and the limited number of employees at the site. Drug costs are lower due to the tightly controlled inventory and the tendency to stock generic drugs.

There are also several disadvantages to telepharmacy. One disadvantage is the cost associated with setting up a remote telepharmacy site, including the purchase or rental of the space, utilities, equipment such as automated dispensing machines, and telecommunication and information technology. Special training in this new technology is also required; that is, both pharmacy staff and patients must learn how to use it. For some pharmacists and patients, a disadvantage of telepharmacy is the lack of physical presence between them during counseling. There also may be insurance reimbursement issues related to a telepharmacy practice.

## TYPES OF TELEPHARMACY MODELS

There are several types of telepharmacies or telepharmacy models. All of them use the telepharmacy concept, but they may vary in location and services. For the remainder of the chapter, the discussion will focus on the traditional telepharmacy model, since it is the only telepharmacy model in which the pharmacy technician is involved.

## TRADITIONAL TELEPHARMACY MODEL

A traditional telepharmacy model involves prescription preparation, pickup, and patient consultation at a remote site that is a pharmacy. Prescriptions are prepared by a pharmacy technician at the remote pharmacy under the supervision of a pharmacist at a base pharmacy. Patient consultation is done in privacy by means of an audio and visual link. It is a retail pharmacy practice where prescriptions are prepared and picked up at the same site. Patient counseling is done at the point of sale of the prescription.

## HOSPITAL TELEPHARMACY MODEL

A hospital telepharmacy model involves a licensed pharmacist providing pharmacy services from a base hospital pharmacy to a remote hospital site. The pharmacist is usually located in the pharmacy in the base hospital. However, medications are not dispensed from the pharmacy in the remote hospital, but are dispensed outside of the pharmacy by means of automated dispensing machines located at various sites within the hospital.

In the hospital telepharmacy model, there is no pharmacy technician present. A medication, usually in a unit-dose form as used by hospitals, is dispensed to a nurse by means of an automated dispensing machine after clinical services are performed by the pharmacist at the base hospital. These services consist of a review of the medication order, computer order entry, and drug information to the nursing staff. The medications are then administered to the patient, which is within the nurse's scope of practice. Computer, audio, and video equipment for communication between the pharmacist and nurse is usually located at or near the nursing stations at the remote hospital.

## REMOTE CONSULTATION SITE MODEL

A remote consultation site model involves prescription pickup and patient consultation at a remote site that is *not* a pharmacy. Prescriptions are filled by a pharmacist at a base pharmacy and delivered to the remote site. There is no pharmacy technician or drug inventory at this site. Patient counseling is done in privacy by means of a video and audio link, as in a traditional telepharmacy. It is not a retail pharmacy practice, since the remote site is not a pharmacy. This model is used when it is not possible for a base pharmacy to staff, stock, or manage another pharmacy site for financial or other reasons.

## AUTOMATED DISPENSING MACHINE MODEL

An automated dispensing machine model involves prescription preparation, pickup, and patient consultation at a remote site that is *not* a pharmacy. This site may be in a rural health clinic, physician office, or emergency care center. Prescriptions are dispensed by means of an automated dispensing machine, usually a small model that has a very limited drug inventory, under the direction of a pharmacist at a base pharmacy. There is no pharmacy technician present at this site. Patient consultation in this model is also done in privacy by means of an audio and video link to the pharmacist. It is *not* a retail pharmacy

**TABLE 14–1**   Types of Telepharmacy Models

| | TRADITIONAL TELEPHARMACY MODEL | HOSPITAL TELEPHARMACY MODEL | REMOTE CONSULTATION SITE MODEL | AUTOMATED DISPENSING MACHINE MODEL |
|---|---|---|---|---|
| Prescription Preparation? | Yes | Yes | No | Yes |
| Prescription Pickup? | Yes | No | Yes | Yes |
| Patient Consultation? | Yes | No | Yes | Yes |
| Pharmacy Technician Present? | Yes | No | No | No |
| Drug Inventory? | Yes | Yes | No | Yes |

practice, since the automated dispensing machine is *not* located in a pharmacy. This model is usually used to deliver an urgent medication, such as a pain medication, or the first doses of a medication, such as an antibiotic, to get the patient started on her therapy.

The types of telepharmacy models are summarized in Table 14–1.

# ELEMENTS OF A TRADITIONAL TELEPHARMACY

There are many elements that make up a traditional telepharmacy. Most of these elements are the same elements that are found in a traditional community retail pharmacy practice. However, some elements are unique to a traditional telepharmacy.

## PERSONNEL

A traditional telepharmacy must be staffed by a trained pharmacy technician. Under no condition can a traditional telepharmacy be open for business without a pharmacy technician on duty. There also may be other personnel at this location, such as store clerks, to address the retail portion of the business.

## INVENTORY

The inventory in a traditional telepharmacy site usually consists of the most commonly prescribed prescription drugs in the most frequently used strengths. Medications are pre-packaged in commonly dispensed sizes and are usually stocked in an automatic dispensing machine. The inventory may include pre-packaged tablets and capsules, syrups and suspensions, oral contraceptives, oral and nasal inhalers, ophthalmic and otic drugs, and rectal, vaginal, and topical drugs. The drug inventory is limited by the capacity of the automated dispensing machine on site. Drug selection is made usually on the basis of a formulary and/or physician prescribing habits. Medications that are not stocked in the automated dispensing machine are available through a mail-order pharmacy by means of a computer link between the base pharmacy site and a mail-order pharmacy. The traditional telepharmacy may also stock a small or complete line of over-the-counter drugs and health and beauty aids.

## PHARMACY DESIGN

The physical design of a traditional telepharmacy is unique in several ways. The traditional telepharmacy is usually small compared to a traditional community retail pharmacy due to the small inventory, the compact size of automated dispensing machines, and the small number of employees working in the space. There are usually no open shelves stocked with medications in the original manufacturers' packaging as in a traditional community retail pharmacy, as medications are stocked in an automated dispensing machine. There should be adequate counter space on which to work. The traditional telepharmacy also has a separate patient consultation room adjacent to the pharmacy.

## EQUIPMENT AND SUPPLIES

Some of the equipment and supplies found in a traditional telepharmacy are the same as those in a traditional community retail pharmacy, such as a computer, printer, and facsimile machine and a refrigerator and sink. Special equipment includes an automated dispensing machine; special computer hardware, such as a bar code scanner and an inspection camera; special software for inspection and verification; a video camera for visual communication; a headset or telephone handset for voice or audio communication; and dial-up phone or DSL service.

## THE PRESCRIPTION-FILLING PROCESS IN A TELEPHARMACY PRACTICE

The prescription-filling process in a traditional telepharmacy practice is different from the process used in a traditional community retail pharmacy practice. In a traditional telepharmacy practice, new prescriptions are received by a pharmacist or a pharmacy technician at the base pharmacy by way of the phone, facsimile machine, or electronically. Prescriptions can also be accepted by the pharmacy technician at the remote pharmacy site. Each prescription is scanned, and the data are entered into the computer by the pharmacist or by the pharmacy technician at either site. All new prescription hard copies must be filed at the base pharmacy. Refill requests can be entered into the computer in the usual way.

The prescription is screened by the pharmacist through the use of the computerized patient medication profile for the appropriate dose, drug interactions, allergies, or other contraindications. Once the pharmacist determines that the prescription is appropriate and the prescription claim is adjudicated, a label is generated, checked for accuracy, and then transmitted to the remote pharmacy site.

The prescription is prepared at the remote site by the pharmacy technician, usually through the use of an automated dispensing machine. The pharmacy technician scans the bar code on the prescription label, which corresponds to the correct drug inside the machine. The drug package is then released, and the bar code on the package is scanned to verify that the correct drug has been delivered. The drug package is labeled by the pharmacy technician, and once labeling is completed, the pharmacy technician communicates with the pharmacist at the base pharmacy site by means of teleconferencing (Figure 14–1). Though the use of a two-way video camera, called an inspection camera, and an audio link to the pharmacy technician, the pharmacist reviews the prescription

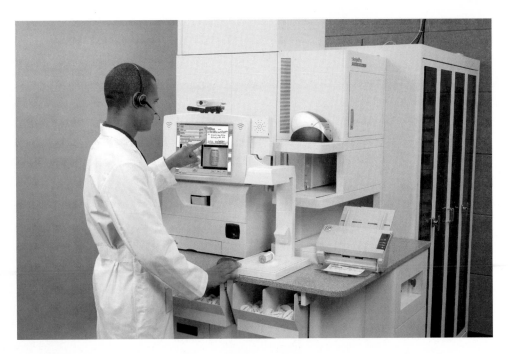

**FIGURE 14–1**    The Pharmacy Technician in a Telepharmacy Practice. (Courtesy of ScriptPro.)

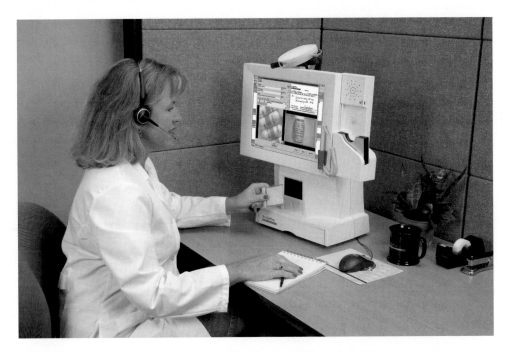

**FIGURE 14–2**    The Pharmacist in a Telepharmacy Practice. (Courtesy of ScriptPro.)

order, examines the prescription label, and examines the drug dispensed to make sure that the label is attached to the correct drug package (Figure 14–2). Once this final check has been performed, the prescription is released by the pharmacist for dispensing to the patient. The release is electronically documented at the base pharmacy.

The pharmacy technician escorts the patient into the consultation room and connects the patient to the pharmacist at the base site by means of a video

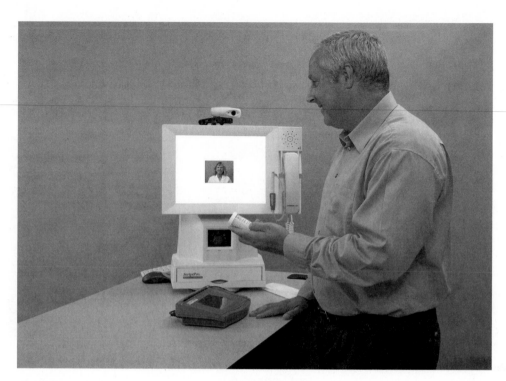

**FIGURE 14–3**    The Patient in a Telepharmacy Practice. (Courtesy of ScriptPro.)

camera and an audio link. It is at this point that the filled prescription is dispensed to the patient and placed in front of her. The patient then receives face-to-face counseling from the pharmacist by way of this video and audio link. This counseling is provided in privacy, unlike in a traditional community retail setting, where other patients are often standing nearby (Figure 14–3). Following consultation, the financial transaction is completed, the prescription is bagged, and the patient may leave the pharmacy.

When needed, the automated dispensing machine at the remote site is stocked by a pharmacist who may visit the remote site to perform this duty or by a pharmacy technician under the supervision of a pharmacist. A bar code on the medication is scanned upon loading into the automated dispensing machine to assure accurate stocking.

It should be noted that a traditional telepharmacy cannot operate and must be closed for business if there is an interruption in the computer, video, or audio link with the base pharmacy. In most states, traditional telepharmacy practice also does not allow any medication to be counted or repackaged by the pharmacy technician from a manufacturer's bulk container into a unit of use package or prescription vial, nor the dispensing of unit of use packaging in partial quantities.

## LEGISLATION AND REGULATIONS FOR TELEPHARMACY

A telepharmacy is licensed and regulated by its individual state board of pharmacy. A traditional telepharmacy is usually licensed as a retail pharmacy. It must comply with all state and federal pharmacy laws and regulations, including the supervision of pharmacy technicians and patient counseling. Telepharmacy satisfies the requirements of pharmacy technician supervision and patient counseling by way of a computer, video, and audio link. Currently there are no federal regulations that govern telepharmacy. However, the National Association of Boards of Pharmacy (NABP) has issued model telepharmacy regulations, and some states have adopted these model regulations. Several states with underserved areas in pharmacy, such as Iowa, Montana, Texas, Vermont, Wyoming, North Dakota, and Wisconsin, currently allow telepharmacy and have telepharmacy legislation and regulations in place. Several additional states are actively investigating or are currently working on telepharmacy regulations.

## OMNIBUS BUDGET RECONCILIATION ACT OF 1990

OBRA 90 mandates patient counseling. A pharmacist is required to counsel the patient about the safe and effective use of medications. This counseling may be accomplished by the use of printed information in the form of a computer-generated printout, in addition to consultation over the phone. OBRA requires the pharmacist to *offer* counseling, giving the patient the option to decline. However, telepharmacy exceeds this counseling requirement. As part of the legislation and regulations established for telepharmacy by state boards of pharmacy, patient consultation *must* be provided to a patient at a remote site by a pharmacist at the base site, or the patient cannot receive her medication. This process is assured by escorting the patient into the consultation room and dispensing the prescription to her immediately before she is counseled by the pharmacist. Telepharmacy satisfies this requirement of patient counseling by means of a video camera and audio link and thus exceeds the standards set for a traditional retail pharmacy practice in this respect.

## DRUG ENFORCEMENT AGENCY REGULATIONS

A remote telepharmacy must register with the Drug Enforcement Administration and obtain its own controlled substance registration, separate from the base pharmacy with which it is associated. As for any pharmacy, the DEA requires that controlled substances be kept in a locked cabinet or dispersed throughout the noncontrolled drug stock to prevent their diversion. Telepharmacy uses automated dispensing machines that are secure and thus DEA compliant for the storage and dispensing of controlled substances in this setting.

## PRIVACY REGULATIONS

Health and Insurance Portability and Accountability Act (HIPAA) regulations require the privacy of personal health information by health care organizations, including telepharmacies. Telepharmacy practice involves the transmission of personal and health-related information over the Internet. Remote telepharmacy software systems are an extension of base pharmacy software systems and are similarly designed for patient confidentiality. Confidentiality is assured by using systems that encrypt information transmitted over the Internet.

## THE ROLE OF THE PHARMACIST IN TELEPHARMACY

Telepharmacy offers a variety of roles for the pharmacist. These can be divided into the dispensing, clinical, and administrative roles. In general, the pharmacist in a telepharmacy practice must possess traditional retail or hospital pharmacy knowledge and skills in addition to clinical skills. The pharmacist must also possess telecommunication and information technology skills, and excellent communication and listening skills in order to communicate and interact with the patient or nurse over a distance.

### DISPENSING ROLE

The dispensing role of the pharmacist in a traditional telepharmacy does not relate to the actual physical dispensing of a prescription. It relates to the final steps in the overall process of filling a prescription for a patient, that is, the final check of the finished prescription order and the subsequent dispensing to the patient at the time of patient counseling. In a traditional telepharmacy, this final check of the prescription and patient counseling is performed in a unique way, that is, by means of a video camera and audio link to the remote telepharmacy.

### CLINICAL ROLE

The clinical role of the pharmacist in telepharmacy involves pharmaceutical care activities, which include screening the prescription order, conducting the drug utilization review, and counseling the patient. Of these clinical activities, patient counseling is performed in a unique way, again by means of a video camera and an audio link to the patient in the traditional telepharmacy. The fact that it is conducted in an area of the remote telepharmacy that is separate from the dispensing area acknowledges the importance of this clinical activity in this type of practice.

Another clinical activity may involve designing and managing a formulary for use in a telepharmacy practice, due to the limited inventory of medications available at a remote telepharmacy site. This is usually done in cooperation with the practicing physicians in the area. The pharmacist may also be involved in other clinical activities, such as monitoring patient compliance and participating in disease management and pain management programs.

### ADMINISTRATIVE ROLE

The administrative role of the pharmacist in telepharmacy is related to the management of both the base pharmacy site and the remote telepharmacy. The pharmacist oversees and supervises all remote telepharmacy operations. The stocking of medications in the automated dispensing machine is supervised by the pharmacist through the use of bar code technology. Video and audio links, in addition to the computer, telephone, and facsimile machine, allow for communication between the pharmacist and the pharmacy technician on all other aspects of pharmacy operations. Administrative tasks include hiring and training pharmacy technicians, overseeing equipment and computer maintenance, developing policies and procedures that pertain to the telepharmacy practice, assuring compliance with pharmacy laws and regulations, and maintaining records.

## THE ROLE OF THE PHARMACY TECHNICIAN IN TELEPHARMACY

The role of the pharmacy technician in a traditional telepharmacy is a very important one. In general, the pharmacy technician assists the pharmacist in providing pharmacy services by physically preparing prescriptions. Due to the significant amount of responsibility that the technician has, it is critical that she has the appropriate qualifications and training for the position. The pharmacy technician must possess traditional retail pharmacy knowledge and skills as well as knowledge and skills specific to telepharmacy, such as:

- A basic knowledge of the telepharmacy concept
- A working knowledge of a traditional community retail pharmacy and the prescription-filling process
- A knowledge of commonly prescribed medications
- A knowledge of the translation and interpretation of prescription orders
- A thorough knowledge of automated pharmacy systems
- An understanding of the legislation and regulations pertaining to telepharmacy practice
- Excellent communication skills
- Excellent computer skills
- Pharmacy management skills

There are many activities that the pharmacy technician can perform in the remote pharmacy. However, the pharmacy technician may not perform any task that involves the professional judgment of a pharmacist, and the pharmacy technician must work under the supervision, although off-site, of the pharmacist. The role of the pharmacy technician in a traditional telepharmacy may be divided into three areas: dispensing, pharmacy maintenance, and computer functions.

### DISPENSING ROLE

The dispensing role for the pharmacy technician in a traditional telepharmacy is unique. The pharmacy technician is responsible for physically preparing prescription orders at the remote pharmacy, with the appropriate medication in the appropriate amount, without a licensed pharmacist being present. This preparation involves removing the correct medication from the automated dispensing machine and affixing the prescription label and the appropriate auxiliary labels to the container before verification by the pharmacist at the base pharmacy. A pharmacy technician may only perform those duties as allowed by the board of pharmacy in that state. The pharmacist at the base site is ultimately responsible for the correct dispensing of a prescription order.

## PHARMACY MAINTENANCE ROLE

As in a traditional community retail pharmacy, the pharmacy technician in a traditional telepharmacy has several duties that relate to the overall running of the pharmacy. These duties include ordering and receiving medications, performing inventory control functions, returning outdated or recalled medications, ordering and stocking pharmacy supplies, generating reports, and performing general housekeeping duties. All of these activities, however, are done without the direct supervision of a pharmacist; that is, these activities are monitored indirectly and off-site by the supervising pharmacist. The most important pharmacy maintenance role for the technician is the restocking of medications in the automated dispensing machine. This activity is monitored for accuracy by the pharmacist at the base pharmacy by means of bar code verification of the drug as it is loaded into the machine.

## COMPUTER ROLE

The pharmacy technician can perform many computer functions in the traditional telepharmacy. These computer functions are similar to those performed in a traditional community retail pharmacy and include maintaining patient demographic records, doing additional third-party billing, and printing reports.

## KEY CONCEPTS

- Telepharmacy involves the dispensing of prescriptions and clinical pharmacy services at a remote location without the physical presence of a pharmacist.
- Telepharmacy has emerged in response to the shortage of pharmacists and the lack of pharmacy services in remote areas.
- Telepharmacy has several advantages, such as access to pharmacy services, patient convenience, and personal care, but it also has several disadvantages, such as the cost of operating a remote site, special training in new technologies, and the lack of the physical presence of the pharmacist.
- There are four types of telepharmacy models: the traditional telepharmacy model, the hospital telepharmacy model, the remote consultation site model, and the automated dispensing machine model.
- A traditional telepharmacy has many unique elements, including its design; prepackaged, limited inventory; and the equipment required to link the remote pharmacy site to the base pharmacy site.
- The prescription-filling process in a traditional telepharmacy is different from the process in a traditional community retail pharmacy.
- Specific legislation and regulations that pertain to a telepharmacy practice continue to emerge.
- Telepharmacy does not include a physical dispensing role for the pharmacist at the base pharmacy site.

- The pharmacy technician performs many tasks in the traditional telepharmacy, the most important being the accurate physical preparation of prescriptions in the absence of the pharmacist.

## SELF-ASSESSMENT QUESTIONS

**MULTIPLE CHOICE**

1. A pharmacy from which prescriptions are dispensed without the presence of the pharmacist is called:
   a. a parent pharmacy
   b. a remote pharmacy
   c. a central pharmacy
   d. a control pharmacy

2. In order to visually communicate with a pharmacist, a remote pharmacy must have a:
   a. facsimile machine
   b. telephone
   c. video camera
   d. printer

3. A disadvantage of telepharmacy is:
   a. access to medications
   b. the lack of the physical presence of the pharmacist
   c. patient convenience
   d. low overhead costs associated with the remote site

4. A traditional telepharmacy provides pharmacy services to patients in:
   a. rural areas
   b. urban areas
   c. large cities
   d. foreign countries

5. Telepharmacy is being used in areas such as:
   a. the Department of Veterans Affairs
   b. rural outpatient clinics
   c. the Indian Health Service
   d. all of the above

6. A unique feature of a traditional telepharmacy is:
   a. a unit-dose packaging machine
   b. a cash register
   c. a private consultation room
   d. a waiting area

7. In a hospital telepharmacy model, the pharmacist performs all of the following duties except:
   a. computer order entry
   b. patient consultation

    c. medication order review

    d. drug information

8. In a traditional telepharmacy model, the pharmacist performs:

    a. drug utilization review

    b. prescription verification

    c. patient counseling

    d. all of the above

9. A duty of a pharmacy technician in a traditional telepharmacy is:

    a. prescription verification

    b. repackaging medications

    c. prescription labeling

    d. patient counseling

10. The telepharmacy model in which a pharmacy technician is present is:

    a. the traditional telepharmacy model

    b. the hospital telepharmacy model

    c. the remote consultation site model

    d. the automated dispensing machine model

## TRUE/FALSE (CORRECT THE FALSE STATEMENTS)

1. _____ A traditional telepharmacy may be found in the same area as other retail pharmacies.

2. _____ The pharmacy technician in a remote pharmacy may dispense a prescription without a final check by the pharmacist, since the pharmacist is not present.

3. _____ Over-the-counter drugs and health and beauty aids can be found in a traditional telepharmacy.

4. _____ In a hospital telepharmacy model, drugs are dispensed from the hospital pharmacy after hours by a nurse.

5. _____ A remote pharmacy does not need a separate pharmacy license from the base pharmacy with which it is associated.

6. _____ A base pharmacy is defined as a pharmacy authorized to operate a remote site by means of a computer, audio, and visual link.

7. _____ The dispensing role of the pharmacist in telepharmacy does not relate to the actual physical dispensing of a prescription.

8. _____ A separate patient consultation room is adjacent to the pharmacy in a traditional telepharmacy.

9. _____ Telepharmacy practice uses the same quality standards as traditional pharmacy practice.

10. _____ A telepharmacy practice is possible between a rural hospital and an urban hospital.

## FILL-IN

1. In a hospital telepharmacy model, medications are dispensed by means of an automated dispensing machine to a _____.

2. In a traditional telepharmacy, the final check of a prescription as well as _____ _____ is performed using an audio/visual link.

3. In telepharmacy, the pharmacist is located in a _____ pharmacy, also referred to as a central pharmacy.
4. The _____ requirement for patient counseling is met in a traditional telepharmacy by means of a video camera and an audio link.
5. A _____ _____ _____ model is the only telepharmacy model in which prescriptions are not prepared.
6. A traditional telepharmacy must be staffed by a _____ _____.
7. There is no prescription pickup or patient consultation in the _____ _____ model.
8. The _____ _____ model is a retail pharmacy practice.
9. A remote telepharmacy must register with the _____ and obtain its own controlled substance registration.
10. In the traditional telepharmacy, prescription dispensing is performed in the _____ _____ immediately before patient counseling by the pharmacist.

## CRITICAL THINKING

1. Why would a traditional telepharmacy not be found in a densely populated area?
2. Compare and contrast the types of telepharmacy models.
3. Compare and contrast pharmacy operations in a traditional telepharmacy with those in a traditional community retail pharmacy.
4. Apply *structure, process,* and *outcomes* to a traditional telepharmacy.
5. Compare and contrast the duties of a pharmacy technician in a traditional telepharmacy with those in a traditional community retail pharmacy.

## ■ BIBLIOGRAPHY

Brugger, A., & Jannicelli, J. (2006). Telepharmacy addresses pharmacy shortage. *U.S. Pharmacist, 31*(2), 84.

Gebhart, F. (2005). Telepharmacy spreading in the community setting. *Drug Topics, 149*(21), 58.

Mosquera, M. (2005, November 29). Washington in the market for a telepharmacy system, *Washington Technology.*

National Association of Boards of Pharmacy. (2006). *NABP Model State Pharmacy Act and model rules.* [On-line] NABP. Available: www.nabp.net.

Stubbings, T., Miller, C., Humphries, T., Nelson, K., & Helling, D. (2005). Telepharmacy in a health maintenance organization. *American Journal of Health-System Pharmacy, 62*(4), 406–410.

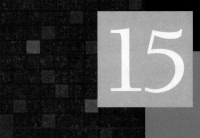

# 15 Advanced Pharmacy Technician Roles

## Learning Objectives

Upon completion of this chapter, the student should be able to:

- Explain advanced pharmacy technician roles and their requirements.
- Describe expanded pharmacy technician roles.
- Describe specialized pharmacy technician roles.
- Describe innovative pharmacy technician roles.
- Discuss pharmacy technician liability in advanced roles.
- List some of the benefits of advanced pharmacy technician roles.

## Key Terms

certified fitter

doctrine of contribution

doctrine of respondeat superior

expanded pharmacy
  technician roles

innovative pharmacy
  technician roles

intellectual error

joint liability

joint tortfeasors

malpractice

mechanical error

negligence

orthosis

prosthesis

specialized pharmacy
  technician roles

tech-check-tech

tortfeasor

## Introduction

The pharmacy profession continues to expand. Pharmacists have moved into pharmaceutical care roles in all practice settings. Pharmacy technicians likewise have moved into greater roles in the medication-dispensing process and are now moving into more advanced roles in other areas. Today, well-trained and highly motivated pharmacy technicians are performing various activities once performed exclusively by pharmacists. These advanced activities involve increased responsibilities and challenges. There are also legal implications, as well as several benefits, that are associated with advanced pharmacy technician roles. This chapter focuses on some of the most recent advanced roles for pharmacy technicians and the increased liability pharmacy technicians may face in these new roles. ∎

## OVERVIEW OF ADVANCED PHARMACY TECHNICIAN ROLES

The roles of the pharmacist and the pharmacy technician have changed. Pharmacists in all practice settings have expanded their involvement in pharmaceutical care and have delegated most of the tasks related to the dispensing of medications to pharmacy technicians. In addition, pharmacy technicians are now being utilized in areas other than medication dispensing, in what are considered to be advanced roles, in order to free pharmacists for more patient care activities. These advanced roles involve increased responsibilities and challenges for the pharmacy technician. Many of these advanced roles are performed outside of the pharmacy, on hospital floors or in various hospital departments, or in nursing facilities and other settings. In performing advanced activities, pharmacy technicians are becoming active and contributing members of the health care team.

For the most part, pharmacy technicians who assume advanced roles are technicians who have already successfully worked in traditional pharmacy technician roles. They are pharmacy technicians who possess qualifications such as the ability to work independently, good organizational and communication skills, the ability to change, the willingness and ability to learn new skills, and comfort with their new roles. In other words, these are committed and capable pharmacy technicians.

Advanced pharmacy technician roles require a higher level of experience and training than traditional pharmacy technician roles. Pharmacy technicians performing advanced activities and having advanced responsibilities should receive additional training and education, through on-the-job training, formal educational programs, or a combination of both. With the proper level of experience and training, pharmacy technicians can then be given the opportunity to *specialize,* or they may be given *expanded* or *innovative* roles. It should be mentioned that pharmacy technicians who are nationally certified are much more likely to be entrusted with greater responsibilities than those who are not.

Pharmacy technicians in advanced roles should not perform activities beyond their training or experience. In fact, their activities and responsibilities should correspond to their training and education. Pharmacy technicians should act within defined and specific protocols. Protocols help to guide the activities of a pharmacy technician, because technicians lack in-depth pharmacy knowledge. Therefore, the advanced roles of pharmacy technicians should be controlled to protect themselves as well as the patients. We are reminded that pharmacy technicians play a supportive role in pharmacy and do not assume all of the responsibilities of a pharmacist. They are meant to support, not replace, the pharmacist. The pharmacist maintains control over all pharmacy activities. Furthermore, the ultimate responsibility rests with the licensed pharmacist in authority.

The roles and responsibilities of pharmacy technicians, including advanced roles and responsibilities, are limited by state board of pharmacy regulations. These regulations vary from state to state. In some states, pharmacy technicians cannot phone a physician's office for refill authorization or enter prescription data into a computer. In other states, pharmacy technicians can check the work performed by another pharmacy technician or accept a verbal order for a new prescription. In a few states, pharmacy technician activities are not even addressed. In reality, few states actually have laws that clearly define the role of the pharmacy technician. As a result, the advanced knowledge and skills of some pharmacy technicians are often underutilized. In the future, state boards of pharmacy may reassess the limitations on pharmacy technician roles. Such a reassessment would allow pharmacists to use pharmacy technicians in advanced roles without compromising patient safety.

## EXPANDED PHARMACY TECHNICIAN ROLES

There are several pharmacy technician roles that are considered to be expanded roles. **Expanded pharmacy technician roles** are defined as roles that are an expansion of current traditional pharmacy technician duties in the preparation and dispensing of medications. Expanded pharmacy technician roles are the result of the advancement of pharmaceutical care by the pharmacist. Expanded pharmacy technician roles free pharmacists to perform activities related to patient care. In many cases, pharmacy technicians are given autonomy to resolve certain problems without the need for a pharmacist's intervention, for example, resolving third-party billing problems or obtaining authorization for refills. It is important to remember that many expanded pharmacy technician roles, as well as specialized and innovative roles, are not permitted in some states and that it is up to each individual pharmacist to determine which activities allowed by law will be delegated to the pharmacy technician.

One expanded role for pharmacy technicians in the hospital setting is **tech-check-tech,** which is defined as a pharmacy technician's performing the final check of another pharmacy technician's work in the same situation, such as the filling of unit-dose cassettes or the restocking of floor-stock drugs in hospitals. There are opposing viewpoints on this practice. Proponents of this practice believe that tech-check-tech can be done safely and effectively. Studies have shown that accuracy rates for pharmacy technicians versus pharmacists in performing the final check are statistically the same. Tech-check-tech is purely a nonjudgmental activity that is clearly separate from any clinical activity. A pharmacist has already checked the prescription order entry and the appropriateness of the medication. Also, medications are not dispensed directly to patients, as in the retail setting. Before a filled and checked medication is administered to the patient, it is verified by an additional health care professional—a nurse. Also, tech-check-tech frees pharmacists to perform more clinical activities. Opponents of this practice are concerned about the pharmacist's lack of control over the drug distribution process. They believe that the practice of tech-check-tech can lead to additional errors in the pharmacy. They also are concerned about

## BOX 15–1    Expanded Pharmacy Technician Roles

Performing tech-check-tech
Accepting new prescriptions
Obtaining refill authorization
Transferring prescriptions
Purchasing drugs and supplies
Training pharmacy technicians
Serving on committees
Maintaining narcotic inventory
Providing drug information
Resolving insurance problems
Managing pharmacy automation and technology

the pharmacist's liability in this practice, because the responsibility for a pharmacy technician's error falls on the pharmacist in charge. Tech-check-tech is currently allowed in several states, and additional states are reviewing the practice.

Another expanded pharmacy technician role is accepting a prescription over the phone. Trained technicians are capable of safely and accurately accepting a verbal order for a new prescription from a physician's office in light of the fact that an untrained agent for the physician, often a receptionist who cannot pronounce drug names, can call a prescription to a pharmacy. In performing this expanded role, the pharmacy technician usually follows a designated protocol to ensure the accuracy of the prescription. There can be some limitations to this practice; for example, only a pharmacist may be allowed to receive an oral prescription for a controlled drug.

Another expanded pharmacy technician role is calling a physician's office to obtain refill authorization. A pharmacy technician can request and accept a verbal refill authorization from an agent of the physician. This role also is performed according to a designated protocol, and there can be limitations; for example, if there are any changes to the prescription or if consultation is involved, a pharmacist must handle the call.

The pharmacy technician can request a prescription transfer or answer the request for a transfer from another pharmacy. In performing this role, the technician usually follows a designated protocol to assure the accuracy of the required information necessary to transfer a prescription according to state law.

Many other expanded pharmacy technician roles have been identified. Some involve time-consuming tasks, whereas others involve clerical tasks. Examples of these roles are found in Box 15–1.

## SPECIALIZED PHARMACY TECHNICIAN ROLES

There are several pharmacy technician roles that are considered to be highly specific roles. **Specialized pharmacy technician roles** are defined as roles that concentrate on one aspect of pharmacy practice. Usually, only highly qualified pharmacy technicians are promoted into specialized positions. These positions are considered to be advancements in the career ladders that are being created in many pharmacy practices for pharmacy technicians. Pharmacy technicians in specialized roles are usually removed from performing the multiple day-to-day tasks within a pharmacy practice; instead, they concentrate on a specific activity within a specific area for which they have been properly trained. Specialized roles usually do not involve the medication-dispensing process but involve increased administrative or clinically oriented activities.

One highly specialized role for a pharmacy technician is that of a clinical pharmacy technician. In this role, the pharmacy technician performs routine clinical activities that do not involve the professional judgment of a pharmacist. The technician receives clinical training that enables her to support the pharmacist in providing pharmaceutical care. In a clinical pharmacy technician role, the pharmacy technician may collect and manage clinical data and laboratory results, perform patient screening according to preset protocols, take patient drug histories, manage clinical projects, generate reports of clinical activities, and even go on routine daily rounds with pharmacists and other interdisciplinary health care team members. A clinical pharmacy technician may perform quality assurance activities such as tracking medication errors, adverse drug reactions, and outcomes. A clinical pharmacy technician also may assist a pharmacist in performing federally mandated drug regimen reviews by gathering information and clinical data and checking compliance with approved criteria according to the federal indicators. As pharmacists find opportunities to expand their clinical pharmacy roles, clinical pharmacy technicians allow them the time and assistance to perform them.

Another specialized pharmacy technician role is that of an ambulatory clinic assistant. In this role, the pharmacy technician directly supports the pharmacist in the provision of pharmaceutical care, where pharmacists provide a level of care traditionally provided by physicians for a variety of diseases and conditions. Ambulatory clinics improve the outcomes of drug therapy through patient education, screening, evaluation, and drug and dosage adjustments. Pharmacy technicians can be found in outpatient clinics, such as anticoagulation clinics, smoking cessation clinics, hyperlipidemia clinics, diabetes clinics, asthma clinics, immunization clinics, and refill clinics. The technician may be responsible for patient communication and education, assisting in patient care, maintaining accurate patient information and clinical patient data, handling referrals, preparing correspondence to referring physicians, and billing.

Another specialized pharmacy technician role is that of an operating room or anesthesia pharmacy technician. This role involves the placement of a pharmacy technician in the operating room or the anesthesia department of a hospital in order to improve drug distribution and accountability. The operating room is one of the most intensive areas of drug use within a hospital. The technician is responsible for maintaining an adequate floor stock of the drugs used in this department; monitoring the use of certain drugs, especially controlled substances; inspecting drug storage areas for proper storage conditions and expired drugs; controlling drug costs by eliminating waste; switching manufacturers and obtaining drugs on contract; collecting data and maintaining records; and acting as a liaison between the pharmacy and the operating room. An operating room or anesthesia pharmacy technician helps control drug costs and reduce drug waste in these departments.

## BOX 15–2    Specialized Pharmacy Technician Roles

Clinical pharmacy technician
Ambulatory clinic assistant
Operating room/anesthesia pharmacy technician
Extemporaneous compounding technician
Oncology pharmacy technician
Investigational drug service pharmacy technician
Pharmacy reimbursement specialist
Quality assurance technician
Pharmacy technician trainer
Pharmacy purchasing technician
Narcotic control technician
Pharmacy technician manager

Several other specialized pharmacy technician roles in various pharmacy practice areas have been identified. Examples of these roles are found in Box 15–2.

## INNOVATIVE PHARMACY TECHNICIAN ROLES

There are several pharmacy technician roles that are considered to be innovative or new. **Innovative pharmacy technician roles** are defined as roles that involve new areas for pharmacy technicians, areas in which they have never been previously involved and areas that are outside of traditional pharmacy practice. These roles are usually found in very progressive pharmacy practices.

One innovative role for pharmacy technicians is that of a certified fitter. A **certified fitter** is a person who is trained and qualified to fit orthotic and prosthetic devices and mastectomy supplies as prescribed by a physician. An orthotic device, or **orthosis,** is a support or brace for weak or ineffective joints or muscles. A prosthetic device, or **prosthesis,** is an artificial device used to replace a missing part of the body. A pharmacy technician wishing to become a certified fitter must attend a fitter education seminar approved by the American Board for Certification in Orthotics and Prosthetics Incorporated. These training seminars are usually sponsored by the manufacturers of these products, for example, the Trulife Institute of Applied Technology through Trulife (800-788-2267). In these intensive courses, the student learns basic anatomy, physiology, terminology, conditions for which orthotic and prosthetic devices are prescribed, the range of available products, proper fitting techniques, the use of specialized fitting tools, and marketing techniques. To maintain certification, the certified fitter must complete 30 hours of continuing education (35 hours if also certified to fit a breast prosthesis) every 5 years. Examples of these products, which are often referred to as surgical supplies, include supports, breast prostheses, cervical collars, traction equipment, and support stockings (Figure 15–1). Many retail pharmacies specialize in surgical supplies as an extension of their professional service.

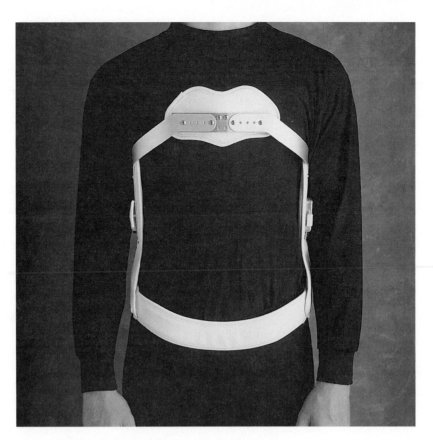

**FIGURE 15–1** Rigid Orthosis. (Courtesy of Trulife.)

Another innovative pharmacy technician role is that of a pharmacy technician instructor in a formal pharmacy technician education program. This role goes beyond the training of a new pharmacy technician by an experienced pharmacy technician within a pharmacy. In this role, the pharmacy technician may teach at a local community college or a career school, in a certificate program or 2-year associate degree program for pharmacy technicians. This role requires a pharmacy technician with extensive knowledge, experience, and excellent communication skills and is one of the most rewarding of all advanced pharmacy technician positions.

Innovative pharmacy technician roles are found not only in pharmacy but also in other nontraditional work environments, where the knowledge and skills of pharmacy technicians are recognized. Pharmacy technicians may be utilized by medical insurance companies, medical software companies, health care information systems companies, drug wholesale companies, medical supply companies, pharmacy supply companies, physician practices, biotechnology companies, and food and beverage companies. For example, a pharmacy technician may be employed by a medical insurance company as a pharmacy insurance specialist because of her knowledge of medications and the operations of a retail pharmacy and her computer experience. A pharmacy technician may work for a medical software company or a health care information systems company because of her knowledge of pharmacy software systems as well as medications and pharmacy terminology. A pharmacy technician may be employed by a drug wholesale company, a medical supply company, or a pharmacy supply company in a sales, customer service, or service technician position because of her experience in dealing with customers and her overall pharmacy or medical knowledge. A pharmacy technician may also be employed by a physician practice as a prescription technician to handle patient prescriptions because of her pharmacy background and computer experience. Finally, a pharmacy technician may work for a biotechnology company or a food and beverage company because of her knowledge of sterile product preparation and aseptic technique. The opportunities are endless.

## PHARMACY TECHNICIAN LIABILITY

The pharmacist is legally responsible for the safe and accurate dispensing of medications and for the education, monitoring, and care of patients. Part of this responsibility is accountability for all activities performed by a pharmacy technician. The pharmacist assumes responsibility for a pharmacy technician's actions under the legal **doctrine of respondeat superior.** According to the doctrine of respondeat superior, an employer is responsible for the actions of her employee. A pharmacist who supervises a pharmacy technician is responsible for any negligent act committed by the pharmacy technician while performing her duties. For example, if a pharmacy technician places the wrong prescription label on a prescription vial, and as a result the patient takes the wrong medication and suffers some harm, the pharmacist is held liable. In addition to this legal doctrine, some state boards of pharmacy regulations specifically hold the pharmacist liable for the actions of a pharmacy technician and can impose a disciplinary action, such as revoking the pharmacist's license.

A pharmacy technician may be exposed to liability under the doctrine of *negligence per se.* **Negligence** is broadly defined as the failure to do something that a reasonable person might do, or doing something that a reasonable person might not do. As it applies to the practice of pharmacy, it is the failure to provide a reasonable standard of care that is expected of a pharmacist. According to the doctrine of negligence per se, a pharmacist or pharmacy technician working under the supervision of a pharmacist who violates a law or regulation that establishes a standard of care and that is designed to protect the patient may be guilty of negligence. For example, if a pharmacy technician incorrectly accepts a verbal order for a new prescription in a state that does not allow this practice, and some harm occurs to the patient as a result, the pharmacy technician may be guilty of negligence.

**Malpractice** is defined as negligence performed by a professional, such as a pharmacist or a pharmacy technician who is working under the supervision of a pharmacist. The majority of malpractice claims in pharmacy are for errors. There are two types of pharmacy errors: mechanical errors and intellectual errors. A **mechanical error** is an error that is mechanical in nature; that is, it involves activities related to the physical dispensing of a medication (Fink, Vivian, & Bernstein, 2005). Examples of mechanical errors are when an incorrect drug or the incorrect strength of a drug is dispensed, or when the wrong directions are placed on the prescription label. The majority of pharmacy malpractice claims are for mechanical errors. An **intellectual error** involves an error in judgment on the part of the pharmacist (Fink, Vivian, & Bernstein, 2005). Examples are when a pharmacist gives incorrect advice, fails to perform a prospective drug regimen review to check for drug interactions or inappropriate drug use, or fails to warn the patient concerning potential side effects. Pharmacists may be exposed to more intellectual errors as they perform more pharmaceutical care activities. Pharmacy technicians may be involved in more mechanical errors as they perform more dispensing activities and assume more advanced roles. Pharmacy technicians can also be involved in intellectual errors, such as overriding a drug interaction warning during prescription processing, giving inaccurate advice to patients, or counseling patients when doing so is not permitted by law.

Finally, a pharmacy technician may face a lawsuit from a supervising pharmacist under the doctrine of contribution. According to the **doctrine of contribution,** a **tortfeasor,** defined as a person who commits a wrong or harm, may bring a lawsuit against a joint tortfeasor to collect a portion of the damages awarded to the injured party. **Joint tortfeasors** are two or more persons who share liability in committing a wrong or harm. As the concept applies to our discussion, joint tortfeasors would be a pharmacist and a pharmacy technician. The pharmacist who faces a lawsuit for an error performed by a pharmacy technician under her supervision can initiate a lawsuit against the pharmacy technician, even though the pharmacist shares liability for the error. This sharing of liability is referred to as **joint liability.** For example, a pharmacy pays damages to a patient as a result of a dispensing error. The pharmacy then sues the pharmacist to recover the damages. The pharmacist, in turn, can sue the pharmacy technician.

Pharmacy technicians can be exposed to liability for violating patient confidentiality laws. As they pertain to pharmacy, confidentiality laws are designed to limit the unauthorized access to patient information that is collected and stored in the pharmacy and to protect the confidentiality of that information. A pharmacy technician has access to confidential patient information. She can be sued by a patient for discussing or releasing information about the patient's medical condition or drug use. Pharmacy technicians can also be prosecuted for engaging in deceptive business practices, for example, dispensing a generic drug and labeling it as a brand-name drug or knowingly dispensing outdated or adulterated drugs.

Pharmacy technicians must be aware of the legal consequences of their actions, especially as they accept more advanced roles with greater responsibilities. In order to lessen their risk of liability, pharmacy technicians must be clear about their roles and how to perform their duties as guided by their supervising pharmacist or specific protocol. Pharmacy technicians must not perform activities beyond their training or experience. They must be aware of their limitations and know when to refer a patient to a pharmacist. They must be aware that they face legal consequences and that there is legal responsibility if their activities are performed in an inaccurate or negligent manner. Finally and most important, they must place the welfare of the patient first in all that they do.

Several insurance companies have introduced individual liability insurance policies for pharmacy technicians. A pharmacy technician liability policy provides coverage for a pharmacy technician's activities. This opportunity for coverage has resulted from the recognition that pharmacy technician roles and responsibilities have changed. Most insurance companies require that a pharmacy technician have completed a recognized pharmacy technician training program to qualify for pharmacy technician insurance coverage. Some states do not allow pharmacy technician liability coverage.

## BENEFITS OF ADVANCED PHARMACY TECHNICIAN ROLES

The use of pharmacy technicians in advanced roles has many benefits. First, pharmacists are able to use their time more efficiently. Pharmacists have more time to counsel patients about their medications; respond to questions from patients and health care professionals; screen for duplicate drug therapies, drug interactions, adverse reactions, and inappropriate drug use; attend rounds with physicians; and develop clinical programs. The increased time for pharmaceutical care activities by pharmacists results in more and better patient care services and, therefore, improved patient care. The use of pharmacy technicians in advanced roles also decreases health care costs. Decreased health care costs result from preventing drug-related problems through pharmaceutical care services provided by pharmacists. Decreased costs also result from decreasing pharmacist staff levels by utilizing more pharmacy technicians and from increasing the productivity of the pharmacy department as a whole. Pharmacy technicians also help the pharmacist improve payment from third parties for pharmacy services. Finally, expanded, specialized, and innovative pharmacy technician roles increase the employment opportunities available to highly trained and motivated pharmacy technicians. These advanced roles ultimately lead to increased job satisfaction and performance, as well as increased respect and higher salaries.

## KEY CONCEPTS

- Advanced roles for pharmacy technicians have emerged as a result of increased pharmaceutical care activities being performed by pharmacists, and involve increased responsibility and require advanced training and experience.
- Expanded pharmacy technician roles are an expansion of current traditional pharmacy technician duties in the preparation and dispensing of medications.
- Specialized pharmacy technician roles concentrate on one aspect of pharmacy practice.
- Innovative pharmacy technician roles involve new areas for the pharmacy technician, areas outside of traditional pharmacy practice.
- Pharmacy technicians face increased liability in performing advanced pharmacy technician roles.
- Benefits associated with advanced pharmacy technician roles include increased time for pharmaceutical care activities by pharmacists, decreased health care costs, and increased employment opportunities and job satisfaction for pharmacy technicians.

## SELF-ASSESSMENT QUESTIONS

### MULTIPLE CHOICE

1.  All of the following are examples of specialized pharmacy technician roles except:
    a. community pharmacy technician
    b. ambulatory clinic assistant
    c. clinical pharmacy technician
    d. operating room pharmacy technician

2.  All of the following are examples of expanded pharmacy technician roles except:
    a. accepting new prescriptions over the phone
    b. obtaining refill authorization
    c. repackaging medications
    d. transferring prescription copies

3.  All of the following are examples of innovative pharmacy technician roles except:
    a. pharmacy technician instructor in a formal training program
    b. hospital pharmacy technician
    c. certified fitter
    d. prescription technician in a physician's office

4.  The legal doctrine that makes a pharmacist responsible for the negligence of a pharmacy technician is:
    a. negligence per se
    b. contribution
    c. respondeat superior
    d. joint tortfeasor

5.  The legal doctrine that allows a pharmacist to sue a pharmacy technician to collect a portion of the damages awarded to the injured party is:
    a. negligence per se
    b. contribution
    c. respondeat superior
    d. joint tortfeasor

6.  An example of a mechanical error is:
    a. the wrong drug is dispensed
    b. the wrong strength of a drug is dispensed
    c. the wrong directions are printed on the prescription label
    d. all of the above

7.  Nontraditional work settings for pharmacy technicians include:
    a. medical insurance companies
    b. drug wholesale companies
    c. medical computer software companies
    d. all of the above

8. A clinical pharmacy technician may perform all of the following duties except:

   a. take patient drug histories
   b. make clinical judgments
   c. track medication errors
   d. assist the pharmacist in performing drug regimen reviews

9. The most important way for pharmacy technicians to lessen their risk of liability is:

   a. to perform activities per protocols
   b. not to perform activities beyond their training or experience
   c. to refer patients to the pharmacist when necessary
   d. to place the welfare of the patient first

10. Advanced roles benefit pharmacy technicians by:

   a. increasing salaries
   b. increasing job satisfaction
   c. increasing respect
   d. all of the above

## TRUE/FALSE (CORRECT THE FALSE STATEMENTS)

1. _____ Pharmacy technicians performing advanced roles face increased liability.
2. _____ The majority of pharmacy lawsuits involve intellectual errors.
3. _____ The checking of one technician's work by another technician does not involve professional judgment.
4. _____ Pharmacy technicians in specialized roles perform multiple day-to-day pharmacy tasks.
5. _____ Pharmacy technicians can be found in outpatient clinics.
6. _____ One benefit of having an operating room technician is better accountability for controlled substances.
7. _____ Innovative pharmacy technician roles can be found in work environments other than pharmacy.
8. _____ Pharmacy technicians are more likely to make mechanical errors than intellectual errors.
9. _____ Pharmacy technicians should not perform any activities beyond their training and experience.
10. _____ State boards of pharmacy regulations limit the roles of pharmacy technicians.

## FILL-IN

1. The final checking of the work of one pharmacy technician by another pharmacy technician is referred to as _____.
2. A _____ _____ is a person who is trained and qualified to fit orthotic and prosthetic devices as prescribed by a physician.
3. _____ pharmacy technician roles are an extension of current traditional pharmacy technician roles.
4. _____ pharmacy technician roles concentrate on one aspect of pharmacy practice.

5. _____ pharmacy technician roles involve new areas of involvement for pharmacy technicians.
6. A support or brace for a weak or ineffective joint or muscle is an _____.
7. The type of error that involves professional judgment is an _____ error.
8. A _____ is a person who commits a wrong or harm.
9. As it pertains to pharmacy, _____ is the failure to provide a reasonable standard of care that is expected of a pharmacist.
10. An artificial device that is used to replace a missing body part is called a _____.

## CRITICAL THINKING

1. Why are the advanced knowledge and skills of some pharmacy technicians often underutilized, and what are some possible solutions to this problem?
2. Can expanded, specialized, and innovative pharmacy technician roles be found in all pharmacy practice settings?
3. Why is it important for pharmacy technicians to perform their duties within the level of their training and experience?
4. Select an example of an expanded pharmacy technician role and compare it to the traditional pharmacy technician role.
5. Why can failing to do something result in a criminal charge of negligence?

## BIBLIOGRAPHY

Andalo, D. (2005). Cancer services benefit from a clinical liaison technician. *Hospital Pharmacist, 12*(12), 452–453.

Arnold, N. (2005). Delivering CPD support—A role for pharmacy technicians. *Hospital Pharmacist, 12*(9), 327–330.

Baker, K. (2005). What responsibilities can be delegated to techs? *Drug Topics, 149*(1), 45–46.

Banzon, S., & Vue, T. (2004). Technician career ladders. *Journal of Pharmacy Technology, 20*(6), 353–355.

Buglass, A. (2006). Emergency department—A role for pharmacy technicians. *Hospital Pharmacist, 13*(4), 139–140.

ContinuingEducation.com. (2005). *The pharmacy technician and professional liability, Program I.D. Number:312-000-05-024-H03.* [On-line] ContinuingEducation.com. Available: www.continuingeducation.com.

Daly, K. (2005). FMEA and the technician's role. *Journal of Pharmacy Technology, 21*(3), 171.

Eckel, F. (2006). Expand the role of pharmacy techs? *Pharmacy Times, 72*(7), 13.

Faulkner, B., Bateman, S., Marren, M., & Harrison, I. (2006). Medicines management technicians in mental health. *Hospital Pharmacist, 13*(2), 58–60.

Fink, J., Vivian, J., & Bernstein, I. (Eds.). (2005). *Pharmacy law digest* (40th ed.). St. Louis, MO: Facts and Comparisons.

Fitzgerald, D. (2005). Opportunities for technicians. *Journal of Pharmacy Technology, 21*(5), 299.

Gebhart, F. (2006). California accepts "tech-check-tech" in hospitals. *Drug Topics, 150*(11), 19.

Lloyd, S. (2005). "Educational pearls": 2005 Pharmacy Technician Educators Council annual meeting report. *Journal of Pharmacy Technology, 21*(5), 281–282.

Oyekan, E. (2005). Population management support coordinators: Pharmacy technicians in population care management. *Journal of Pharmacy Technology, 21*(5), 299–300.

Rose, D., Evans, S., & Williams, R. (2005). Introducing a technician discharge prescription transcribing service. *Hospital Pharmacist, 12*(6), 233–236.

Telford, J. (2005). Developing technician-focused controlled drug management. *Hospital Pharmacist, 12*(3), 113–116.

University of the Sciences in Philadelphia. (2005). *Remington: The science and practice of pharmacy* (21st ed.). Easton, PA: Mack Publishing Company.

Wilson, D., Brushwood, D., & Kimberlin, C. (2006). Regulation and Florida pharmacy technicians. *Journal of Pharmacy Technology, 22*(1), 63–67.

Woods, A., Currie, M., Scott, M., & McElnay, J. (2005). Introducing a technician-led inhaler counseling service. *Hospital Pharmacist, 12*(11), 417–418.

# Apparent Irregularities

An apparent irregularity is a drug therapy circumstance that may constitute an irregularity.

> *Source:* Indicators for Surveyor Assessment of the Performance of Drug Regimen Review, State Operations Manual, Provider Certification, Department of Health and Human Services, Health Care Financing Administration, Transmittal No. 242, September 1990.

- Multiple orders of the same drug for the same patient by the same route of administration
- Drugs administered in disregard of established stop order policies
- As needed (p.r.n.) drug orders administered as directed every day for more than 30 days
- Patients receiving three or more laxatives concurrently
- Use of antipsychotic or antidepressant drugs for fewer than 3 days
- Continuous use of hypnotic drugs (sleep medications) for more than 30 days
- Use of two or more hypnotic drugs at the same time or administered in excess of maximum doses (based on patient age)
- Use of two or more antipsychotic drugs at the same time
- Use of antipsychotic drugs in excess of maximum daily doses (based on patient age)
- Use of antipsychotic drugs unless the clinical record documents that specific conditions exist (that justify their use)
- Use of antipsychotic drugs in the absence of gradual dose reduction attempted every 6 months after therapy was initiated
- Use of antipsychotic drugs when one or more specific behaviors (that do not warrant their use) are the only indication for use
- Use of a p.r.n. antipsychotic drug more than five times in any 7-day period without a review of the resident's condition by a physician
- Use of anxiolytic (antianxiety) drugs in excess of maximum doses (based on patient age)
- More than two changes of an antidepressant drug within a 7-day period
- Use of antidepressant drugs in excess of maximum daily dosages (based on patient age)
- Patients who repeatedly lose seizure control while taking anticonvulsant drugs

- Patients who are taking thyroid drugs and have not had some assessment of thyroid function
- Patients who are taking antihypertensive drugs and have not had a blood pressure recorded at least weekly
- Patients who are taking anticoagulant drugs and have not had some assessment of blood clotting function at least monthly
- Patients who are taking cardioactive drugs and have not had a pulse rate recorded daily in the first month of therapy and weekly thereafter, or if the chart shows a pulse consistently below 60 or above 100
- Patients who are taking insulin or oral hypoglycemic drugs and have not had a urine sugar test at least daily or a blood sugar test at least every 60 days
- Patients who are taking iron preparations, folic acid, or vitamin $B_{12}$ and have not had a red blood cell assessment during the first month of therapy
- Use of urinary tract antibiotics in chronic urinary tract infections if urinalysis has not been performed at least once, 30 days after therapy was initiated
- Patients who are taking Mandelamine or Hiprex (drugs that require an acidic urine to produce an effect) and have not had a urine pH determination within 30 days after therapy was initiated
- Use of nitrofurantoin for conditions other than treatment or prophylaxis of urinary tract infections
- Three or more orders for analgesics used at the same time
- Patients who are taking diuretic drugs and have not had a serum potassium level determination within 30 days after therapy was initiated
- Patients who are taking certain diuretic drugs and cardioactive drugs at the same time and have not had a serum potassium level determination within 30 days after initiation of the cardioactive drug and every 6 months thereafter
- Use of cardioactive drugs without documentation of specific diagnoses (that justify their use)
- Use of anticholinergic drugs with antipsychotic drugs in the absence of recorded extrapyramidal side effects
- Continuous use of an antibiotic/steroidal ophthalmic preparation for more than 14 days
- Use of aminoglycoside drugs without a serum creatinine determination when therapy was initiated
- Orders for drugs for which there is a known allergy as documented in the resident's chart
- Crushing solid dosage forms when the result may be patient discomfort or undesired blood levels

# Material Safety Data Sheet

## 1. IDENTIFICATION OF THE SUBSTANCE/ PREPARATION

NAME: TAMOXIFEN CITRATE

**Alternative Names**

ICI 46,474
Nolvadex
Tamoxifen citrate
(Z)-2-(4(1,2-Diphenylbut-1-enyl)phenoxy)ethyldimethylamine citrate

## 2. COMPOSITION/INFORMATION ON INGREDIENTS

CAS No.:    054965-24-1
EC No.:    259-415-2
Use:    treatment of breast cancer and infertility

| Hazardous Ingredient(s) | CAS No. | Symbol | R Phrases |
|---|---|---|---|
| Tamoxifen citrate | 054965-24-1 | T,N | R45 R48/25 |
| | | | R60 R61 |
| | | | R50/53 |
| | | | Carc. Cat. 1 |
| | | | Repr. Cat. 1 |

## 3. HAZARDS IDENTIFICATION

**Toxic:** Danger of serious damage to health by prolonged exposure if swallowed. May impair fertility. May cause harm to the unborn child. May cause cancer. Very toxic to aquatic organisms; may cause long-term adverse effects in the aquatic environment. Can form flammable dust clouds in air.

## 4. FIRST AID MEASURES

**Inhalation:**    Remove patient from exposure. Obtain medical attention.
**Skin Contact:**    Remove contaminated clothing. Wash skin with water.
**Eye Contact:**    Irrigate with eyewash solution or clean water, holding the eyelids apart, for at least 10 minutes. Obtain medical attention.
**Ingestion:**    Wash out mouth with water. Obtain medical attention.

**Further Medical Treatment**

Symptomatic treatment and supportive therapy as indicated. There is no specific antidote.

## 5. FIRE-FIGHTING MEASURES

Burns with flames. It is sensitive to ignition by electrostatic discharge. The material can form flammable dust clouds in air.

**Extinguishing Media:** Water spray, foam, dry powder or $CO_2$.

## 6. ACCIDENTAL RELEASE MEASURES

Do not scatter the dry material. Moisten spillages with water.

## 7. HANDLING AND STORAGE

### 7.1 HANDLING

Avoid exposure. Obtain special instructions before use. Do not breathe dust. Avoid contact with skin and eyes. Take precautionary measures against static discharges.

### 7.2 STORAGE

Keep container tightly closed. Protect from light.

## 8. EXPOSURE CONTROLS/PERSONAL PROTECTION

Wear suitable respiratory protective equipment if exposure to levels above the occupational exposure limit is likely. Wear suitable protective clothing and gloves.

### OCCUPATIONAL EXPOSURE LIMITS

|  | LTEL 8hr TWA | | STEL 15min | |
| --- | --- | --- | --- | --- |
| **Hazardous Ingredient(s)** | **ppm** | **mg/m³** | **ppm** | **mg/m³** |
| Tamoxifen | – | 0.01 | – | – COM |

## 9. PHYSICAL AND CHEMICAL PROPERTIES

| | |
| --- | --- |
| Form: | crystalline powder |
| Color: | white to almost white |
| pH (Value): | no data |
| Boiling Point (Deg C): | no data |
| Melting Point (Deg C): | 140 |
| Vapor Pressure (Pascals): | |
| Solubility (Water): | sparingly soluble |
| Solubility (Other): | sparingly soluble in acetone; soluble in methanol; freely soluble in aqueous ethanol |
| Partition Coefficient (Log Pow): | 3.9–4.5 |
| Flammable Powder Class: | A |
| Specific Gravity: | no data |
| Vapor Density (Air = 1): | no data |
| Dissociation constant: | 5.67–7.73 |

## 10. STABILITY AND REACTIVITY

Stable at room temperature.

| | |
| --- | --- |
| **Hazardous Reactions:** | none known |
| **Hazardous Decomposition Product(s):** | none known |

# 11. TOXICOLOGICAL INFORMATION

**Inhalation:** Atmospheric concentrations in excess of the occupational exposure limit may lead to adverse effects, as described under long term.

**Skin Contact:** Slight/mild irritant following repeated applications to rat skin. May cause skin irritation in sensitive individuals. It is not a strong skin sensitizer in animal tests. Unlikely to cause skin sensitization.

**Eye Contact:** No evidence of irritant effects from normal handling and use.

**Ingestion:** May cause adverse effects, as described under long term. Oral Median Lethal Dose 2000–3000 mg/kg (rat).

**Long-Term Exposure:** Toxic: danger of serious damage to health by prolonged exposure if swallowed. Repeated exposure may produce adverse effects on eyes and liver. May impair fertility. May cause harm to the unborn child. May cause cancer. Chronic ingestion studies in animals have shown that high doses of tamoxifen produce cancer (liver tumors) observed in rats dosed at 5, 20, and 35 mg/day in a 2-year carcinogenicity study. Epidemiological studies have shown that repeated exposures are associated with increased incidence of endometrial cancer. None of these effects are likely to occur in humans, provided exposure is maintained at or below the occupational exposure limit.

# 12. ECOLOGICAL INFORMATION

## ENVIRONMENTAL FATE AND DISTRIBUTION

The substance is soluble in water. It should be noted that this solubility is different from that quoted in Section 9. Solid with low volatility. The product has high potential for bioaccumulation. The substance has low mobility in soil.

## PERSISTENCE AND DEGRADATION

The substance shows no evidence for biodegradability in water. Biological oxygen demand (BOD 28 day) 0.18 g $O_2$/g. Chemical oxygen demand (COD) 1.74 g $O_2$/g. Biological oxygen demand (BOD 28 day/COD) 10%. There is evidence of hydrolysis in water (pH7, pH9). There is no evidence of hydrolysis in water (pH5).

## TOXICITY

Very toxic to aquatic organisms; may cause long-term adverse effects in the aquatic environment. LC50 (rainbow trout) (96 hour) (flow through) 0.41 mg/l. The no effect concentration was 0.15 mg/l. LC50 (bluegill sunfish) (96 hour) (flow through) 0.23 mg/l. The no effect concentration was 100 mg/l. EC50 (nitrifying bacteria) >100 mg/l. No observed effect concentration (cell density) (green algae) (14 days) 0.012 mg/l. No observed effect concentration (growth rate) (green algae) (14 days) 0.049 mg/l. No observed effect concentration (cell density) (blue-green algae) (21 days) 0.098 mg/l. No observed effect concentration (growth rate) (blue-green algae) (21 days) 0.098 mg/l.

**EFFECT ON EFFLUENT TREATMENT**

This substance was not shown to be biodegradable under anaerobic conditions.

## 13. DISPOSAL CONSIDERATIONS

Disposal should be in accordance with local, state, or national legislation.

This material and/or its container must be disposed of as hazardous waste.

## 14. TRANSPORT INFORMATION

| | |
|---|---|
| UN No.: | 3077 |
| UN Pack. Group: | III |

**Air**

| | |
|---|---|
| ICAO/IATA Class—primary: | 9 |

**Sea**

| | |
|---|---|
| IMDG Class—primary: | 9 |
| Marine Pollutant: | Classified as a marine pollutant |
| UN Packing Group Sea: | III |
| Proper Shipping Name: | ENVIRONMENTALLY HAZARDOUS SUBSTANCES, SOLID, N.O.S. |

**Road/Rail**

| | |
|---|---|
| ADR/RID Class—primary: | 9 |
| ADR/RID Item No.: | 12(c) |
| CDG Road Class—primary: | 9 |

## 15. REGULATORY INFORMATION

Users should ensure that they comply with any relevant local, state or national legislation. EC category 1 Carcinogen. EC category 1 Toxic for Reproduction

| | |
|---|---|
| EC Classification: | TOXIC, DANGEROUS FOR THE ENVIRONMENT |
| Hazard Symbol: | T, N |
| Risk Phrases: | R45: May cause cancer. R48/25: Toxic: danger of serious damage to health by prolonged exposure if swallowed. R60: May impair fertility. R61: May cause harm to the unborn child. R50/53: Very toxic to aquatic organisms, may cause long-term adverse effects in the aquatic environment. |
| Safety Phrases: | S22: Do not breathe dust. S28: After contact with skin, wash immediately with plenty of water. S45: In case of accident or if you feel unwell, seek medical advice immediately (show the label when possible). S53: Avoid exposure. Obtain special instructions before use. S60: This material and/or its container must be disposed of as hazardous waste. S61: Avoid release to the environment. Refer to special instructions/Safety data sheet. |

## 16. OTHER INFORMATION

This data sheet was prepared in accordance with Directive 91/155/EEC (93/112/EC).

The following sections contain revisions or new statements: 3,8

## GLOSSARY

OES: Occupational Exposure Standard (UK HSE EH40)
MEL: Maximum Exposure Limit (UK HSE EH40)
COM: The company aims to control exposure in its workplace to this limit
LTEL: Long-term exposure limit (8-hour TWA)
STEL: Short-term exposure limit (15-minute)
TLV: The company aims to control exposure in its workplace to the ACGIH limit
TLV-C: The company aims to control exposure in its workplace to the ACGIH Ceiling limit
MAK: The company aims to control exposure in its workplace to the German limit
Sk: Can be absorbed through skin
Sen: Capable of causing respiratory sensitization

(Revision: 12 Date: 0505)

(UK00)
UK02
(PH130/15)

*(Reprinted with permission of AstraZeneca)*

# Professional Organizations

## ■ LONG-TERM CARE PHARMACY

American Society of Consultant Pharmacists (ASCP)
1321 Duke Street
Alexandria, Virginia 22314-3563
(703) 739-1300 or (800) 355-2727
(703) 739-1321 or (800) 220-1321 Fax
www.ascp.com

## ■ HOME INFUSION PHARMACY

American Society for Parenteral and Enteral
    Nutrition (ASPEN)
8630 Fenton Street, Suite 412
Silver Spring, Maryland 20910
(301) 587-6315 or (800) 727-4567
(301) 587-2365 Fax
www.nutritioncare.org

Board of Pharmaceutical Specialties (BPS)—
    (Nutrition Support Pharmacy)
1100 15th Street, NW, Suite 400
Washington, D.C. 20005-1707
(202) 429-7591
(202) 429-6304 Fax
www.bpsweb.org

National Home Infusion Association (NHIA)
205 Daingerfield Road
Alexandria, Virginia 22314
(703) 549-3740
(703) 683-1484 Fax
www.nhianet.org

Institute for Safe Medical Practices (ISMP)
1800 Byberry Road, Suite 810
Huntingdon Valley, Pennsylvania 19006
(215) 947-7797
(215) 914-1492 Fax
www.ismp.org

## ■ MANAGED CARE PHARMACY

Academy of Managed Care Pharmacy (AMCP)
100 North Pitt Street, Suite 400
Alexandria, Virginia 22314
(703) 683-8416 or (800) 827-2627
(703) 683-8417 Fax
www.amcp.org

National Council for Prescription Drug Programs,
    Inc. (NCPDP)
9240 E. Raintree Drive
Phoenix, Arizona 85260-7518
(480) 477-1000
(480) 767-1042 Fax
www.ncpdp.org

International Society for Pharmacoeconomics and
    Outcomes Research (ISPOR)
3100 Princeton Pike, Building 3, Suite E
Lawrenceville, New Jersey 08648
(609) 219-0773 or (800) 992-0643
(609) 219-0774 Fax
www.ispor.org

National Committee for Quality Assurance (NCQA)
2000 L Street, NW, Suite 500
Washington, D.C. 20036
(202) 955-3500
(202) 955-3599 Fax
www.ncqa.org

## ■ MAIL-ORDER PHARMACY

Pharmaceutical Care Management Association
    (PCMA)
601 Pennsylvania Avenue, NW, Suite 740
Washington, D.C. 20004
(202) 207-3610
(202) 207-3623 Fax
www.pcmanet.org

# ■ NUCLEAR PHARMACY

Board of Pharmaceutical Specialties (BPS)—
    (Nuclear Pharmacy)
1100 15th Street, NW, Suite 400
Washington, D.C. 20005-1707
(202) 429-7591
(202) 429-6304 Fax
www.bpsweb.org

American Pharmacists Association
Academy of Pharmacy Practice and Management
    (APhA-APPM)
Section on Nuclear Pharmacy Practice
1100 15th Street, NW, Suite 400
Washington, D.C. 20005-1707
(202) 628-4410 or (800) 237-2742
(202) 783-2351 Fax
www.aphanet.org

Society of Nuclear Medicine (SNM)
1850 Samuel Morse Drive
Reston, Virginia 20190-5316
(703) 708-9000
(703) 708-9015 Fax
www.snm.org

# ■ HOSPICE PHARMACY

National Hospice and Palliative Care Organization
    (NHPCO)
1700 Diagonal Road, Suite 625
Alexandria, Virginia 22314
(703) 837-1500
(703) 837-1233 Fax
www.nhpco.org

# ■ FEDERAL PHARMACY

Society of Air Force Pharmacists (SAFP)
Scott AFB Pharmacy
375th Medical Group
310 Losey Street
Scott AFB, Illinois 62225
(618) 256-7345
www.af-pharmacists.org

# ■ PHARMACEUTICAL INDUSTRY

Pharmaceutical Research and Manufacturers of
    America (PhRMA)
950 F Street, NW
Washington, D.C. 20004
(202) 835-3400
(202) 835-3414 Fax
www.phrma.org

Certified Medical Representatives Institute, Inc.
    (CMR Institute)
4423 Pheasant Ridge Road, Suite 100
Roanoke, Virginia 24014-5274
(540) 989-4596 or (800) 274-2674
(540) 989-4710 Fax
www.cmrinstitute.org

Generic Pharmaceutical Association (GphA)
2300 Clarendon Boulevard, Suite 400
Arlington, Virginia 22201
(703) 647-2480
www.gphaonline.org

Biotechnology Industry Organization
1225 I Street, NW, Suite 400
Washington, D.C. 20005
(202) 962-9200
www.bio.org

# ■ ADVANCED PHARMACY TECHNICIAN ROLES

American Board for Certification in Orthotics
    and Prosthetics (ABC)
330 John Carlyle Street, Suite 210
Alexandria, Virginia 22314
(703) 836-7114
(703) 836-0838 Fax
www.abcop.org

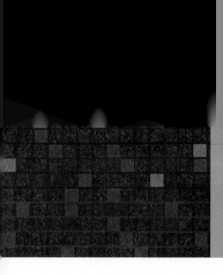

# Professional Publications

## LONG-TERM CARE PHARMACY

*The Consultant Pharmacist*
American Society of Consultant Pharmacists
1321 Duke Street
Alexandria, Virginia 22314-3563
(703) 739-1300 or (800) 355-2727
(703) 739-1321 or (800) 220-1321 Fax
www.ascp.com

## HOME INFUSION PHARMACY

*Nutrition in Clinical Practice* and *Journal of Parenteral and Enteral Nutrition*
American Society for Parenteral and
    Enteral Nutrition
8630 Fenton Street, Suite 412
Silver Spring, Maryland 20910
(301) 587-6315 or (800) 727-4567
(301) 587-2365 Fax
www.nutritioncare.org

*Infusion*
National Home Infusion Association
205 Daingerfield Road
Alexandria, Virginia 22314
(703) 549-3740
(703) 683-1484 Fax
www.nhianet.org

## MANAGED CARE PHARMACY

*Journal of Managed Care Pharmacy*
Academy of Managed Care Pharmacy
100 North Pitt Street, Suite 400
Alexandria, Virginia 22314
(730) 683-8416 or (800) 827-2627
(730) 683- 8417 Fax
www.amcp.org

*Value in Health*
International Society for Pharmacoeconomics
    and Outcomes Research
3100 Princeton Pike, Building 3, Suite E
Lawrenceville, New Jersey 08648
(609) 219-0773 or (800) 992-0643
(609) 219-0774 Fax
www.ispor.org

*Formulary*
7500 Old Oak Boulevard
Cleveland, Ohio 44130
(800) 225-4569
(440) 891-2683 Fax
www.formularyjournal.com

*Drug Benefit Trends*
330 Boston Post Road, P.O. Box 4027
Darien, Connecticut 06820-4027
(203) 662-6599
(203) 662-6777 Fax
www.cmpmedia.com

*Managed Care Interface*
66 Palmer Avenue, Suite 49
Bronxville, New York 10708
(914) 337-7878
(914) 337-5023 Fax
www.medicomint.com

## NUCLEAR PHARMACY

*Journal of Nuclear Medicine*
Society of Nuclear Medicine
1850 Samuel Morse Drive
Reston, Virginia 20190-5316
(703) 708-9000
(703) 708-9015 Fax
www.snm.org

## ■ HOSPICE PHARMACY

*Journal of Pain and Symptom Management*
National Hospice and Palliative Care Organization
1700 Diagonal Road, Suite 625
Alexandria, Virginia 22314
(703) 837-1500
(703) 837-1233 Fax
www.nhpco.org

*International Journal of Pharmaceutical Compounding*
122 N. Bryant
Edmond, Oklahoma 73034
(800) 757-4572
(405) 330-5622 Fax
www.ijpc.com

## ■ FEDERAL PHARMACY

*The Journal of Air Force Pharmacy*
Society of Air Force Pharmacists
Scott AFB Pharmacy
375th Medical Group
310 Losey Street
Scott AFB, Illinois 62225
(618) 256-7345
www.af-pharmacists.org

*Federal Practitioner*
7 Century Drive, Suite 302
Parsippany, New Jersey 07054-4609
(973) 206-8950
(973) 206-9378 Fax
www.fedprac.com

*VA Practitioner*
P.O. Box 3085
Princeton, New Jersey 08543
(908) 874-8550
(908) 874-5611 Fax
www.publist.com

## ■ PHARMACEUTICAL INDUSTRY

*Pharmaceutical Formulation and Quality*
208 Floral Vale Boulevard
Yardley, Pennsylvania 19067
(215) 860-7800
(215) 860-7900 Fax
www.pharmaquality.com

*Pharmaceutical Representative*
2 Northfield Plaza, Suite 300
Northfield, Illinois 60093-1219
(847) 441-3700 or (800) 451-7838
(847) 441-3701 Fax
www.pharmrep.com

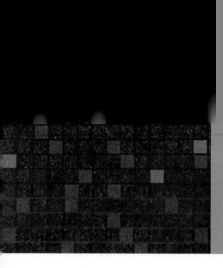

# Answers to Self-Assessment Questions

## CHAPTER 1 PHARMACY AND THE U.S. HEALTH CARE SYSTEM

### MULTIPLE CHOICE

1. d. all of the above
2. b. patient outcomes
3. b. institutions
4. d. surgery centers
5. d. all of the above
6. d. all of the above
7. b. it is provided to a patient in a bed
8. d. nursing home
9. d. health care is available to every American
10. d. all of the above

### TRUE/FALSE

1. TRUE
2. TRUE
3. FALSE – The foundation of a managed care organization is the primary care physician.
4. TRUE
5. TRUE
6. FALSE – Funding for the U.S. health care system comes from public *and* private sources.
7. FALSE – In a three-party system, a payment is made directly to a health care provider by the payer.
8. TRUE
9. FALSE – A preferred provider organization provides health care services to members on a fee-for-service basis.
10. TRUE

### FILL-IN

1. emergency services
2. out-of-pocket
3. retrospective
4. prospective
5. network

6. gatekeeper
7. drug-related problem
8. primary
9. tertiary
10. interdisciplinary

## CHAPTER 2    INTRODUCTION TO LONG-TERM CARE
### MULTIPLE CHOICE

1. b. donations
2. a. acute care facility
3. d. all of the above
4. d. all of the above
5. d. they do not require a good income
6. b. housing but not medical, nursing, or personal care services
7. c. it is the same as home health care
8. a. young-old
9. d. multiple medications
10. d. nursing care

### TRUE/FALSE

1. FALSE – Long-term care is defined as care provided for an extended period of time.
2. TRUE
3. TRUE
4. FALSE – Medicaid is the primary source of publicly funded long-term care.
5. TRUE
6. FALSE – The elderly consume a larger percentage of drugs than younger people.
7. TRUE
8. FALSE – The majority of people who receive long-term care are in the community and home-based settings.
9. TRUE
10. TRUE

### FILL-IN

1. seven
2. nursing home
3. board and care home
4. respite care
5. old-old
6. adverse drug reactions
7. community-based care
8. resident
9. subacute care
10. instrumental activities of daily living

## CHAPTER 3 THE LONG-TERM CARE PHARMACY

### MULTIPLE CHOICE

1. b. multiple vitamin
2. d. 24-hour cassettes
3. a. decreased inventory of medications in the pharmacy
4. d. an intravenous compounding record
5. d. all of the above
6. c. modified unit-dose system
7. a. the nursing facility administrator decides the contents of the emergency box
8. d. it is not necessary to lock a medication cart
9. b. hourly delivery
10. c. the resident's nightstand

### TRUE/FALSE

1. FALSE – An open-shop pharmacy can fill prescriptions for any patient, including long-term care residents.
2. TRUE
3. TRUE
4. FALSE – The emergency medication supply cannot be used as a routine source of medications for long-term care residents. Emergency medications are to be used only for a medical emergency until a delivery from the long-term care pharmacy can be made.
5. TRUE
6. TRUE
7. TRUE
8. TRUE
9. FALSE – The goals of any drug distribution system are safety and efficiency.
10. TRUE

### FILL-IN

1. unit-dose
2. emergency drug
3. in-house
4. turn-around
5. drug distribution system
6. blended
7. multiple medication package
8. security container
9. configuration
10. treatment administration record

## CHAPTER 4   LEGISLATION AND REGULATIONS FOR LONG-TERM CARE PHARMACY

### MULTIPLE CHOICE

1. a. OBRA
2. d. all of the above
3. d. all of the above
4. d. wrong place
5. d. normal saline irrigation
6. a. the administration of drugs
7. d. an optional survey
8. c. renting medication carts to the facility at fair market value
9. a. the facsimile copy does not have to be retained
10. d. all of the above

### TRUE/FALSE

1. FALSE – The Joint Commission will accredit any organization that provides pharmaceutical care and pharmacy services to residents in a long-term care facility.
2. TRUE
3. TRUE
4. FALSE – Current DEA regulations permit controlled substances to be returned only between DEA registrants. Since most long-term care facilities do not have their own pharmacy and are therefore not DEA registrants, they are not permitted to return controlled substances to their contract pharmacy.
5. TRUE
6. TRUE
7. TRUE
8. TRUE
9. TRUE
10. TRUE

### FILL-IN

1. CMS
2. safe harbor
3. 60
4. drug holiday
5. USP
6. seven
7. irregularity
8. five
9. standards
10. chemical

## CHAPTER 5 THE ROLE OF THE PHARMACIST AND THE PHARMACY TECHNICIAN IN LONG-TERM CARE

### MULTIPLE CHOICE

1. b. are usually performed in the long-term care facility
2. d. all of the above
3. a. drug information
4. a. penicillin
5. d. all of the above
6. d. all of the above
7. d. emergency medication supply
8. d. it is performed on an occasional basis
9. c. decrease hospitalizations
10. d. all of the above

### TRUE/FALSE

1. FALSE – There are currently no federal regulations for the provision of consultant pharmacist services in assisted living facilities.
2. TRUE
3. TRUE
4. TRUE
5. TRUE
6. FALSE – The role of the consultant pharmacist in board and care homes is not legally required at this time.
7. TRUE
8. TRUE
9. TRUE
10. FALSE – Pharmacy technicians cannot perform tasks involving professional judgment regarding medication therapy in any pharmacy practice setting; however, they may assist the pharmacist in nonjudgmental activities.

### FILL-IN

1. care planning
2. consultant pharmacist
3. chart review
4. educational
5. cognitive
6. problem-centered
7. appropriate drug use
8. drug regimen review
9. 3
10. inspections

## CHAPTER 6    HOME HEALTH CARE
### MULTIPLE CHOICE

1. b. personal care services
2. a. it is more expensive than in-patient care
3. d. all of the above
4. c. diabetes
5. b. elderly
6. d. all of the above
7. c. hospitals
8. c. long-term care facilities
9. d. all of the above
10. d. dental products

### TRUE/FALSE

1. TRUE
2. TRUE
3. TRUE
4. FALSE – Functional limitations can be physical *or* mental in nature.
5. FALSE – An admission assessment is not the same as an initial assessment. An initial assessment determines if a patient is an appropriate candidate for home care and if home care is the right choice for the patient. It is performed prior to intake. An admission assessment is more extensive than an initial assessment and contains detailed information about the patient and her medical history. It is performed after intake and is the first step in the home health care process.
6. FALSE – Patient monitoring is an important step in the home health care process.
7. TRUE
8. TRUE
9. TRUE
10. TRUE

### FILL-IN

1. homebound
2. durable medical equipment
3. care plan
4. functional limitation
5. discharge summary
6. rehabilitation service
7. iontophoresis
8. intake
9. private health insurance
10. respiratory therapist

# CHAPTER 7    HOME INFUSION PHARMACY

## MULTIPLE CHOICE

1. c. carbohydrate, protein, and lipids in the same bag
2. b. includes a pharmaceutical care plan
3. c. cleaning and tracking infusion devices
4. d. all of the above
5. d. b and c only
6. b. parenteral nutrition therapy
7. c. can remain in place for weeks to months
8. c. sterilizing
9. b. peripheral catheter
10. d. all of the above

## TRUE/FALSE

1. TRUE
2. FALSE – Intravenous infusion pumps cannot be used to deliver enteral therapy. Enteral infusion pumps are used to deliver enteral formulas. They are different from and not interchangeable with intravenous infusion pumps.
3. TRUE
4. TRUE
5. FALSE – The drug inventory in a home infusion pharmacy is a limited and specialized inventory and does not include oral and IV dosage forms of medications.
6. FALSE – Enteral nutrition is less involved than parenteral nutrition. It is the next approach to feeding when oral nutrition is not appropriate or possible. Enteral nutrition formulas are not compounded in the home infusion pharmacy but are commercially available. Parenteral nutrition is highly complex therapy and must be compounded in the home infusion pharmacy. There are several compounding and stability concerns associated with parenteral nutrition solutions.
7. FALSE – The Joint Commission *does* recognize the home infusion pharmacist as an important member of the home health care team. There are specific activities that the Joint Commission expects the home infusion pharmacist to perform or to be involved in.
8. TRUE
9. TRUE
10. TRUE

## FILL-IN

1. anti-infective
2. enteral nutrition therapy
3. medical record
4. vascular access
5. compounding record
6. flushed
7. therapy-specific
8. syringe pump
9. elastomeric balloon system
10. patient additives

## CHAPTER 8    MANAGED CARE PHARMACY

### MULTIPLE CHOICE

1. c. a formulary exception process
2. b. the drug benefit can include tiered co-pays and can exclude certain drugs
3. b. source
4. b. day supply limit
5. d. unit-dose repackaging
6. b. increased calls to help desks
7. d. it is a formulary exception process
8. c. acute medical problems are managed in this way
9. d. all of the above
10. d. all of the above

### TRUE/FALSE

1. TRUE
2. TRUE
3. TRUE
4. TRUE
5. TRUE
6. FALSE – Member satisfaction is an important consideration in prescription drug plans. Managed care organizations work to maintain member and employer satisfaction with the drug benefit while lowering costs and assuring the best possible outcomes of drug therapy.
7. TRUE
8. FALSE – The administrative role of the managed care pharmacist involves drug *benefit* management through various administrative activities. The clinical role of the managed care pharmacist involves drug *therapy* management through clinical activities.
9. FALSE – A managed care organization may not give prescription benefit information to a member's employer without the member's consent. Regulations issued under HIPAA limit the use and release of health information, which includes prescription drug benefit records, restrict the disclosure of information to the minimum needed for the intended purpose, and establish new requirements for access to records by researchers and others.
10. FALSE – Formulary drugs do not require an exception process to be covered. Formulary drugs are drugs already approved for use or reimbursement under a prescription drug plan.

### FILL-IN

1. formulary
2. prior authorization
3. network
4. co-payment
5. disease management
6. Freedom of Choice
7. dispensing fee
8. fixed
9. utilization
10. pharmacy benefit manager

## CHAPTER 9    MAIL-ORDER PHARMACY
### MULTIPLE CHOICE

1. b. distractions
2. d. all of the above
3. d. not disclose its location
4. c. limited patient monitoring
5. c. indirect contact between patient and pharmacist
6. d. counting trays
7. d. all of the above
8. b. adjudication support
9. a. ability to do many tasks at the same time
10. b. facsimile machines

### TRUE/FALSE

1. TRUE
2. TRUE
3. TRUE
4. FALSE – Most prescription drug benefit plans *do* offer a mail-order pharmacy option.
5. TRUE
6. TRUE
7. FALSE – The majority of prescriptions in a mail-order pharmacy are received by mail.
8. FALSE – Pharmacist screening of prescriptions before adjudication is part of the prescription-filling process in a mail-order pharmacy. The pharmacist verifies that all prescription information is correct and performs a prospective drug utilization review before the prescription order is forwarded to adjudication, the next step in the workflow.
9. TRUE
10. FALSE – Despite the large volume of prescriptions dispensed in a mail-order pharmacy, there are fewer dispensing errors than in a traditional retail pharmacy. This is due to the use of automation, employees performing specialized tasks, and fewer distractions in addition to strict quality and safety checks for every prescription filled.

### FILL-IN

1. VIPPS™
2. traditional
3. rogue
4. workflow
5. nonresident
6. task specialization
7. screening
8. TTD
9. certificate of origin
10. filling

## CHAPTER 10    NUCLEAR PHARMACY

### MULTIPLE CHOICE

1. c. carrier drugs
2. d. all of the above
3. d. temperature changes
4. d. all of the above
5. b. a vertical laminar airflow hood
6. d. all of the above
7. c. it is distributed to all areas of the body
8. d. all of the above
9. d. all of the above
10. a. placarding the delivery vehicle

### TRUE/FALSE

1. TRUE
2. FALSE – A centralized nuclear pharmacy operates out of a centralized site in the community. An institutional nuclear pharmacy operates within a nuclear medicine department in an institution.
3. TRUE
4. FALSE – Adverse reactions to radiopharmaceuticals are rare, since the quantities involved are so small.
5. FALSE – The drug inventory in a nuclear pharmacy is completely different from the drug inventory in any other type of pharmacy. It consists of radionuclides and carrier drugs, both unique to the preparation of radiopharmaceuticals
6. TRUE
7. FALSE - A pharmacy technician may accept a verbal order for a radiopharmaceutical for diagnosis. A prescription for a radiopharmaceutical for treatment may be accepted only by a licensed nuclear pharmacist or a pharmacist intern.
8. TRUE
9. TRUE
10. TRUE

### FILL-IN

1. radionuclide
2. technetium
3. carrier drug
4. fume hood
5. Department of Transportation
6. just-in-time
7. breakdown
8. decay
9. eluant
10. half-life

## CHAPTER 11    HOSPICE PHARMACY

### MULTIPLE CHOICE

1. c. manage symptoms
2. b. antibiotics
3. d. all of the above
4. d. all of the above
5. a. burial services
6. c. mail order
7. d. all of the above
8. a. dispensing medications
9. c. elderly
10. a. cholesterol-lowering medications

### TRUE/FALSE

1. TRUE
2. FALSE – Joint Commission accreditation is not awarded to a hospice pharmacy but is awarded to the hospice organization.
3. TRUE
4. TRUE
5. TRUE
6. TRUE
7. TRUE
8. TRUE
9. FALSE – Hospice does not use aggressive treatment to cure disease. Hospice provides palliative care that treats the symptoms associated with a disease to provide comfort and relieve suffering rather than cure the disease.
10. TRUE

### FILL-IN

1. breakthrough
2. opioids
3. pain management
4. starter kit
5. hospice
6. cancer
7. inpatient hospice facility
8. inventory
9. constipation
10. addiction

## CHAPTER 12   FEDERAL PHARMACY

### MULTIPLE CHOICE

1. d. it does not involve patient counseling
2. d. all of the above
3. d. all of the above
4. c. is a highly competent pharmacy technician
5. b. a career ladder for pharmacy technicians
6. c. the same equipment available as in a civilian pharmacy
7. a. the U.S. Navy
8. b. counsel patients
9. c. perform minor surgery
10. c. a mobile field hospital

### TRUE/FALSE

1. FALSE – Military pharmacy technicians have been given greater responsibility than their civilian counterparts.
2. TRUE
3. TRUE
4. TRUE
5. FALSE – A military pharmacy may employ civilian pharmacists and pharmacy technicians. Although the majority of pharmacists and pharmacy technicians in all three branches of the military are active members of the military, they are supported by a small number of civilian pharmacists and pharmacy technicians.
6. TRUE
7. TRUE
8. FALSE – Pharmacy technicians are not found in all of the agencies of the Public Health Service. Pharmacists are found in all of the divisions of the Public Health Service, but pharmacy technicians are found only in the Indian Health Service.
9. TRUE
10. TRUE

### FILL-IN

1. field hospital
2. basic training
3. medical readiness
4. Indian Health Service
5. federal
6. expeditionary medical deployment system
7. networks
8. National Institute of Health
9. electronic record
10. Naval Laboratory

# CHAPTER 13  PHARMACEUTICAL INDUSTRY

## MULTIPLE CHOICE

1. c. packaging and shipping
2. a. provide kickbacks to customers
3. d. detailing is not a marketing strategy
4. d. all of the above
5. d. all of the above
6. d. all of the above
7. a. undergoing clinical trials
8. c. a pharmacy license
9. d. all of the above
10. d. the Kefauver-Harris Amendment

## TRUE/FALSE

1. TRUE
2. TRUE
3. TRUE
4. FALSE – A new drug application is submitted to the FDA to request approval for marketing a new drug. An investigational new drug application is submitted to the FDA to request authorization to begin testing a new drug in humans.
5. TRUE
6. FALSE – Direct distribution involves the sale of a drug to the outlet for the drug, such as a pharmacy retailer, hospital, or government agency. Indirect distribution involves the sale of a drug to an intermediary between the drug manufacturer and the outlet for the drug, which is a drug wholesaler.
7. TRUE
8. TRUE
9. TRUE
10. FALSE – Pharmaceutical manufacturers can provide information on the unapproved use of a drug under the Food and Drug Administration Modernization Act of 1997.

## FILL-IN

1. orphan drug
2. detailing
3. abbreviated new drug application
4. therapeutic equivalent
5. pharmaceutical biotechnology
6. adulterated
7. unapproved use
8. master batch record
9. Prescription Drug Marketing Act
10. good manufacturing practices

# CHAPTER 14   TELEPHARMACY

## MULTIPLE CHOICE

1 b. a remote pharmacy
2 c. video camera
3 b. the lack of the physical presence of the pharmacist
4 a. rural areas
5 d. all of the above
6 c. a private consultation room
7 b. patient consultation
8 d. all of the above
9 c. prescription labeling
10 a. the traditional telepharmacy model

## TRUE/FALSE

1. FALSE – A traditional telepharmacy may be found in remote or sparsely populated areas where there are no traditional retail pharmacies.
2. FALSE – The pharmacy technician in a remote pharmacy may *not* dispense a prescription without a final check by the pharmacist at the base pharmacy site.
3. TRUE
4. FALSE – In a hospital telepharmacy model, drugs are dispensed from an automated dispensing machine located outside of the pharmacy *to* a nurse.
5. FALSE – A remote pharmacy does require its own license as well as its own controlled substance registration, separate from the base pharmacy with which it is associated.
6. TRUE
7. TRUE
8. TRUE
9. TRUE
10. TRUE

## FILL-IN

1. nurse
2. patient counseling
3. base
4. OBRA
5. remote consultation site
6. pharmacy technician
7. hospital telepharmacy
8. traditional telepharmacy
9. DEA
10. consultation room

## CHAPTER 15    ADVANCED PHARMACY TECHNICIAN ROLES

### MULTIPLE CHOICE

1. a. community pharmacy technician
2. c. repackaging medications
3. b. hospital pharmacy technician
4. c. respondeat superior
5. b. contribution
6. d. all of the above
7. d. all of the above
8. b. make clinical judgments
9. d. to place the welfare of the patient first
10. d. all of the above

### TRUE/FALSE

1. TRUE
2. FALSE – The majority of pharmacy lawsuits involve mechanical errors.
3. TRUE
4. FALSE – Pharmacy technicians in specialized roles are removed from performing multiple day-to-day pharmacy tasks, but concentrate on a specific activity within a specific area for which they have been properly trained.
5. TRUE
6. TRUE
7. TRUE
8. TRUE
9. TRUE
10. TRUE

### FILL-IN

1. tech-check-tech
2. certified fitter
3. expanded
4. specialized
5. innovative
6. orthosis
7. intellectual
8. tortfeasor
9. negligence
10. prosthesis

# Glossary

**abbreviated new drug application (ANDA)**—an application submitted to the FDA for the approval of a generic drug

**access**—a patient's ability to obtain medical care

**accreditation**—recognition that an organization meets certain standards

**activity of daily living (ADL)**—an activity that is related to personal care functions

**actual acquisition cost (AAC)**—the actual cost of a drug to a pharmacy

**acute care**—health care needed on an urgent basis for an acute condition

**acute medication**—a medication that is needed on an urgent basis for an acute condition

**addiction**—a psychological and physiological dependence on a drug to obtain a psychic effect

**admission assessment**—the first step in the home health care process once the patient is admitted for care

**adjudication**—electronic submission of a claim to verify insurance coverage and payment

**adult day care**—personal care and social services provided to adults who need supervision while their caregiver works

**adulterated drug**—a drug that is not pure

**adverse drug reaction (ADR)**—a response to a drug that is unexpected, unintended, undesired, or excessive when used in appropriate doses

**allied health personnel**—workers in health-related areas who assist, facilitate, or complement the work of a physician

**alternative medicine**—therapies used instead of traditional medical therapies

**ambulatory care institution**—a health care institution that provides health care services to ambulatory patients

**ambulatory infusion pump**—an infusion device that is portable and worn by the patient

**ambulatory patient**—a patient who is able to walk in to a health care institution for services

**antipsychotic drug**—a drug used in the treatment of psychotic disorders

**apparent irregularity**—a drug therapy circumstance that may constitute an irregularity

**assisted living**—a long-term care setting that provides a homelike environment and some support services

**authorized user**—a person who has met specialized requirements for training and experience in the handling of radioactive materials

**average wholesale price (AWP)**—the average cost of a drug to a pharmacy

**base pharmacy**—a base site that is an actual pharmacy

**base site**—the site at which a supervising pharmacist is located in a telepharmacy practice

**behavior monitoring form**—a form used to document behaviors and information relevant to them

**benefit**—a form of compensation other than wages paid to an employee

**bioequivalent**—delivering the same amount of active ingredient into the bloodstream in the same amount of time by different drugs

**biologics license application (BLA)**—an application submitted to the FDA for the approval of marketing a biotechnology drug

**biotechnology**—the use of biology and technology to solve problems concerning living organisms

**biotechnology drug**—a naturally occurring drug product that produces specific biological changes in the body

**blended unit-dose system**—a drug distribution system that combines a unit-of-use medication package with a non-unit-dose drug distribution system

**board and care home**—a nonmedical living arrangement of two or more people not related to the owner or operator of the home

**breakdown area**—the area in a nuclear pharmacy where empty or unused containers of radiopharmaceuticals are returned and dismantled for reuse

**breakthrough pain**—an episode of acute pain that occurs spontaneously or as a result of a stimulus

**bundling**—the practice of providing a group of goods and services together at no charge or below fair market value in order to obtain or keep business

**capitation**—a health care reimbursement system in which a flat, prepaid fee is paid for a range of health care services

**capitation fee**—a fixed, prepaid fee per person paid to a health care provider to provide a range of health care services

**care plan**—a plan that identifies all of the identified problems being treated and the strategies for treatment

**care planning**—the process that uses information about a long-term care resident to form an individual plan of care for the resident

**carrier drug**—a pharmaceutical that delivers a radionuclide to the desired area of the body for study or treatment

**carve out**—to separate one benefit from a group of benefits

**catheter**—a tube used to inject or infuse fluids into a vein

**central fill pharmacy**—a high-volume pharmacy that fills prescriptions for a number of individual pharmacies

**central vascular access**—access to the bloodstream through a large vein in the chest that empties into the superior vena cava

**central venous catheter**—a rigid intravenous catheter that is surgically inserted into a large vein in the chest

**certification**—formal recognition of meeting certain qualifications for pharmacy technicians

**certified fitter**—a person who is trained and qualified to fit orthotic and prosthetic devices as prescribed by a physician

**chart review**—a drug regimen review

**chemical impurity**—the presence of a foreign chemical in a radiopharmaceutical

**chemical restraint**—a pharmacologic method of restricting a nursing facility resident's physical movement

**clinic services**—ongoing health care services provided for routine or nonemergency medical problems

**clinical trials**—the testing of a new drug in humans

**closed formulary**—a formulary in which a limited list of drugs is covered

**closed-shop pharmacy**—a pharmacy that dispenses medications only for long-term care facility residents

**complementary medicine**—therapies used in conjunction with traditional medical therapies

**compliance**—following the prescribed directions for a specific drug therapy

**compounding record**—the form used in a home infusion pharmacy to document compounding activities

**confidentiality**—restriction of unauthorized access to patient information

**consultant pharmacist**—a pharmacist specially trained to provide pharmaceutical care services to long-term care facility residents

**consultant pharmacy practice**—the practice of pharmacy in which pharmacists provide pharmaceutical care services to achieve definite outcomes of drug therapy and to improve the quality of life for the long-term care resident

**continuity of care**—the continuation of health care services from one health care setting to another

**continuous care retirement community (CCRC)**—a residential arrangement that offers future health care services

**continuum of care**—the movement through continuous levels of care as the patient's needs change

**cost shifting**—shifting the cost of a service from one group to another

**covered drug**—a drug that will be reimbursed under a prescription drug plan

**cycle fill**—a system for obtaining refill medications that occurs automatically by means of a computer program

**day supply limit**—the amount of drug that can be dispensed according to a certain day supply

**direct-to-consumer (DTC) advertising**—the promotion of a new drug directly to patients instead of to health care professionals

**disability**—any medical condition that results in a functional limitation

**disease management**—a coordinated approach to treating a specific disease that involves the entire health care team

**dispensing fee**—a fixed dollar amount added to the ingredient cost in the reimbursement formula

**displacement**—the movement of a feeding tube or intravenous catheter out of the proper position

**doctrine of contribution**—the legal principle that a tortfeasor may bring a lawsuit against a joint tortfeasor

**doctrine of respondeat superior**—the legal principle that an employer may be held responsible for the actions of an employee

**dollar limit**—the maximum dollar amount of prescriptions that can be dispensed for a member over a particular period of time

**dose calibrator**—an instrument used to measure the radioactivity of a sample of radionuclide during the compounding of a radiopharmaceutical

**dosimeter**—a personal monitoring device used to measure the radiation exposure of an individual

**drug distribution system**—a safe and economical method of distributing a drug

**drug holiday**—the temporary discontinuation of a drug to test the need for its continued use

**drug interaction**—when one drug interferes with the working of another drug

**drug regimen review (DRR)**—the process of reviewing a resident's medications and corresponding medical information, formulating a clinical recommendation, and communicating that recommendation

**drug-related problem**—an event or situation involving drug therapy that actually or potentially interferes with an optimum outcome for the patient

**drug repackager**—a company that buys drugs in bulk and repackages them in small units for resale

**drug sample**—a prescription drug that is not sold but is provided by a pharmaceutical manufacturer without charge as a way to promote the use of a drug

**drug utilization review (DUR)**—the process that examines whether prescription drugs are being used efficiently and appropriately within a prescription drug benefit

**durable medical equipment**—medical equipment that can be reused

**e-prescribing**—the transmission of a prescription between a physician and a pharmacist by way of an electronic medium

**e-prescription**—a prescription transmitted by an electronic medium

**elderly population**—persons 65 years of age or older

**electronic medical record**—an electronic patient chart that is stored in a computer

**eluant**—the solvent that washes a daughter radionuclide from a parent radionuclide

**elution**—the process of separating a daughter radionuclide from a parent radionuclide

**emergency drug**—a drug that can result in discomfort, distress, or an acute or life-threatening condition if not administered within a reasonable length of time

**emergency services**—immediate health care services provided for serious or acute illness or injury that may be life-threatening

**enteral nutrition**—nutrition delivered into the gastrointestinal tract through a tube

**excluded drug**—a drug whose cost will not be reimbursed under a prescription drug plan

**expanded pharmacy technician roles**—roles that are an expansion of current traditional pharmacy technician duties in the preparation and dispensing of medications

**federal pharmacist**—a licensed pharmacist who works within the federal government

**federal pharmacy**—the practice of pharmacy within the federal government

**fee-for-service**—a health care reimbursement system in which a separate fee is paid for each type of health care service provided

**feeding tube**—a hollow tube that provides access to the GI tract

**fixed co-payment**—a co-payment that is a fixed dollar amount

**focused review**—a drug regimen review that concentrates on a specific medication, medication class, medication problem, or medical problem within the long-term care facility

**formulary**—a list of medications approved for use or reimbursement under a prescription drug plan

**formulary drug**—a drug that is included for coverage in a formulary

**formulary exception process**—a process that provides access to nonformulary drugs and certain formulary drugs when necessary

**formulary override**—a formulary exception process that involves obtaining authorization to use a nonformulary drug

**freedom of choice**—the concept in which patients have the freedom to choose their health care provider

**fume hood**—a laminar airflow hood adapted for compounding radiopharmaceuticals

**functional limitation**—a condition that limits a person's ability to function in a normal manner

**gatekeeper**—a primary care physician who coordinates and authorizes all health care services

**Geiger-Müller counter**—an instrument used to measure low-level radiation of an area

**general review**—a drug regimen review that involves an overview of a resident's medication therapy

**generic substitution**—the substitution of a generic drug for a brand-name drug

**glove box**—a type of laminar airflow hood in which an operator works by inserting his hands through special gloves that allow access to the inside of the hood

**good manufacturing practices (GMPs)**—regulations that set minimum standards for the manufacturing of drugs

**group practice**—three or more physicians who practice medicine together

**half-life**—the time required for one-half of a radionuclide to decay

**hazardous chemical**—a chemical substance that poses a threat to health or safety

**health care**—deals with the promotion of health and the treatment of disease

**health maintenance organization (HMO)**—a managed care organization that provides health care services to enrolled members for a fixed, prepaid fee

**hemotherapy**—the treatment of a medical condition through the administration of blood products

**home care pharmacy practice**—the practice of pharmacy that provides medications, home health care products and services, and pharmaceutical care to patients at home

**home health care**—health care services and health-related products provided to a patient at home

**home infusion pharmacy**—a pharmacy that prepares and dispenses infusion therapies to patients in the home and alternative sites

**homebound**—the inability to leave the home under normal conditions

**hospice**—an organized program of services to meet the physical, emotional, spiritual, and social needs of a patient who is terminally ill

**hospice pharmacy**—a pharmacy that dispenses medications to hospice patients at home or in institutions

**independent practice association (IPA)**—a health maintenance organization in which individual physicians enter a nonexclusive contract to see both HMO and non-HMO patients

**indicator**—a tool used by a surveyor to assess the performance of a pharmacist in performing a drug regimen review

**infusion device**—a device that regulates the infusion of an intravenous therapy

**ingredient cost**—the raw cost of a drug

**in-house pharmacy**—a closed-shop pharmacy located inside a long-term care facility

**initial assessment**—a process that evaluates whether a patient is an appropriate candidate for home health care

**innovative pharmacy technician roles**—roles that involve areas outside of traditional pharmacy practice

**inpatient**—a patient who is treated inside of a traditional health care institution

**inpatient care institution**—a health care institution that provides health care services to a patient who is confined to a bed in that institution

**instrumental activity of daily living (IADL)**—an activity that is related to household and social functions

**intellectual error**—an error in judgment on the part of the pharmacist

**interdisciplinary**—different health care personnel working together

**Internet pharmacy**—an established commercial Web site that enables a patient to obtain medications by way of the Internet

**interpretive guidelines**—guidelines published by CMS to help in the interpretation of the regulations regarding Medicare and Medicaid Conditions of Participation for long-term care facilities

**investigational new drug application (INDA)**—an application submitted to the FDA to begin the testing of a new drug in humans

**iontophoresis**—the delivery of small doses of drugs through the skin

**irregularity**—a potential drug therapy problem

**joint liability**—the sharing of liability by two or more persons

**joint tortfeasors**—two or more persons who share liability in committing a wrong or harm

**kickback**—a portion of a payment returned to another party according to a secret agreement

**lead barrier shield**—a lead shield used to protect a worker from radioactivity during the compounding of a radiopharmaceutical

**lifestyle drug**—a drug that enhances the quality of a patient's life but is not considered medically necessary

**long-term care**—care that is provided for an extended period of time

**long-term care facility**—an inpatient care institution that provides care for patients over a longer period of time than would be provided in an acute care hospital

**long-term care pharmacy**—a pharmacy that dispenses medications to residents in a long-term care facility

**mail-order pharmacy**—a pharmacy that dispenses maintenance medications to members through mail delivery

**maintenance medication**—a medication that is taken on an ongoing basis for a chronic condition

**malpractice**—negligence performed by a professional

**managed care**—a system of health care delivery that provides both the financing and delivery of health care

**managed care organization (MCO)**—a health care organization that both insures and provides health care services

**managed care pharmacy practice**—the practice of pharmacy that involves clinical and administrative activities performed in a managed care organization by a pharmacist

**master batch record**—a set of specifications for manufacturing a new drug

**material safety data sheet (MSDS)**—a document that provides detailed information on the hazards associated with a particular chemical substance

**maximum allowable cost (MAC)**—the maximum cost that a plan will pay for a generic drug that is available from many sources

**mechanical error**—an error that involves activities related to the physical dispensing of a medication

**medical readiness**—being prepared for any medical emergency as a result of a wartime or peacetime military mission

**medication administration record (MAR)**—a form used to document medications administered to a patient

**medication error**—the difference between what a physician orders and what is administered to a resident

**medication pass observation**—the observation of the medication administration process in a nursing facility by a consultant pharmacist

**member**—a participant in a health care benefit

**member co-payment**—the portion of the total cost of a prescription that the member must pay

**midline catheter**—a long, flexible intravenous catheter that is inserted into a peripheral vein in the arm

**military pharmacist**—a pharmacist who practices in the U.S. Army, U.S. Navy, or U.S. Air Force

**misbranding**—false and misleading information concerning a drug

**modified unit-dose system**—a drug distribution system that combines unit-dose medications blister-packaged onto a multiple-dose card

**modular cassette**—a combination of a cassette exchange system with unit-dose or blister-packaged medications

**multidisciplinary**—different health care personnel working independently

**multiple medication package**—a medication package in which all medications for a specific administration time are packaged together

**multiple-therapy pump**—an ambulatory infusion pump that can infuse a variety of infusion therapies

**multispecialty group practice**—a group practice of physicians in different medical specialties

**negligence**—the failure to do something that a reasonable person might do or doing something that a reasonable person might not do

**network**—a group of health care providers linked through a contract to provide health care services

**new drug application (NDA)**—an application submitted to the FDA for the approval of marketing a new drug

**noncoring needle**—a needle that does not produce a core or rubber plug with each insertion through a diaphragm

**nonformulary drug**—a drug that is not included for coverage in a formulary

**nonresident pharmacy**—a pharmacy that is located outside of a particular state that mails, ships, or delivers prescriptions to patients inside that particular state

**nuclear pharmacist**—a pharmacist who has specialized training in the handling of radioactive compounds

**nuclear pharmacy**—a pharmacy that prepares, stores, and dispenses radiopharmaceuticals

**nuclide**—the composition of the nucleus of an atom

**number limit**—the maximum number of prescriptions that can be dispensed for a member over a particular period of time

**nursing facility**—a type of institutional long-term care facility

**nutritional assessment**—an evaluation of a patient's nutritional status

**occlusion**—the blockage of a feeding tube or intravenous catheter

**open formulary**—a formulary in which a broad range of drugs are covered

**open-shop pharmacy**—a pharmacy that dispenses medications for long-term care facility residents and regular retail patients

**organized ambulatory care setting**—an outpatient care institution identified by the type of service provided

**orphan drug**—a drug that treats a disease that affects fewer than 200,000 people

**orthosis**—a support or brace for weak or ineffective joints or muscles

**out-of-house pharmacy**—a closed-shop pharmacy that is located outside of a long-term care facility

**out-of-pocket payment**—a direct payment to a health care provider by a patient

**outcome**—a change in a patient's health status resulting from a health care service

**outcomes research**—the process of collecting information to determine the effectiveness of a therapy

**outpatient**—a patient who is treated outside of a traditional health care institution

**outpatient care institution**—a health care institution that provides health care services to patients without an overnight stay

**outpatient clinic**—an organized ambulatory care setting where clinic services are provided

**outpatient pharmacy**—a pharmacy that provides pharmaceutical products and services to outpatients

**pain management**—the pharmacologic management of pain

**palliative care**—care that treats the symptoms associated with a disease to provide comfort and relieve suffering rather than to cure the disease

**parenteral nutrition**—nutrition provided directly into the bloodstream through a vein

**partnership practice**—two physicians who practice medicine together

**pedigree law**—legislation that requires wholesalers to track a drug's movement through the supply chain

**percentage co-payment**—a co-payment that is a fixed percentage of the total cost of a prescription

**peripheral catheter**—a short, flexible intravenous catheter that is inserted into a peripheral vein in the arm

**peripheral vascular access**—access to the bloodstream through a peripheral vein

**peripherally inserted central venous catheter (PICC)**—a flexible central venous catheter that is inserted peripherally into a vein in the arm and threaded into a large vein in the chest

pharmaceutical biotechnology—the application of biology to the development of drugs

pharmaceutical care—the responsible provision of drug therapy for the purpose of achieving definite outcomes that improve a patient's quality of life

pharmaceutical care plan—a part of the overall care plan that sets goals for each medication prescribed for a patient

pharmacoeconomics—the evaluation of the cost as well as the outcomes of drug therapy

pharmacy benefit management (PBM) company—a managed care organization that designs, administers, and manages only the prescription drug benefit

pharmacy network—a group of pharmacies that sign a contract to provide pharmacy benefits to members in exchange for a specified reimbursement

pharmacy practice acts—state laws that govern the functions and responsibilities of pharmacy technicians

pharmacy technician—an individual who assists in pharmacy activities that do not require the professional judgment of a pharmacist

physician order form—a complete list of all of the physician's orders for a long-term care resident

postmarketing studies—studies conducted during the general use of a drug following FDA approval

preclinical trials—testing a new drug in the laboratory and on animals before testing it on humans

preferred provider organization (PPO)—a managed care organization that provides health care services to enrolled members for a discounted fee

prescription drug benefit—the portion of a health care benefit that provides prescription drug coverage to a member

primary care—preventative health care and routine medical care provided by a primary care practitioner

primary care practitioner—the first health care professional that a patient sees for a condition or illness

prior authorization—a formulary exception process that involves obtaining authorization to use certain formulary drugs

private practice—the practice of medicine in which services are provided directly to the patient in return for a fee

problem-centered review—a drug regimen review that concentrates on a particular medical problem and its medication therapy for an individual resident

process—how structures are used to provide health care

prospective payment—a payment made for a health care service before it is provided

prosthesis—an artificial device used to replace a missing part of the body

provider—health care personnel or a health care institution that provides health care services

psychotropic medication—a drug that alters a patient's behavior

quantity limit—the maximum quantity of a drug that can be dispensed at one time

quasi-legal standard—a standard that is voluntary and not legally required

radiation—excess internal energy released from a radionuclide as it decays

radioactive—having the property of releasing radiation

radioactive decay—the disintegration of a radionuclide to return to a stable state

radiochemical impurity—the presence of a radionuclide in a different chemical form

radionuclide—an atom that has an unstable nucleus

radionuclide generator—a device in which a daughter radionuclide is produced from a parent radionuclide through the principle of radioactive decay

radionuclide impurity—the presence of a foreign radionuclide

radiopharmaceutical—a radioactive drug used for the diagnosis and treatment of disease

reagent kit—a commercially available bulk supply of a carrier drug

recombinant DNA technology—combining DNA from different sources to produce a new DNA product with a different function

referral—a request for care made by a health care professional on behalf of a patient

reimbursement formula—the formula used to calculate the reimbursement to a pharmacy for filling a prescription remote pharmacy—a remote site that is an actual pharmacy

remote site—the site at which prescriptions are dispensed in a telepharmacy practice

remote telepharmacy—a remote pharmacy

remuneration—a payment made directly or indirectly in the form of cash or free or discounted goods or services

resident—a patient in a nursing facility

respite care—short-term, temporary care provided to an individual so that a family caregiver can take a break from the daily routine of caregiving

restraint—any method of restricting a nursing facility resident's physical movement

restricted formulary—a formulary in which some nonformulary drugs are covered

retrospective payment—a payment made for a health care service after it is provided

rogue site—an illegitimate Internet pharmacy site

safe harbor—a practice that is not considered unlawful under the Anti-Kickback Act

secondary care—specialized health care services beyond primary care

single-specialty group practice—a group practice of physicians in the same medical specialty

solo practice—the practice of medicine by a single physician

specialist—a physician who specializes in one area of medicine

specialized pharmacy technician roles—roles that concentrate on one aspect of pharmacy practice

specialty mail-order pharmacy—a mail-order pharmacy that concentrates on specific areas of the prescription drug market

standard—an established guideline for providing quality health care services

stationary infusion pump—an infusion device that attaches to an IV pole

structure—the resources, personnel, and policies and procedures available to provide health care

subacute care—inpatient care that lies between acute hospital care and nursing facility care

subcutaneous port—a vascular access device that is surgically implanted into a large vein in the chest with all parts of the device under the skin

surveyor—a trained individual who evaluates a health care organization for its compliance with established standards

symptom management—the pharmacologic management of symptoms

task specialization—the performing of an individual task in the pharmacy

tech-check-tech—a pharmacy technician's performing the final check of another pharmacy technician's work in the same situation

telepharmacy—the provision of pharmaceutical care through the use of telecommunication and information technology to patients at a distance

terminally ill patient—a patient who has an illness that is likely to result in death within 6 months

tertiary care—highly specialized health care beyond primary and secondary care

therapeutic equivalent—causing the same effect in the body by different drugs

therapeutic equivalent drug—a drug with a different chemical structure but in the same therapeutic or drug class, that can be expected to have the same outcome when used in therapeutically equivalent doses

therapeutic interchange—the authorized substitution of a prescribed drug with a therapeutic equivalent drug

therapy-specific pump—an ambulatory infusion pump that infuses a specific type of infusion therapy

three-party payment system—a health care payment system that involves three parties

time limit—the maximum amount of time in which a prescription can be filled for a member

tortfeasor—a person who commits a wrong or harm

treatment administration record (TAR)—a form used to document external treatments administered to a patient

tunneled catheter—a central venous catheter that is tunneled under the skin for a short distance before being inserted into a large vein in the chest

**turn-around system**—a system for obtaining refill medications that requires reordering at a specific, predetermined time

**unapproved use**—the use of a drug for a disease or a condition that it has not been approved to treat

**unit-dose system**—a drug distribution system that provides medication in its final unit-of-use form

**unnecessary drug**—a drug whose use should be reduced or discontinued on the basis of monitoring data or an adverse drug reaction

**variable co-payment**—a co-payment that is a variable or different dollar amount depending on the type of drug dispensed

**vascular access**—access to the bloodstream

**vascular access device**—a catheter placed directly into a vein through which intravenous medication is infused

**wholesaler**—an intermediary between a drug manufacturer and the outlet for the drug

**workflow**—an organized way of filling prescriptions

# Index